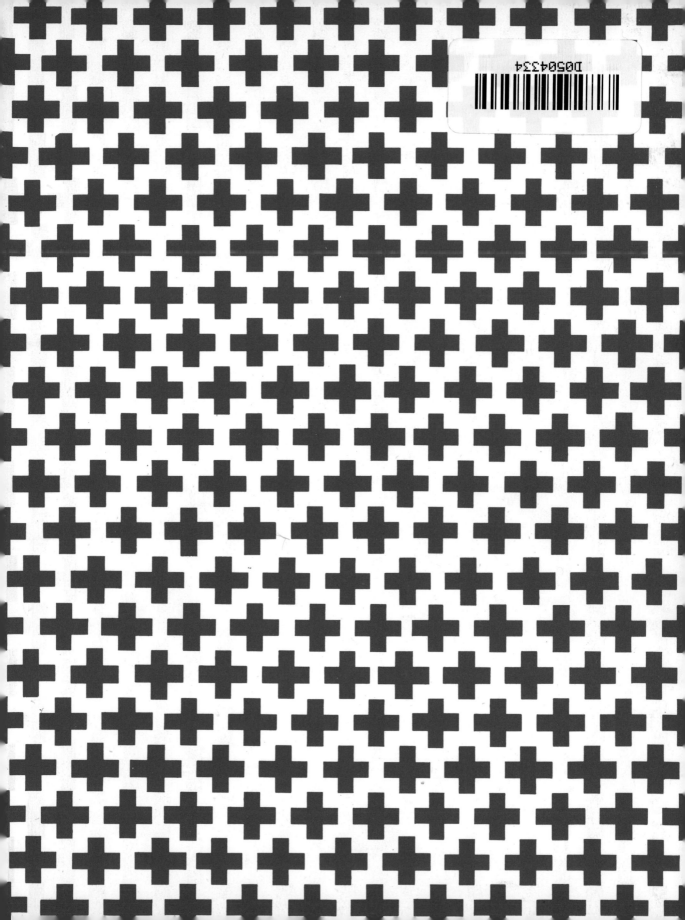

THE WHICH? GUIDE
TO
FAMILY HEALTH

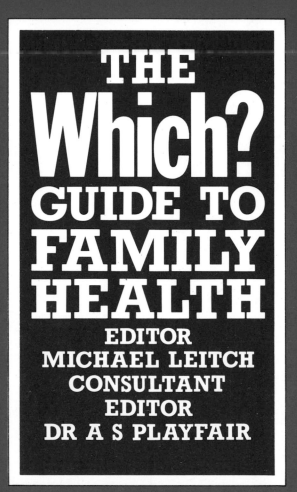

THE Which? GUIDE TO FAMILY HEALTH

EDITOR
MICHAEL LEITCH
CONSULTANT
EDITOR
DR A S PLAYFAIR

Published by
Consumers' Association and
Hodder & Stoughton

The Which? Guide to Family Health is
published in Great Britain
by Consumers' Association, 14 Buckingham Street,
London WC2N 6DS
and Hodder & Stoughton

© Consumers' Association 1980

ISBN 0 340 25051 8

Printed and bound in Yugoslavia by
Mladinska Knjiga, Ljubljana

ACKNOWLEDGEMENTS
Editor Michael Leitch
Consultant Editor Dr A S Playfair
Art Director David Pocknell
Designers Michael Cavers, Barry Lowenhoff
and Duncan Moore
Production Reynolds Clark Associates Ltd
Contributors
John Bryant, Dr David Muller, Dr Norman Pollitt,
Jenny Salmon, Robert Watkins
Illustrations Mike Lynn, Tony Swift
and David Pocknell
Photographs Camera Press, Mark Edwards,
Dr Lionel Fry, Graves Medical
Audiovisual Library, Ikon, Lisa Mackson,
Andrea Nelki, Christopher Steele-Perkins,
Homer Sykes and John Walmsley

CONTENTS

INTRODUCTION
The purpose of this *Guide*
is to equip the family bookshelf with an all-round
source of reference on the various aspects of health that seem to
concern us most. Most of us suffer in the course of a year from one or
more of the common ailments discussed in the *Guide's* longest section.
Even if we do not, it is likely that others close to us, our children for
example, will be less fortunate and help will be needed. Many such
illnesses are minor and short-lived, and we need no deep fund of
medical knowledge to deal effectively with them. Reference to Part 3 of
the *Guide* can then take the place of a time-wasting trip to the doctor
for similar words of advice, with the possible extra burden of an
expensive prescription.

At other times it will be necessary to seek professional
help, and we hope that the information in the *Guide* will help readers to
explain with greater clarity to the doctor the nature of their problem.
The principle is much the same when someone has an accident. First
aid is needed and the *Guide,* which deals with the most likely
emergencies, should prove reassuring and helpful. Sometimes first aid
is all that is needed: the bleeding may be mild, for instance, and the
cut can be dressed and left to heal. But not always, and the *Guide*
stresses that 'first aid aims to stop your patient's condition from
worsening and perhaps to save life. It is not treatment proper, which is
second aid and a matter for a nurse or doctor.'

Nowhere is the need for self-help more obvious than
when personal survival is at stake and no outside help can be
summoned. The *Guide's* closing chapter is about survival – the need to
act if you are to stay alive. Your house catches fire and people in it are
trapped, or you are alone in deep water after a sailing accident, or
marooned for hours in a snowdrift. You may think such crises could
never happen to you, that they are other people's nightmares. The
reality, though, is that they and many other incidents are everyday
killers, and it is surely worthwhile to be forewarned, to have the
knowledge to curtail a developing crisis and to deal swiftly with one
that has already arisen. For when it does arise, there is *never* any time
to spare. It takes only seconds for someone to drown, or be overcome
by smoke.

THE IMPERFECT BODY Popular medical profiles of modern man
tend to delineate a pitiable creature close to deformity. Partly this is the
fault of the profiler, who in trying to be comprehensive oversteps
reality. His man is all bad: sedentary, obese, unclean, eats the wrong
food, takes no exercise, has forgotten how to relax, smokes
cigarettes, drinks too much, cannot bear the prospect of growing old . . .
the list can be extended all the way to the undertaker's parlour. It is a
dangerous approach because it is so thoroughly discouraging. The

Which? Guide to Family Health takes a longer, less sensational view, inviting the reader to see for himself.

The book begins with a demonstration of the human body. The function of this demonstration is not unlike that of the car manual: to show, in a matter-of-fact way, the nature of the organism. It says: here are the 206 bones of the skeleton, here are the muscles that move them, here is the blood stream that keeps the muscular tissue alive, here is how the blood is pumped round the body. And so on. By clearly stating, in the space of a few amply illustrated pages, how the body has been engineered, the *Guide* seeks to make the reader more aware of its powers, its needs and its limitations.

The second part of the book is called 'Stay Healthy', and isolates six areas of activity where, with a little extra care, most of us can measurably improve our fitness and general well-being. A well-tuned body, refreshed by exercise and a sensible diet, feels not only better but capable of doing more. And while physical fitness is something we need to work at, requiring a small regular investment of time each week, it takes no longer to eat well than it does to eat foolishly.

It may well be, however, that some readers need to make little or no adjustment to their eating and exercise habits. Even so, they may find welcome variety in the choice of exercises proposed, and useful information about special diets – during pregnancy for instance. Other sections in Part 2 offer ideas and guidance on personal hygiene for all the family, with a subsection on sex and sexually transmitted diseases, and on three common areas of stress. These concern our ability to relax, to have an enjoyable social life without reliance on cigarettes, excess alcohol or addictive drugs, and to plan for and enjoy our retirement years.

The remaining parts of the *Guide* deal with the predicaments described earlier: common ailments, accidents and first aid, and survival. It is unfortunate that the lone survivor of an air crash in the Andes will very likely not have his copy of the *Guide* with him when he needs it most. We must only hope that some of the advice about exposure, finding water and food, and preparing rescue signals will have remained in his memory from a previous reading. It is hardly feasible to expect more.

Opportunities to practise first aid occur with much greater frequency, however much we may regret it. Here the *Guide* does ask its readers to learn certain emergency procedures which they can then carry out anywhere and at any time (see page 176). It also suggests that at least one member of the family attends a first aid course. The benefit to the community's health, as well as to the family's, could be beyond calculation.

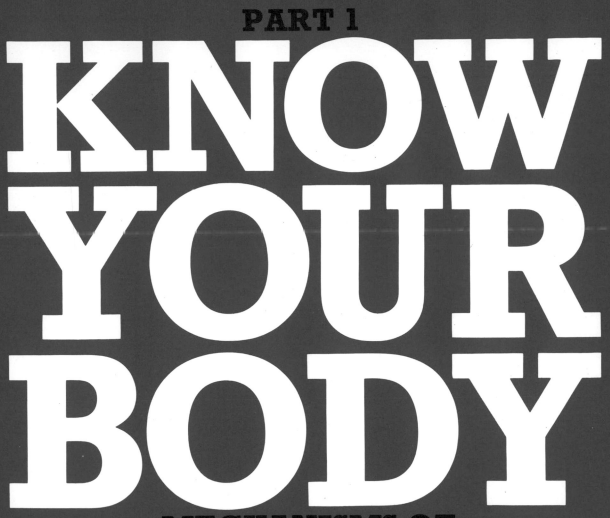

PART 1

KNOW YOUR BODY

MECHANISMS OF THE BODY AND MIND, AND HOW THEY WORK TOGETHER

The **skeleton** with its joints is the chassis upon which the body's stability and potential mobility are based. Movement itself is achieved by **muscles.** Like every other tissue muscles are kept alive by the **blood stream.** Life depends on the blood bringing oxygen from the **lungs** and nutrients from the **digestive system.** Waste material is excreted in great part through the **kidneys.**

All this is coordinated by two messenger services, the **nervous system** and the **endocrines.** Finally the organism achieves if not its own immortality at least that of its kind through its **reproductive organs.** This section of the book will briefly describe each one of these systems.

THE SKELETON

It is unfortunate that custom has associated the skeleton with a concept of death. Bones are extremely alive and it is only because they contain hard firm minerals which remain long after the body around them has died and disintegrated that they have acquired their undeserved macabre connotation.

Bone is constantly undergoing a slow process of breakdown and regeneration. To a great extent its growth and formation is shaped by the pull of muscles attached to it, and by the stresses to which body posture and movement subject it. It contains nerves and blood vessels and is the seat of much chemical activity. The calcium it contains can act as a reservoir to be drawn upon when needed in other parts of the body. Within many bones the marrow is the site of constant formation of new blood cells.

Most bones develop from the softer cartilage which is their precursor in the embryo. Calcification, the deposit of the hard calcium structure, begins in their centres and spreads through the thickness and towards the ends, thickening and lengthening the structure until maturity. Growth of bones continues after birth from cartilage areas near the ends and finally until full maturity, at about 24 years old, when all cartilage is replaced by bone and growth ceases. In some elderly people, the calcium deposits may be depleted so that bones become relatively thinned and brittle.

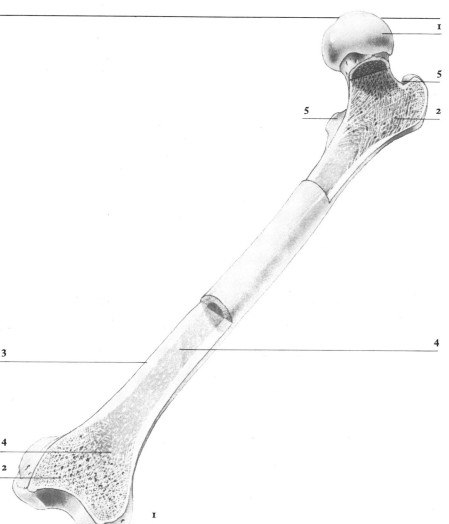

Inside a bone
This adult long bone shows:
1 Over the extremities a thin smooth cap of cartilage allowing easy movements at the joint surfaces.
2 At the extremities the so-called 'spongy bone' which in section looks honeycombed.
3 Over the shaft the 'compact bone', which is denser and uniform, and can take heavy stresses.
4 The marrow. This is a jelly-like substance, with a rich blood supply.
5 Characteristic ridges and projections due to the pull of attached muscle tendons during bone growth.

12

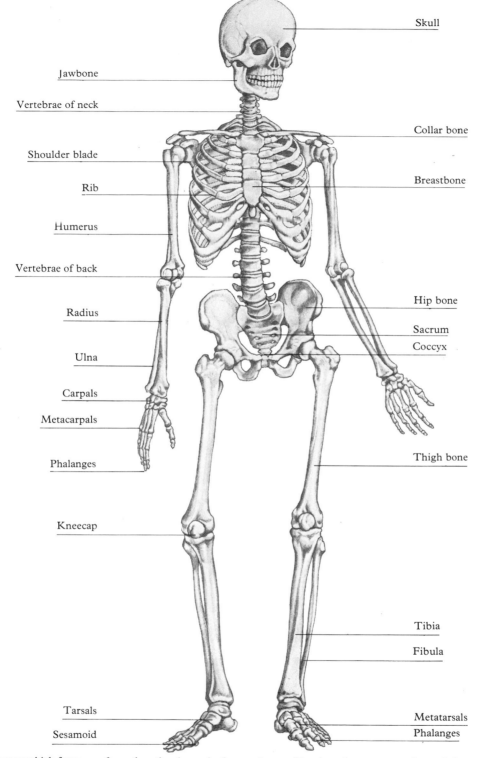

Skull

Jawbone

Vertebrae of neck

Collar bone

Shoulder blade

Breastbone

Rib

Humerus

Vertebrae of back

Hip bone

Radius

Sacrum

Coccyx

Ulna

Carpals

Metacarpals

Phalanges

Thigh bone

Kneecap

Tibia

Fibula

Tarsals

Metatarsals

Sesamoid

Phalanges

The 206 bones which form the skeleton vary from the massive thigh bone to the minute ossicles (less than one centimetre in length) within the ear. The latter have a role quite different from the other bones in the body: they exist to transmit sound vibrations in the ear. Another variation is that sometimes quite small extra nodules of bone are found in tendons attaching muscles to bones of hands or feet. The front view of the skeleton, as seen hanging up in museums, is useful for labelling with the names of individual bones. But we need always to bear in mind that a skeleton belonged to a living person who was constantly moving and changing posture. Some of the ways movement is achieved are shown on pages 16–17.

Though here we need no detailed analysis of skeletal anatomy, we can consider a few of the more interesting points.

The backbone, basic support on which all else depends, consists of 33 vertebrae, superimposed to give a strong yet flexible column. The major component of a typical vertebra consists of a large block sitting on the block of the next vertebra below, and separated from it by a buffering cartilage pad, the intervertebral disc. But each vertebra is continued at its back by a bony arch, so that the whole forms a ring. The spinal cord of nerves passes down within the series of these protective rings.

Finally the ring bears bony outgrowths giving each vertebra its characteristic knobbly appearance. The knobs allow each vertebra to link firmly with its neighbours, and also provide attachments for the muscles which support the back. Some of the vertebrae are modified and rudimentary and may be fused together as in the sacrum, a corrugated triangular plate representing five vertebrae in one. The coccyx has five minute vertebrae in fusion and is all that man has to represent the tail he lost during evolution. Interestingly specialized vertebrae are to be found where the head and neck join. The first vertebra, the atlas, is 'all ring' and lacks its block. The lowest end of the head sits on the ring and can rock back and forth, allowing nodding movement. From the second vertebra, the axis, immediately beneath, a large peg projects up into the ring of the atlas; a man who shakes his head from side to side is rotating both head and atlas around this peg.

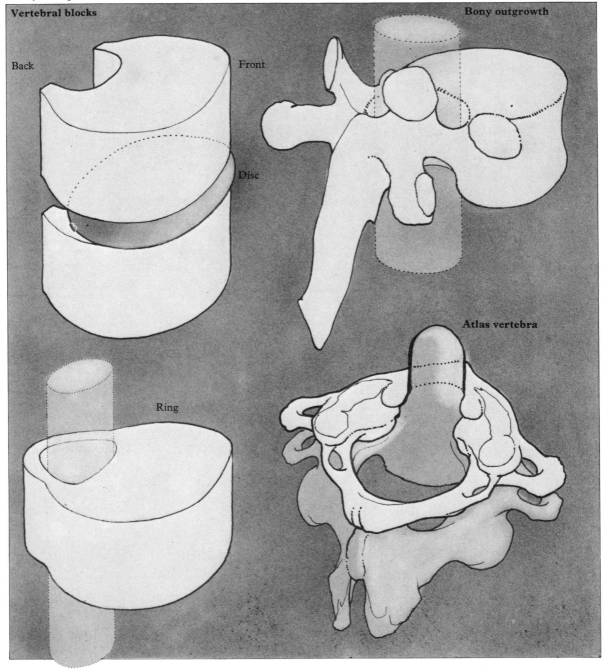

Vertebral blocks

Back

Front

Disc

Ring

Bony outgrowth

Atlas vertebra

SKULL

When they think of the skull many people fail to appreciate just how much there is above the part which delineates the face. The cranium is the large round box above the eyes which contains the brain. All too often the non-anatomist's concept of the head is like the child's simple drawing of a face, below, and ignores that large round box, the cranium, which houses the brain.

The dotted line in the diagrams shows the level of the 'base of the skull', the very irregular shelf of bone upon which the brain rests. It is pitted with large and small holes for the passage of blood vessels, of nerves and of the thick brain stem which will continue into the spinal cord through the rings of the vertebrae.

LIMBS

In many ways the skull and the backbone form the main support for the whole body. To the upper backbone is attached the protective cage of ribs, collar bone and shoulder blade—relatively thin bones from which the upper limbs hang, allowing wide and versatile mobility. Lower down is the balcony-like pelvis to which the lower limbs are attached: here power and stability are more important.

The leg swings far less at the hip than does the arm at the shoulder, fingers curl and close more than toes. The two bones of the lower leg, tibia and fibula, form a stable pillar and do not change position. Whereas the radius of the forearm will rotate around its fellow, the ulna, and so help wrist and hand to twist about.

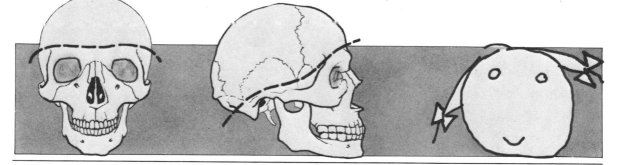

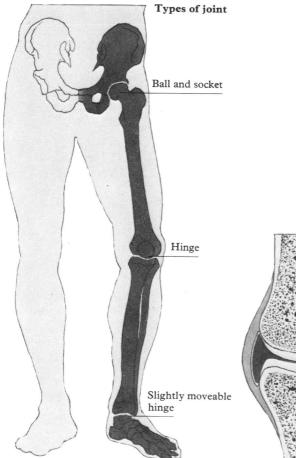

Types of joint

Ball and socket

Hinge

Slightly moveable hinge

JOINTS

Joints are the sites where two bones are in apposition. When we think of joints we tend to think of movement. But many are immoveable. Examples are the finely interlocking bones which form the top of the skull and the tightly fitted but separate bones of the pelvis. Moveable joints are of several types. We have already noted the pivot at the first two vertebrae of the neck, and forearm bones. Gliding movement occurs to a slight extent between the vertebrae. The wider movement of bending and straightening is found in the many hinge joints of the body, as in the fingers or at the knee. The ankle, though also a hinge, has little range of movement but very fine stability. Greatest mobility is found in the ball and socket type, as in shoulder and hip, where a wide swinging arc is possible. A typical moveable joint in a limb shows the features illustrated in the diagram below; these assure both stability and ease of action.

Moveable joint

A typical moveable joint in a limb shows the following features which assure both stability and ease of action

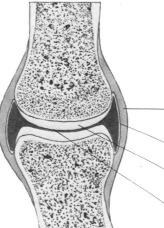

A thick firm capsule or ligament surrounds and encloses the joint, and maintains its stability. This is enhanced by the holding power of the muscles around the joint

Lining the ligament and folding over on to the bone is the smooth slippery synorial membrane

Each end of the bone is covered by smooth cartilage.

Within the joint space a small amount of thin synorial fluid acts as lubricant.

MUSCLES

Muscles are for movement. Very broadly they can be divided into two groups, the 'voluntary' and the 'involuntary'. **Voluntary muscles** are also called 'striped muscles', for microscopic examination shows them to consist of long contractile fibres made up of alternating light and dark materials. They act under the direct influence of the will, of the intention to cause movement. The mind may, for instance, decide to kick a ball: from the brain, nerves are activated to all the many muscles. The impulses are transmitted through complicated, well directed nerve paths along the spinal cord, and thence to each set of relevant nerve fibres. Each individual nerve then ends up within the muscle. A combination of electrical and chemical changes causes the muscles to tense and contract. As we shall see later, some of these voluntary muscles may move automatically in a 'reflex action' without the direct influence of the brain. Many muscles are attached to bones by thick firm tendons at each end. As it contracts, a muscle pulls the bones to which it is attached closer to each other. To let this happen, any other muscle which will perform the opposite movement has to relax.

Not all muscles are linear bands between moving bones. Some are attached to softer areas, as large sheets or as circles. You can see some of these, right, in the muscles which govern facial expressions.

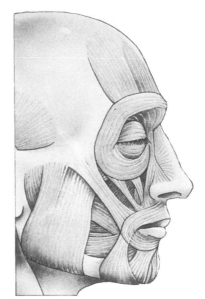

How muscles work together

The accompanying diagram of some of the forearm and hand muscles gives an idea of the finely coordinated actions involved in apparently simple matters such as reaching out to pick up a pencil and then writing with it.

Bends the wrist

Bends the wrist and helps to pull the hand sideways

Deepens the hollow of the palm

Pulls the little finger sideways

Straightens the elbow

Bends the elbow

Turns the forearm to make the palm face forwards

Turns the forearm to make the palm face backwards

Bends the elbow

Bends the wrist and helps to pull the hand sideways

Bends the wrist and the further ends of the fingers

Bends the thumb and the wrist

Bends the thumb

Pulls the thumb sideways

Pulls the thumb into the palm

Hand and finger muscles bring fingers towards each other, and also create positions for use in gripping or writing

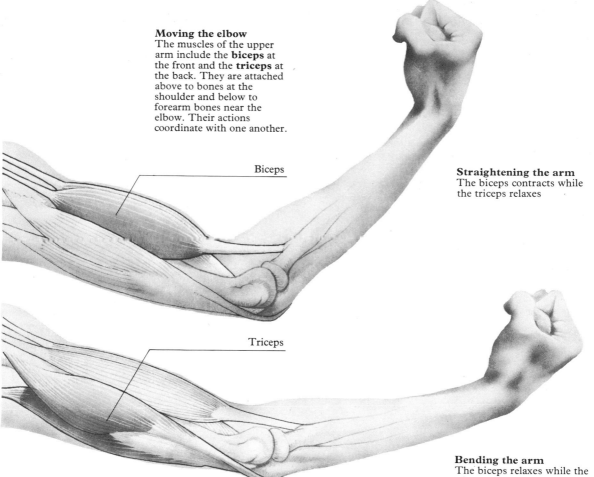

Moving the elbow
The muscles of the upper arm include the **biceps** at the front and the **triceps** at the back. They are attached above to bones at the shoulder and below to forearm bones near the elbow. Their actions coordinate with one another.

Biceps

Straightening the arm
The biceps contracts while the triceps relaxes

Triceps

Bending the arm
The biceps relaxes while the triceps contracts

Involuntary muscles are also called 'smooth muscles' since they do not show the microscopic striations of the voluntary muscles, but consist rather of longitudinally set interconnecting fibres. They are not under voluntary control and work automatically under the influence of the autonomic nervous system (see page 33), without needing the purposeful direction of the mind. Their actions are slower and longer than those of the voluntary muscles, and they govern such things as movements of the bowel, the uterus and the bladder. Involuntary muscles are also found in the walls of the blood vessels, giving them their tone.

A very special type of involuntary muscle is the cardiac muscle, highly specialized to keep the thick heart wall beating. Their fibres contract on their own, constantly and tirelessly. They do not need nervous stimulation for this, though they can be influenced by the autonomic nervous system.

Stomach muscles
In the stomach several layers of muscles encircle the organ with their fibres acting in different directions, giving the slow churning movements which mix the food with digestive juices. At each end a thick ring-like band, a sphincter, controls the entry and exit of the stomach contents.

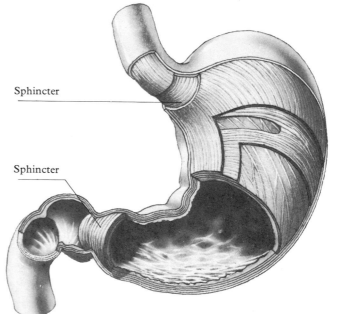

Sphincter

Sphincter

BLOOD AND CIRCULATION

'Blood takes everything everywhere.' This is as valid a statement for the body as saying of a country 'The road and rail traffic take everything everywhere.' If we imagine blood vessels to be roadways then the blood itself would be represented by lorries bringing raw materials to factories, by vans delivering finished products to shops, and by cars, bicycles and pedestrians taking purchases to the home for stores or for immediate use. The simile even extends to refuse processing and disposal if we consider the action of such organs as the kidneys, the liver and the lungs.

The amount of blood we have in the body is very approximately 1 litre for every 10 kilogrammes of body weight (or 1 pint for every stone). It consists of fluid, the plasma, and of many millions of cells floating within it. By far the most numerous of these are the **red blood cells**, whose role is to absorb oxygen from the air breathed into the lungs and carry it to all the tissues. Oxygen, essential for life, is 'burnt up' producing carbon dioxide which is carried back by the red cells, to be given up to and got rid of through the air breathed out of the lungs. The **white blood cells** are of many sorts with varied functions which could be compared to defensive and repair services. Some serve to fight and destroy bacteria and their poisons, some are involved in tissue repair after injury, and others create the chemicals concerned with immunity to infection. Some minute ones called platelets help to form clots where there is bleeding. These blood cells are manufactured mainly in the bone marrow, but some white cells are also produced in the lymph glands and the spleen. They are constantly being broken down: the red blood cells' life in circulation is about four months.

Types of blood cell

Platelets

Red blood cells

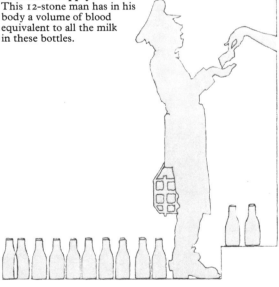

White blood cells

The blood supply

This 12-stone man has in his body a volume of blood equivalent to all the milk in these bottles.

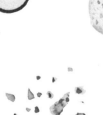

Every cubic millimetre (here illustrated full-size) of his blood contains about:

8 thousand white cells
300 thousand platelets
5 million red cells

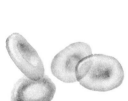

The plasma itself, streaming through all parts of the body, carries the immense number of chemicals involved in life processes, probably more varied and complicated than those transported by roadway traffic, and certainly better regulated. A medical 'blood test' taken from a patient is therefore no one simple thing; in the laboratory it can be used to determine an enormous number of factors concerning the patient's health. Circulation can be said to begin in the heart, which pumps the blood into the aorta, the first large artery, and thence through repeated branching and rebranching of the vessels to pass through the smallest arteries and reach the capillaries. These capillaries, minute microscopically thin vessels form a network of relatively slowly moving blood in all living parts. It is here that the real events of blood take place, the actions and chemical changes between tissues on the one hand and blood fluid and cells on the other. The large powerful organs of the lungs and the heart pump exist to serve this microscopically invisible system of capillaries.

Oxygen for life

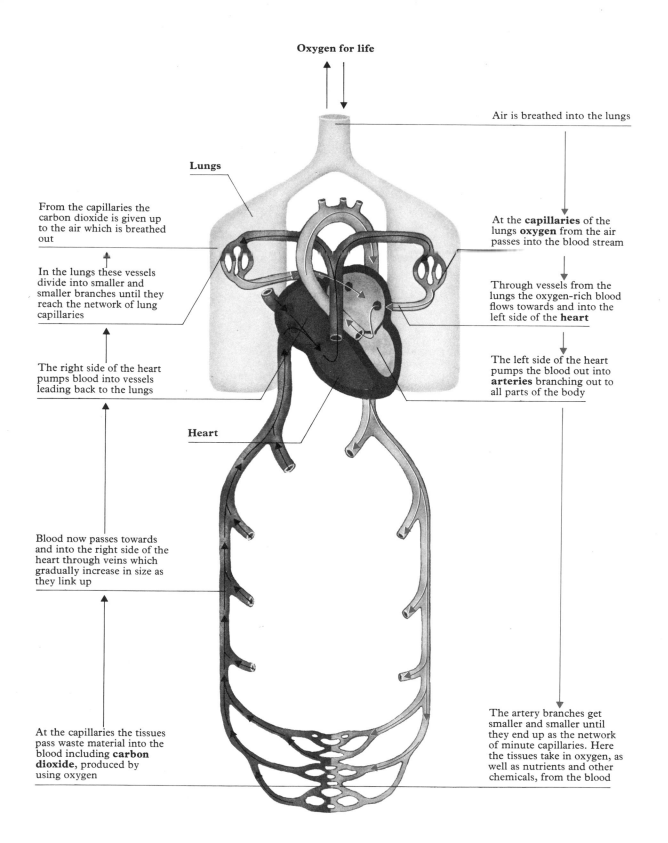

Air is breathed into the lungs

Lungs

From the capillaries the carbon dioxide is given up to the air which is breathed out

At the **capillaries** of the lungs **oxygen** from the air passes into the blood stream

In the lungs these vessels divide into smaller and smaller branches until they reach the network of lung capillaries

Through vessels from the lungs the oxygen-rich blood flows towards and into the left side of the **heart**

The right side of the heart pumps blood into vessels leading back to the lungs

The left side of the heart pumps the blood out into **arteries** branching out to all parts of the body

Heart

Blood now passes towards and into the right side of the heart through veins which gradually increase in size as they link up

At the capillaries the tissues pass waste material into the blood including **carbon dioxide**, produced by using oxygen

The artery branches get smaller and smaller until they end up as the network of minute capillaries. Here the tissues take in oxygen, as well as nutrients and other chemicals, from the blood

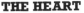

THE HEART

The heart is here drawn in section to show its division into two sides, and that of each side into a collecting chamber (atrium) leading to a pumping chamber (ventricle).

Blood, rich in oxygen, enters the left atrium through veins from the lungs. As the atrium is filling it is relaxed. It now contracts, forcing its contents into the ventricle beneath. The ventricle now contracts, expelling the blood into the first large artery, the aorta, which soon gives off branches leading to all parts of the body. Concurrently, blood low in oxygen comes from other tissues of the body to the heart through veins opening into the right atrium, and so to the right ventricle. With the contraction of the ventricle it passes into arteries leading to the lungs where its oxygen supply is replenished. (An artery is a blood vessel leading away from the heart: it carries oxygen-rich blood from the left side, and oxygen-poor blood from the right. A vein has the reverse role, carrying blood towards the heart.)

An all-important valve, a flap-like opening, lies between the atrium space and the ventricle space on each side, and also at the exit from each ventricle. They ensure that as the heart chambers contract the blood moves in the correct direction only, and also that there is no backflow during relaxation.

As the valves snap shut they produce blood vibrations which make the characteristic clear noises of the heart beat, which can be heard through a stethoscope or by an ear against the chest. A poorly functioning valve, which has difficulty in opening or does not close fully, can cause the extra sounds known as 'heart murmurs'. By no means do all murmurs indicate disease; some of them are of no harmful significance at all. With the body at rest the heart can beat between 60 and 80 times a minute, and in that time can pump out some five litres of blood. These figures increase considerably with exercise.

Blood pressure is the measure of the force with which the blood leaves the left ventricle, and it is measured in terms of the height to which similar pressure would raise a column of mercury in a tube. 'Systolic' is the upper pressure as the heart contracts, and 'diastolic' is the lower one with the heart between contractions.

Position of the heart

The heart is not entirely on the left side of the chest, as is often thought. It is more central, behind the breast bone, but the greater part lies towards the left.

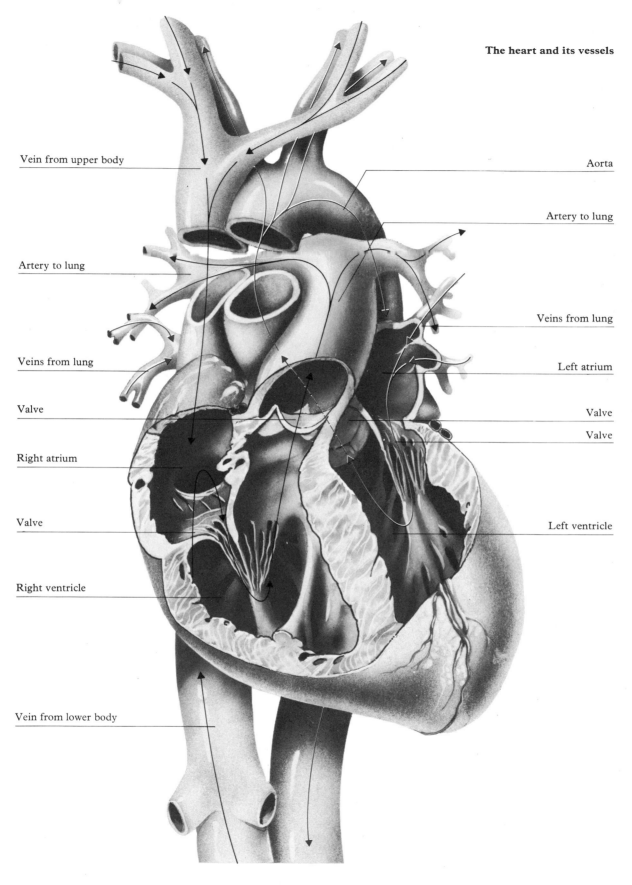

The heart and its vessels

Vein from upper body

Aorta

Artery to lung

Artery to lung

Veins from lung

Veins from lung

Left atrium

Valve

Valve

Valve

Right atrium

Valve

Left ventricle

Right ventricle

Vein from lower body

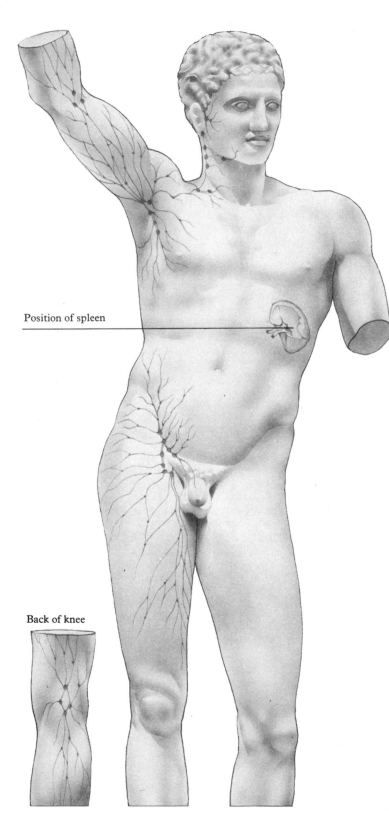

Position of spleen

Back of knee

THE LYMPHATIC SYSTEM

Fluid which forms a large and normal part of the tissues drains into a series of thin lymph vessels set in all parts of the body. The clear lymph fluid thus collected eventually passes into the blood stream where major lymph vessels open into veins at the root of the neck. This system of lymph vessels is punctuated by groups of **lymph glands** (also known as lymph nodes) at various 'meeting points' of the body, rather like junction stations in a railway network. Here the fluid and its contents are subject to the action of certain white blood cells which fight infection and destroy microbes and other foreign matter. In this way they act as a trap and barrier against the spread of infection from tissues, protecting the blood stream from receiving undesirable matter.

The lymph glands lie in many sites deep in the chest and abdomen, as well as superficially. The main surface ones are grouped at the back of the knee, at the groin, at the fold of the elbow, at the armpit, at the neck and by the ear. When they become involved in fights against bacteria they become swollen and tender. The most familiar example of this condition is the development of painful glands in the neck during a severe throat infection.

The **spleen**, a large organ under the lower ribs on the left side, is part of the lymphatic system and takes a large share of its protective role. It also helps to manufacture some of the white cells and to destroy old, spent red cells.

Lymph glands
The diagram shows the main groups of surface lymph glands and lymph vessels on the right side of the body.

THE LUNGS

Imagine a rigid tube fitted into a balloon. Let this balloon hang free within a stout but malleable plastic bottle which has an air-tight seal around the place where the tube sticks through its neck.

Stretch the plastic bottle outwards. Its volume increases but because of the air-tight seal the amount of air within it (between its walls and the balloon) does not alter. Something must fill the extra space created and this is done by air coming in from outside through the tube and blowing up the balloon. Now relax the pull on the plastic bottle, which will regain its original dimensions and thus cause the balloon to flatten and expel the extra air which was inside it. This, quite simply, is the principle by which we breathe through our lungs.

The tube leading from the back of the throat to the lungs is the **trachea** ('windpipe') surmounted by the **larynx** ('voicebox'). The larynx can produce sounds by virtue of two ligaments within it. They vibrate as air passes by them. Alterations in their tension by muscles create different pitches of sound. The adjustment of these sounds into speech is effected by movements of the mouth, the palate, the tongue and the lips.

The trachea divides into a right and left **bronchus**, one for each lung. Each bronchus branches repeatedly through the lung tissue, the tubes growing progressively smaller until the very finest branchings end in microscopically small clusters of air sacs.

During inspiration of air (breathing in), the chest space is expanded partly through the pull of muscles between the ribs and mainly by the downward flattening of the **diaphragm**, the great muscle sheet which separates chest and abdominal cavities. In forced breathing other muscles about the neck also play some part in chest expansion. Air passes down the trachea, the bronchi and its branchings and stretches out the lungs, filling up the air sacs.

These sacs are very thin-walled and surrounded by small capillary blood vessels. Here oxygen from the air

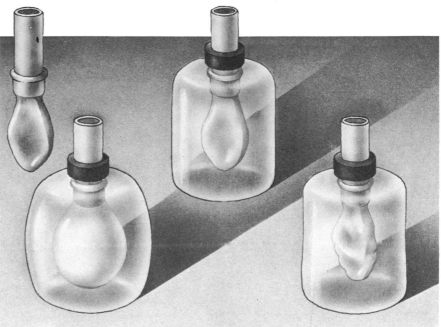

The lung system

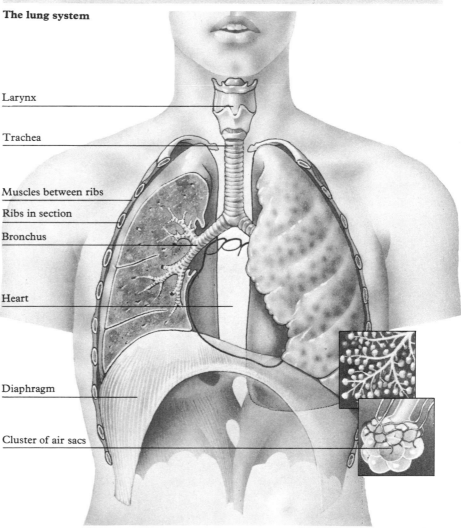

Larynx

Trachea

Muscles between ribs

Ribs in section

Bronchus

Heart

Diaphragm

Cluster of air sacs

passes into the blood, to be taken up by the red cells. And here the unwanted carbon dioxide carried by the blood passes out as gas into the air sacs.

At expiration (breathing out) the muscles concerned relax. The chest narrows back and the diaphragm settles upwards again. The lungs themselves contain elastic-like tissues which have been stretched at inspiration. Now their recoil helps to drive air out, carrying the 'waste' carbon dioxide with it to be breathed out through the nose and mouth.

Breathing in is therefore an active matter due to the work of rib and diaphragm muscles, and breathing out is passive, caused by a slackening of these muscles. However, forced expiration—expelling more air than is usual—can be done by tensing other muscles, between the ribs and those in the abdominal wall, to narrow the chest further than at its usual resting position.

Four-fifths of the volume of air we breathe in is nitrogen—which is inert as far as the body is concerned. Only one-fifth is oxygen, but this is more than enough for normal needs since only a small amount is taken into the blood stream at each breath.

The amount of oxygen needed by the body when it is resting, as in sleep, increases considerably during severe exercise. This can be effected in three ways. The rate of breathing can increase from about 12 times a minute (at rest) to something in the order of 30 times a minute. The depth of breathing will increase so that with each breath the chest may take in up to eight times as much air as it would at rest. And the supply through the blood is speeded up by a heart not only beating at a faster rate but also pumping a much greater volume at each beat. In very strenuous exercise the blood flow may increase to six times its normal rate.

THE DIGESTIVE SYSTEM

The illustration demonstrates the fate of the foods we eat, and the organs involved in their digestion. Crucial to this process are various internal fluids which work to soften and break up the foods as they pass through the body.

The **nose** and **tongue** begin digestion. Savoury smells and tastes trigger off the flow of **saliva** (1) which not only softens foods but also initiates the breakdown of foods. **Teeth** cut and grind the food making it easier to swallow.

The food mass passes (2) down the **oesophagus** (gullet) which pierces (3) the broad **diaphragm** (separating chest and abdominal cavities) before it reaches the **stomach** (4). Here the food is acted on by several kinds of digestive juices and by hydrochloric acid, all secreted by stomach glands.

The mixture now moves into the **duodenum** (5), the first part of the small intestine. Here two 'outsiders' enter. Bile secreted by the liver and stored in the **gall bladder** (6) enters the duodenum through the bile duct at a point where another duct brings digestive juices from the **pancreas** (7). These two work together to break down fats.

The mixture of juices and half-digested foods proceed into the **jejunum** (8) and then into the **ileum** (9), the other two parts of the small intestine whose total length is about five metres.

More digestive juices secreted within the intestines flow in to complete the break-up of food. Nutritionally valuable chemicals are absorbed into the blood stream through vessels in the lining of the intestines. The residue passes into the wide **colon** (10) or large intestine, which is 1½ metres long; near its blind end is the **caecum** (11) from which hangs the thin useless vestigial pouch, the **appendix** (12).

The colon forms a large inverted U and finally ends up at the short **rectum** (13), which leads to the **anus** (14) through which the contents can be expelled in the form of faeces.

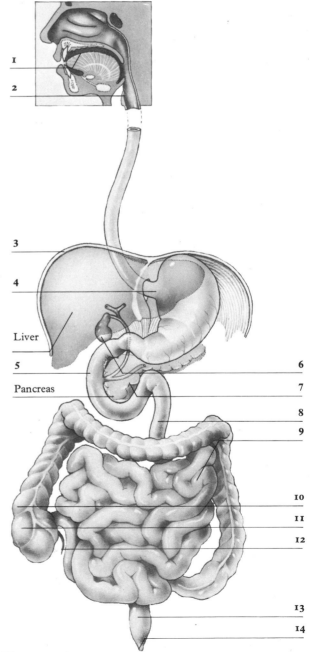

1

2

3

4

Liver

5

Pancreas

6

7

8

9

10

11

12

13

14

INTESTINAL MOVEMENTS

The stomach, the small and the large intestines have strong muscles which keep them in their characteristic churning motion.

This helps to mix up the food with the digestive juices and also to push it along the alimentary tract.

Peristalsis is the name given to the alternating waves of contraction and relaxation of the gut which propel the contents in the right direction on its journey. (When the waves of the oesophagus and stomach work backwards to propel their contents in the opposite direction, this is **antiperistalsis** and causes vomiting.)

The time taken after being swallowed for food to be digested and for its residues to reach the rectum is very variable indeed. It can range from 12 to 48 hours or more according to its nature and the state of the bowels. An average might be about 36 hours, of which some 12 would be spent in travelling through the colon.

Contraction

Relaxation

Peristalsis
The bolus of food is propelled along the gut by alternating waves of contraction and relaxation.

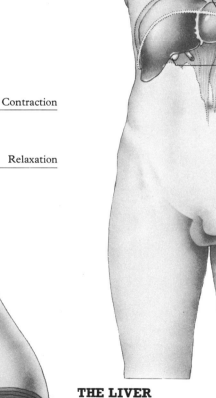

Diaphragm

Gall bladder

THE LIVER

The liver is a fantastic and indefatigable factory with almost five hundred functions. That is the number of actions given it by those who have specialized in its study.

It is the largest single organ in the body and weighs about one and a half kilos. Shaped like a large wedge (above), it is situated below the diaphragm behind the lowest ribs on the right side of the body. Overleaf we look at some of the liver's functions. One of its many

How the liver functions

The liver has its own artery bringing it blood from the heart and its vein taking blood back to the heart. The intestines have their own arteries bringing them blood from the heart. But their veins do not return blood directly to the heart. The blood passes first by the **portal vein** to the liver so that material from the intestines can be processed.

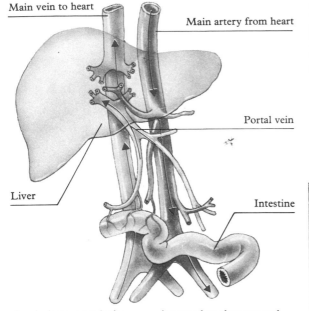

Main vein to heart

Main artery from heart

Portal vein

Liver

Intestine

chemical processes is the manufacture and secretion of bile. This yellow-green fluid passes into the gall bladder where it is stored before moving to the duodenum to help the digestion of fats. Nearly two litres of bile are produced each day.
One of the most important tasks of the liver is the receiving and 'processing' of the many products of digestion which come to it from the intestines. This is achieved by the blood from the intestines not returning to the main circulation at once but only after it has passed through the liver.
The **portal vein** is remarkable since it carries blood from one set of organs (the intestines) to another organ (the liver). All the breakdown products of digestion, all the chemicals absorbed from the intestine have to be 'checked' for storage in or alteration by the liver before they are released to the body. The liver synthesizes some of the most important materials for life.
Of the many actions which happen in this factory-cum-laboratory-cum-depot only some need be listed as examples. Sugar (as glucose)

is turned to glycogen and stored, awaiting a change back to glucose when the body requires it for energy. The breakdown products of fat are held by the liver as sources of energy in the form of sugars and other chemicals. Cholesterol is manufactured by the liver cells. So are many extremely important proteins essential to the blood plasma. These include not only factors concerned in blood clotting but also the anticoagulant, heparin. The liver stores the fat-soluble vitamins of the A, D and B groups, also chemicals of iron and copper. Its chemical processes play a large part in breaking up or neutralizing poisonous substances which may have entered the body. Some of its special cells are scavengers which destroy débris of cells, minute but harmful particles and bacteria which might come through the portal circulation. The liver is also involved in the formation of red blood cells in the foetus, though this task ceases after the baby is born.
With so much constant activity this organ is a source of considerable heat for the body.

THE KIDNEYS

Kidneys are primarily considered as filters which extract unwanted residues of the biochemistry of life, forming urine which they send out by way of the bladder. In fact they do considerably more: by very selective processes they regulate the body's delicate balance of water and of many chemicals.
The kidneys lie high in the abdominal cavity by the lower ribs, tucked beneath the diaphragm and against the back. From each kidney issues the **ureter**, the long tube which takes the urine down to be collected in the **bladder**. This is situated in the lowest part of the abdomen, just behind the bones which form the front of the pelvis. The bladder will empty itself through another tube, the **urethra**, which leads to the outside. The baby's bladder automatically contracts to empty itself as the pressure of urine inside rises.
Training has taught the older

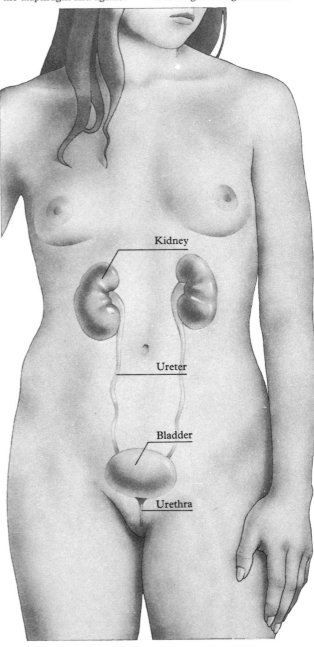

Kidney

Ureter

Bladder

Urethra

child and the adult to acquire conscious, deliberate control to delay emptying until circumstances are correct.

Sliced lengthwise, as in the illustration, the kidney shows a simple structure which belies its microscopical complexity. The tubules are accompanied by a network of capillary vessels which will eventually lead to the vein system, bringing blood back from the kidney to the heart and general circulation. It is within the twists and turns of each tubule that the contents undergo extremely important changes. Here there takes place an active and highly selective reabsorption of water and of salts into the blood of the capillaries. What is reabsorbed (and how much of it is reabsorbed) is variable, according exactly with the chemical needs of the body at the moment. If the body tissues are short of one special chemical, all of that chemical goes back to the blood. If the body has too much, then none of it is reabsorbed; all will go down to the collecting tube, and so through the ureter to the bladder. Those substances, like urea, which are just waste products, are never reabsorbed. By the time the material has passed the second bundle of tubule-twists, the work of the nephron is complete: what now passes into the collecting tube is the formed urine.

In this way the kidneys play an essential regulating role, controlling the concentration of many elements and compounds in the body and guarding the normal composition of blood and other tissues. Though their principal task is to produce urine the kidneys, like so many other organs, have multiple actions. Under special circumstances they can create two chemicals. Renin is produced by a kidney diseased with restricted blood supply; acting with other body chemicals it can raise the blood pressure.

Erythropoietin is made by the kidney as a defensive response to a sustained deficiency of oxygen; it stimulates the bone marrow to a higher production of red blood cells to increase oxygen transport.

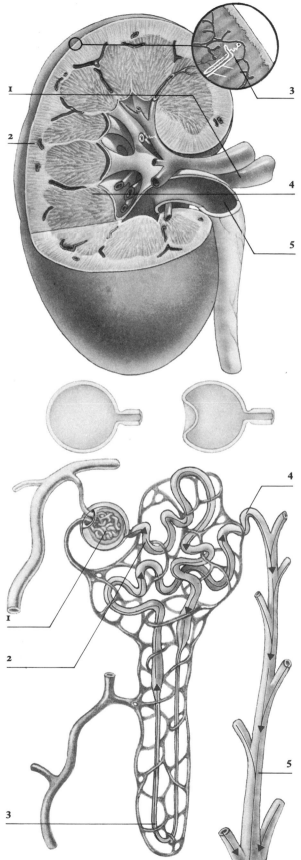

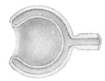

Structure of the kidney

The artery and vein taking blood into the kidney and away from it are at the side (1).

The relatively thin outer part of the kidney (2) contains over a million microscopically small, intertwined filtering units called **nephrons** (see below). The position of one is shown (3). The filtered fluid, the urine, passes through collecting tubes to the thicker inner part of the kidney (4) and so enters the wide funnel-like space which is the beginning of the ureter (5).

Nephrons

The nephron is a tubule which twists and turns in a characteristic way. Its very first part is a blind end, shaped like a thin balloon which has been pressed inwards to give a double-walled spherical cavity.

Into this cavity is tucked a coiled mass of fine capillary vessels (1). Here the first filtration takes place. It is a copious passing-out from the blood into the nephron cavity of a great deal of water and a large number of chemicals.

This is a passive or unselective filtration of more or less everything whose molecular disposition makes it small enough to move through the walls of these structures, and that includes the unwanted wastes (e.g. urea) which have to be got rid of, as well as many chemicals still of potential value to the body.

The fluid brought within the nephron flows along its microscopically fine, but long tubule. At first this is a highly twisted bundle (2), then it straightens out and runs along to a hairpin bend (3), where it runs straight back and reaches a second twisted bundle (4). Finally it turns back again into a widening collecting tube (5), which is joined by tubules from adjoining nephrons.

THE NERVOUS SYSTEM

Just as the circulation of blood has been compared to a nation's stream of traffic so could the nervous system be likened to an extremely complicated computer governing at long distance a series of electrical and telegraphic controls.

The brain is, of course, the headquarters of this process, but peripherally many sub-stations play their own partially independent parts. A severely damaged brain may largely cease to function as a thinking, perceiving and ordering organ but could still act with other parts of the nervous system in such a way as to keep the body 'vegetably' alive.

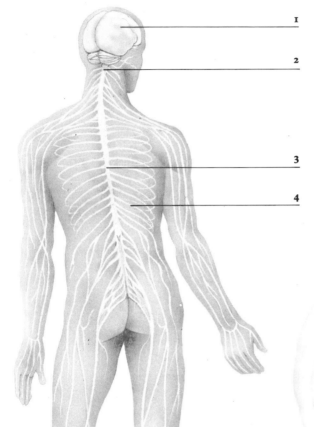

THE BRAIN

The brain's anatomy is so complex that anything beyond some general statements about it is likely to end up as a confusing list of names and structures more suited to the struggling despair of the medical student. To start, not at the top but at the base with what is called the **hind-brain**, we can see from the diagram that a cylinder of nerves passes through the large bony hole at the back of the base of the skull and continues below as the spinal cord. Apart from the nerve fibres leading to and from the brain, the hind-brain holds extremely important centres which achieve the basis of life – breathing, heart beat and circulation. Projecting from its rear and filling the lower space at the back of the skull is the **cerebellum**. It receives messages from joints and muscles and from eyes and ears. Coordinating this information controls posture, balance, some reflex actions and also the ease of fine or skilled movements. It does not initiate motion; that is the work of other parts of the nervous system. But it is essential for supervising efficiency of motion and position.

Moving up to the **mid-brain**, we meet a thick cylinder only two centimetres in length which may not look much when anatomically exposed. However, it holds relay points for cranial nerves connected with eyeball and eyelid muscles, and with hearing and vision. Even more important, it contains a complicated criss-cross of fibres which help to coordinate movement in the body.

Central nervous system
The **brain** (1) fills the cranium, the hard protecting upper part of the skull. It is our body's main communications centre. Here begin and end the major nerve stimulations to and from all parts of the body, receiving sensations, sending messages or controlling movement. The **brain stem** (2), the lowest part of the brain, passes through a large opening at the back of the skull to become the **spinal cord** (3), a thick cord of nerve fibres protected within the bony rings of the vertebral column (shown on page 14).

Peripheral nervous system
From each level of the spine, where vertebrae sit upon each other, **spinal nerves** (4) enter or leave the spinal cord. Their ramifications connect to different parts of the body. Some nerves are 'motor', that is they control muscle actions. Some are 'sensory' in that they carry sensations from different parts. The majority carry both motor and sensory fibres. However, a dozen pairs of nerves, mainly serving the face and back areas, do not arise from the spinal cord but direct from the brain. These are the **cranial nerves**.

Hind-brain

Mid-brain

Cerebellum

Hind-brain and mid-brain
The position and general structure are shown. The fore-brain is omitted.

The **fore-brain,** which is situated above the mid-brain, is remarkably large in comparison, filling the rest of the skull cavity, overlapping and hiding the mid-brain and much of the hind-brain. Its biggest part is the **cerebrum** consisting of two large cerebral hemispheres, arising forward from two stalks at the upper end of the mid-brain. Each is shaped into several large lobes (front, top, base and back). Its whole substance is folded and compressed with deep fissures between the convolutions so formed. This gives an enormous surface area for the total volume. In the three-millimetre thickness below the surface, the 'grey matter' holds the myriads of individual nerve cells which one can consider as the receiving and the initiating points of the major part of brain activity. Beneath this is the 'white matter', packed with long but microscopically slender nerve fibres leading to and from the nerve cells. These are protected in glistening white fatty sheaths.

The fore-brain

Right cerebral hemisphere

Left cerebral hemisphere

Cerebellum

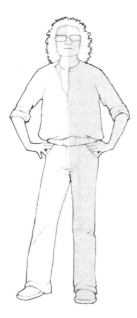

Opposite halves
Each half of the brain is linked to the opposite half of the body. For instance, the left arm muscles are moved by the appropriate part of the right half of the brain; feeling in the right hand is registered in the left half of the brain. As the nerve fibres run from the cortex of one side of the brain there is a point where they cross over to continue their course in the opposite side of the spinal cord. This cross-over is not total, for some nerve fibres remain on their original side, helping to coordinate actions involving both sides of the body.

Special functions

Each zone of the cerebral hemisphere has its special function. Though not all of them are yet known, some fairly definite mapping can be shown.

Moving—working muscles in different parts of the body

Feeling—sensations from different parts of the body

Speech

Hearing

Understanding speech

Writing ability

Reading ability

Vision

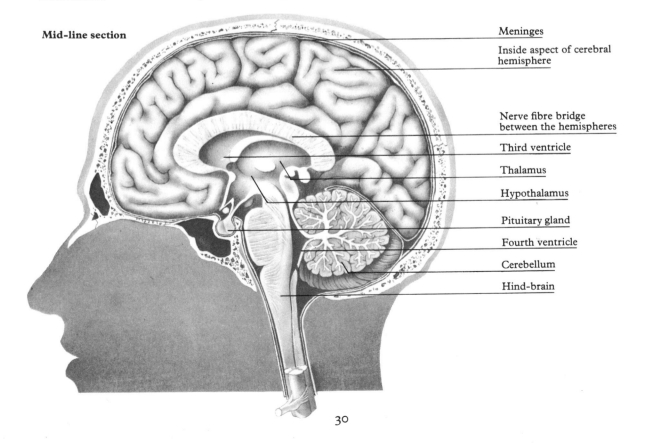

If one cuts through each cerebral hemisphere from back to front it will be seen to contain a large 'ventricle' or cavity. If, however, the cut is made not into a hemisphere itself but between the two hemispheres and down the mid-line of the brain, the picture is as shown below:

The inside aspect of the hemisphere shows a long, broad band of nerve fibres linking the two hemispheres. Below this can be seen a third ventricle which connects with the two ventricles of the cerebral hemispheres. The outer walls of this ventricle are formed by the sides of a big brain

mass, the thalamus, which is an important relay station receiving nerves of fine sensation and having connections controlling muscular activity. Below this a small mass, the hypothalamus, regulates many basic features like temperature, hunger, thirst, body use of fat and sugar,

sleep, primitive emotions and the workings of much of the autonomic nervous system. Damage to this area could cause abnormal overeating and abnormal outbursts of anger. This area is connected to the pituitary gland. Within the hind-brain is the fourth ventricle, continuous with the third.

Mid-line section

Meninges

Inside aspect of cerebral hemisphere

Nerve fibre bridge between the hemispheres

Third ventricle

Thalamus

Hypothalamus

Pituitary gland

Fourth ventricle

Cerebellum

Hind-brain

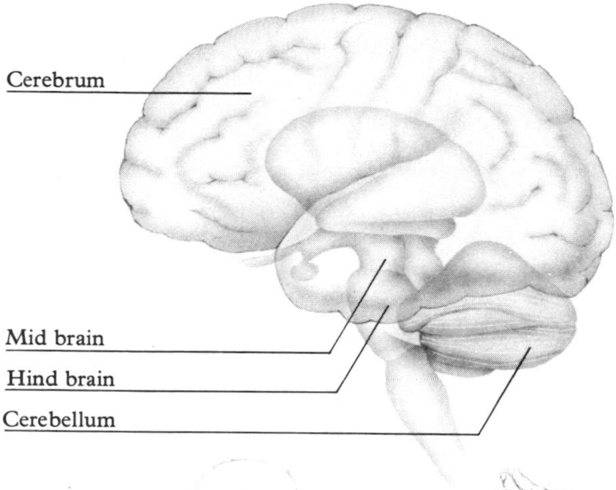

Cerebrum

Mid brain

Hind brain

Cerebellum

So brief an account omits many important structures. It can at least convey the concept that the brain is a tremendously complex system not only for initiating action and receiving sensation but also, through countless interconnections, for integrating and coordinating the whole. Which is the 'thinking' part of the brain? Where are the sites for judgment and creation? Though no specific areas can be confidently marked out for these, they are undoubtedly associated with the forward part of the cerebral hemispheres which are enormously developed in man compared with those in animals.

Wrapped closely round the brain is a treble layer of membranes, the meninges. A thin watery liquid, the cerebrospinal fluid, lies between the membranes. This liquid also fills the ventricles communicating with the meningeal fluid through small openings at the fourth ventricle. It cushions and protects the jelly-like matter of the brain.

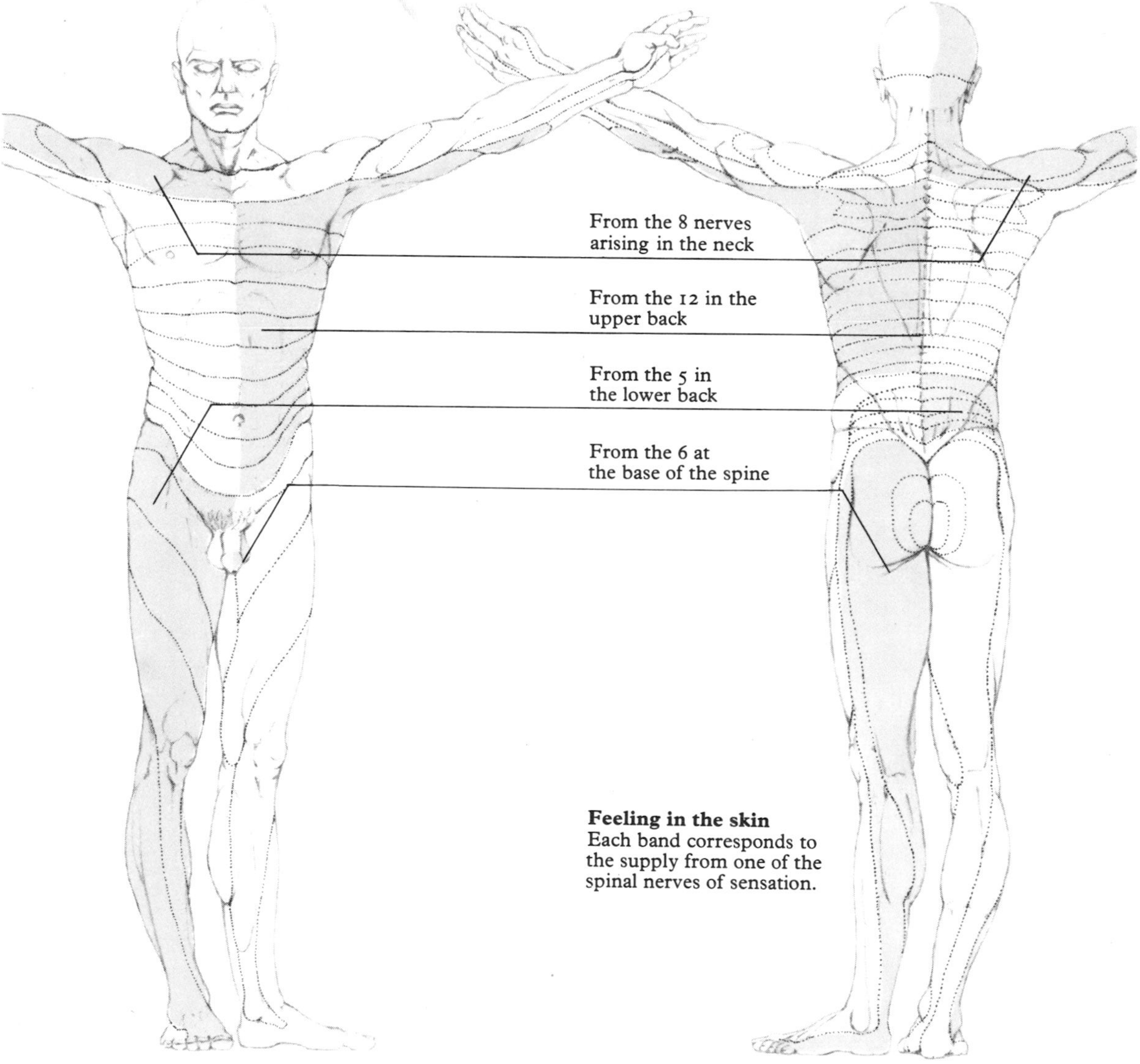

From the 8 nerves arising in the neck

From the 12 in the upper back

From the 5 in the lower back

From the 6 at the base of the spine

Feeling in the skin
Each band corresponds to the supply from one of the spinal nerves of sensation.

THE SPINAL CORD

The spinal cord is well protected in the position it occupies within the bony tunnels of the vertebrae. A spinal nerve comes off the cord on each side, in the spaces between adjacent vertebrae. They go to form nerves supplying almost every part of the body. A pattern of their spread can be shown by skin sensation. One can map out bands of body surface corresponding to the various levels of the

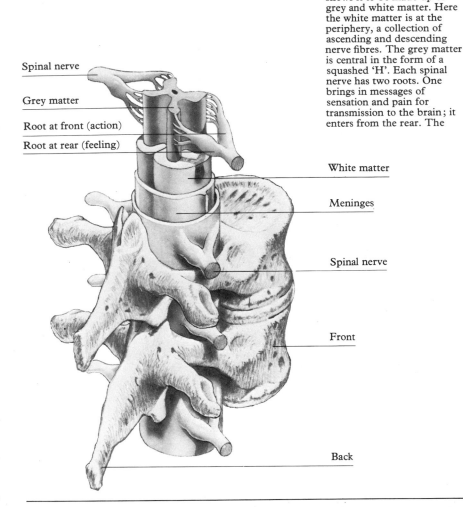

Spinal nerve

Grey matter

Root at front (action)

Root at rear (feeling)

White matter

Meninges

Spinal nerve

Front

Back

vertebral column from which the nerves issue.

A section of the spinal cord shows it to be made up of grey and white matter. Here the white matter is at the periphery, a collection of ascending and descending nerve fibres. The grey matter is central in the form of a squashed 'H'. Each spinal nerve has two roots. One brings in messages of sensation and pain for transmission to the brain; it enters from the rear. The other carries stimulus for muscle action and leaves from the front.

The nerve roots connect up with cells and very short fibres in the grey matter and to the white-matter fibres going to and from the brain. Just as the brain tissue has much interlinking of specific areas, so the spinal cord is not solely a 'pipeline' to the brain. It has its own interconnections.

The **reflex action** is one example. Many muscle actions take place without past training or purposeful direction from the brain. They can be considered as protective. The quick, automatic pull of an arm to withdraw a hand from a burning object is a reflex action. So, in a baby, is the contraction of an overfull bladder to empty itself.

In these cases the sensation messages (heat, bladder distension) do not only travel to the brain. They have also a short-circuiting route across the grey matter of the spinal cord to stimulate nerve cells and fibres which will act on the appropriate muscles.

Side connections also become evident. Nerve links could make the sufferer cry out or jerk other parts of the body not directly involved, like a leg moving as if preparing for flight. Often the brain can override the reflex; the burned person can force himself to keep his hand in position; the adult has learnt to exercise bladder control.

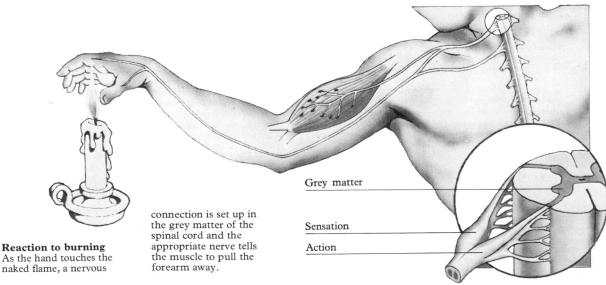

Reaction to burning
As the hand touches the naked flame, a nervous connection is set up in the grey matter of the spinal cord and the appropriate nerve tells the muscle to pull the forearm away.

Grey matter

Sensation

Action

THE AUTONOMIC NERVOUS SYSTEM

This is part of the peripheral nervous system. But it works mainly outside the awareness and control of the conscious brain. It is concerned with regulating such things as digestion, circulation, hormones, smooth muscle action and the sugar in the blood.
It has two very distinct divisions.
The first of these, the **parasympathetic system**, is formed from nerves which arise within various centres of the brain and also, at the other end of the body, from the lower end of the spinal cord. One of its major components is the vagus nerve, a cranial nerve which extends down to many organs such as the stomach, bowels, heart and lungs.
The task of the parasympathetic system is to keep going the routine activities of the body under normal circumstances. It sees to hormone formation, to the tone of smooth muscle in bladder and bowel, to the secretion of digestive juices and to peristalsis. It helps to store sugar in the body. It will maintain a steady quiet heart beat with a lower level of blood pressure.
The **sympathetic system** has nerves which arise from the spinal cord in the chest and back regions. Their actions are the opposite of those of the parasympathetic nerves. They stimulate the body for activity and effort, for coping with difficulties or fear. Under their influence the heart will beat faster and stronger, blood pressure will rise, more air will enter the lungs through widening of the air tubes, sugar will be released from storage for immediate use as body fuel, sweat will be produced, eye pupils will be widened and digestion will be slowed down. Hair also will be made to stand on end.
In the well-regulated body these contrary processes of sympathetic and parasympathetic activity cooperate until an emergency arises, when the sympathetic system takes over.

THE SENSES

Traditionally five senses are described: touch, sight, taste, smell and hearing. This overlooks others like pain, heat and cold, balance, and awareness of the position or movement of different parts of the body. Each has its scheme of reception and reception in the brain. Two organs merit special consideration here, the eye and the ear.
Movements of the eyeball are effected by six muscles set onto the sclera like small straps so that turning towards any direction is possible. Their nerve connections are linked so that when one eye moves the other one, even if covered up, goes the same way.

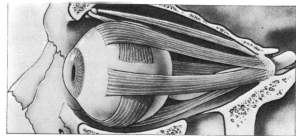

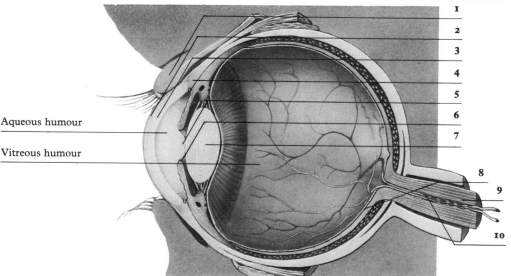

Aqueous humour

Vitreous humour

I
2
3
4
5
6
7
8
9
10

How the eye works

The rays of light must first pass between the **eyelids** (1) through a very thin protective layer, the **conjunctiva** (2) and then through the slightly domed and transparent **cornea** (3). This is a specialized part of the eyeball's general shell which in all parts is opaque and called the **sclera** (4). In front it forms the white of the eye. The light goes through the **pupil** (5), the dark central opening of the **iris** (6). This coloured ring dilates and contracts to the degree of illumination as it tries to even out the amount of light entering, and reaching the **lens** (7). By the pull of muscles around it, the lens adjusts its shape to focus light rays on the **retina** (8) at the back of the eye. The retina contains the first receivers of light, minute nerve cells of two different types: the 'cones' are concerned with colour and the 'rods' deal with darker, black and white registration. Through a complex relay system of nerve cells and fibres the light impulses pass to the **optic nerve** (9) which enters behind the eye. The nerve passes to various points of the brain and so to the visual centres at the back of the cerebral hemispheres. Elements from different parts of the retina 'switch sides' so that each visual centre receives vision from a part of both right and left eye. The **blood supply** (10) to the eye comes through vessels which pass through the centre of the optic nerve and then spread over the retina. The eye is hollow but not empty. The space in front of the lens is filled with the water, **aqueous humour**, which is constantly being secreted and drained. If drainage is impeded pressure builds up to the condition known as glaucoma which carries a real threat to vision. Behind the lens the major part of the eye holds the transparent jelly-like substance called **vitreous humour.**

THE EAR

Our hearing system is devised to turn the air vibrations of sound into nervous impulses which reach the hearing centres of the brain. The ear itself is divided into an outer, a middle and an inner part.

In the inner ear is found a feature common to many organs of the body, that of performing several tasks. Here is not only part of the hearing mechanism but also a means of informing the brain about position and balance.

Hearing begins with the outer ear. Built as a funnel for collecting sound, it cannot twitch and turn like the outer ears of some animals but the shape of its shell helps to inform on the direction from which the sound comes. Air vibrations travel down the **ear canal** to reach the **drum** to which they transmit their movements to the middle ear. Within the middle ear the movements are passed to the **ossicles,** a set of three minute bones linked together. The last bone has a footplate which fits into a small aperture at the wall of the inner ear.

This wall belongs to the **cochlea**, a chamber containing fluid that is surmounted by a spiral and in shape is rather like the shell of a snail. Within the spiralling canals are rows of microscopic membranes whose fibres respond to the vibrations of the fluid and register pitches of sound. This is the starting point of nerve fibres which go to form the **auditory nerve** leading to the hearing centre of the brain.

Just above the cochlea is the organ for balance. Within it hang minute hair-like processes which are tipped with solid particles. Similar processes are found in the adjacent three **semi-circular canals**. Each canal is set in a different plane, at right-angles to the other two.

When the head moves, fluid in the canals is set in motion on to the fine hairs.

In this way information on position and motion is transmitted by nerves to the brain, especially to the cerebellum.

The nerve fibres concerned with balance and movement and those concerned with hearing unite in one **auditory nerve**, and travel to the brain by this route. From the middle ear there passes the narrow **Eustachian tube** which leads to the back of the nose. Being open at both ends it equalizes the air pressure inside the ear and that outside—essential for the working of the ear drum.

Outer ear　　　Middle ear　　　Inner ear

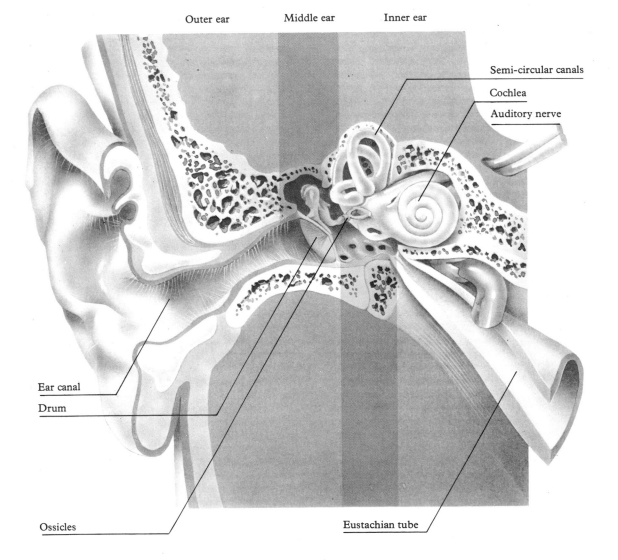

Semi-circular canals

Cochlea

Auditory nerve

Ear canal

Drum

Ossicles

Eustachian tube

REPRODUCTION

Union of a male and a female reproductive cell, each of which carries representative genetic factors, makes the offspring resemble its parents yet retain his or her own particular characteristics.

These reproductive cells are the **ovum** from the mother and the **spermatozoon** from the father. Their formation, their individual travels, their meeting and fusion and the development of this combined cell into a new individual form distinct stages of the reproductive adventure.

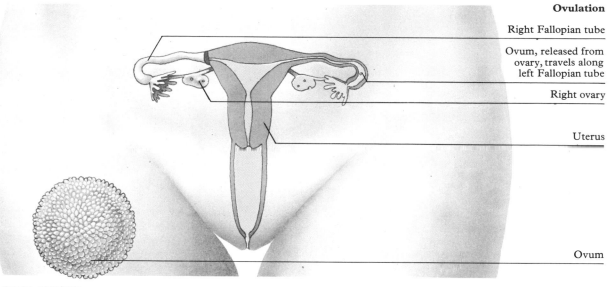

Ovulation

Right Fallopian tube

Ovum, released from ovary, travels along left Fallopian tube

Right ovary

Uterus

Ovum

THE OVUM

The ovum begins its life within the ovary. The two ovaries lie low in the pelvic area of the abdomen; one on each side, they are oval-shaped, about 3 cm long and 2 cm wide. The ovaries of a female child at her birth contain several hundred potential but immature ova, each in its own microscopic pack of membranes called the follicle. During the reproductive life of the woman one, and generally only one, ovum matures each month, the ovaries taking this task in turn. When it has reached its mature form, about two weeks after the onset of the previous menstrual period, the ovum bursts through the surface of the ovary and is released into the abdominal cavity; this is known as ovulation. At this stage the ovum could be just visible to the naked eye; in size it would be about the size of this next full stop.

The ovum does not stay there. Open over each ovary, like a funnel, is the wide end of the **Fallopian tube.** Each of these two tubes, about 12 cm long, leads towards the mid-line and into the top of the cavity of the **uterus** (womb). Almost as soon as it is released, the ovum is wafted through this funnel and begins its travel to the uterus, helped by the movement of fine, hair-like processes within the tube and of the tube's muscle. The ovum is waiting to be fertilized by the spermatozoon.

SPERMATOZOON

The paternal reproductive cells are lavishly produced. Whereas only one ovum is released each month the material ejaculated by a male during intercourse can contain several hundred million spermatozoa. Although this could be justified by the extra travelling that the sperms have ahead of them before one of their number succeeds in uniting with the ovum, this contrast in numbers is awe-inspiring. They are very much smaller than ova, tadpole-shaped and progress by sharp movements of the tail. They are formed in the man's two **testicles**. During the development of the foetus that will become the grown man each testicle begins its life within the abdominal cavity and then migrates downwards to pass into the scrotum. the pouch hanging

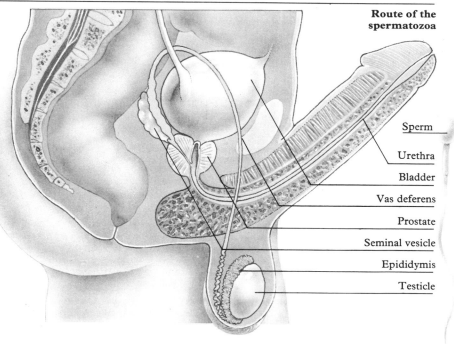

Route of the spermatozoa

Sperm

Urethra

Bladder

Vas deferens

Prostate

Seminal vesicle

Epididymis

Testicle

behind the penis.
The many spermatozoa formed in tubules of the testicle pass into a very long duct called the **epididymis**. This duct is so fine and coiled that its full length (some six or seven metres) is shaped compactly as a small organ sitting over the top of the testicle. It is a transit station for the spermatozoa which fill the duct and then leave the scrotal area through a long tube, the **vas deferens**. This passes into the abdominal cavity to just behind the bladder, where it opens into the **urethra**, the tube leading from the bladder to the outside, via the penis. However, just before doing this, the vas deferens receives a duct from a small gland, the **seminal vesicle**. And in this region the urethra also receives the openings of many ducts from the **prostate gland.**

Spermatozoa are stored within the end of the vas deferens. When sexual activity causes ejaculation they shoot out along the urethra. In themselves they form only a quite small part of the volume of the ejaculated fluid. The greater part is contributed by secretions from the seminal vesicles and from the prostate gland; their chemistry helps to activate the spermatozoa.

FERTILIZATION

The many millions of spermatozoa in the fluid ejaculated into the vagina compete in the journey to find the ovum. The vault of the vagina is surmounted by the 8-cm-long uterus which is roughly triangular in shape. The lower tip of the uterus, the **cervix**, projects a little into the upper end of the vagina. At the time of ovulation the small opening of the cervix is lightly filled with a jelly-like matter, receptive to spermatozoa. Those spermatozoa deposited here have the advantage of easier passage to the inside of the uterus. They ascend its moist lining and so enter the Fallopian tubes. Several hundred of them may reach the ovum which at this stage generally lies within the beginning of the tube, near the ovary. One of them will penetrate and move into the centre of the ovum which is now fertilized and will accept no more spermatozoa.

Fertilization

Meeting point of
spermatozoa and ovum

Uterus

Cervix

Vagina

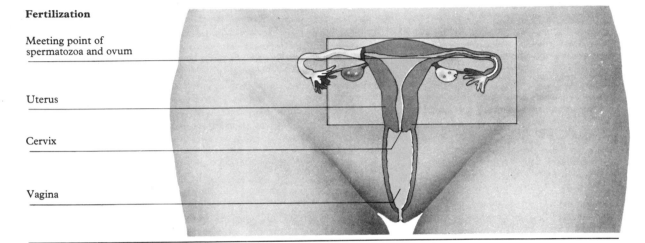

The embryo forms

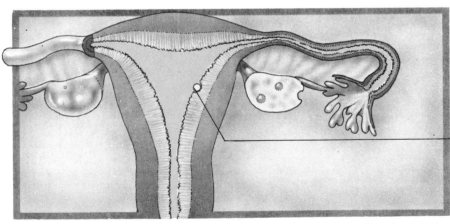

The early embryo becomes embedded in the uterine lining

SECURING PREGNANCY

The fertilized ovum now begins to divide, first into two cells, then into four, then eight and so on. During this time it continues its journey along the Fallopian tube and will enter the cavity of the uterus about one week after ovulation has taken place.
Meantime the lining of the uterus has prepared itself to receive it, becoming thick and spongy and with abundant blood supply. The ovum has by now developed into the very earliest structural collection of cells which can be called an embryo and embeds itself into the soft surface of this lining. Pregnancy proper can be considered to have commenced.
Unless it is fertilized the ovum lives for no more than 24 hours after ovulation. And the spermatozoa themselves survive only about 72 hours within the genital tract of the female. When fertilization has not occurred, the lining of the uterus sheds its extra thickness, with some bleeding, about two weeks after ovulation, thus forming the 'period' or menstrual loss. (For further information on the hormonal activity of the testicle and ovary, see opposite.)

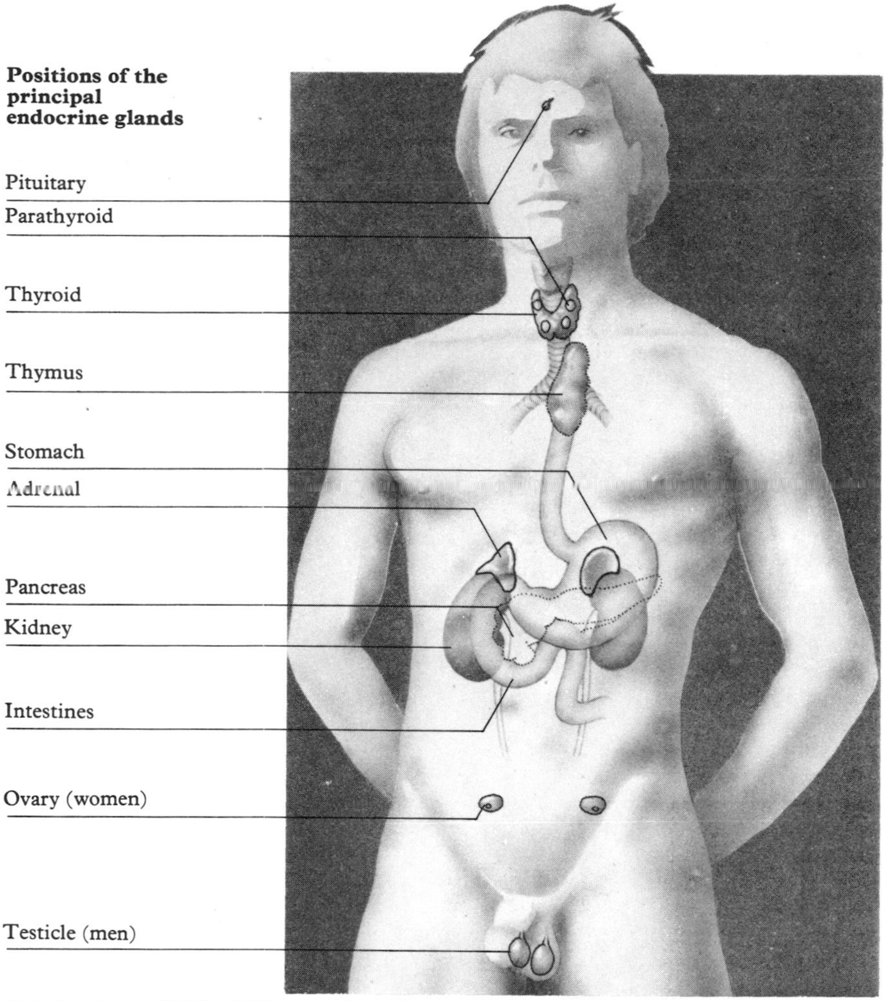

Positions of the principal endocrine glands

Pituitary
Parathyroid

Thyroid

Thymus

Stomach
Adrenal

Pancreas
Kidney

Intestines

Ovary (women)

Testicle (men)

HORMONES

The word 'gland' can be confusing for it is used in three different senses concerning the body. It has been applied to lymph nodes (see page 22) which are part of the circulation. The term is also used for the organs which secrete chemicals to act locally, like the digestive juices of the stomach and intestines. Thirdly, there are the many different **endocrine glands** whose secretions pass into the blood stream to be carried to and influence distant organs. Like messengers sent out from central offices they bring 'personal instructions' to remote agents. As the endocrine glands need no ducts to lead their secretions to their targets they are also called **ductless glands**. Their chemicals are called **hormones**.

In a healthy person hormones are produced in the right quantities automatically in response to the needs of the body. Their influence is slower than the fast immediate messages sent by that other control method, the nervous system, but it is far longer sustained. Some of the endocrine glands have several functions, not only secreting different types of hormones but also coping with completely dissimilar tasks.

Below is a summary of the chief functions undertaken by those endocrine glands located in the diagram.

THE TESTICLES

In addition to creating spermatozoa in their millions the testicles secrete the male sex hormone which appears at puberty. It guides the development of the man's secondary sexual characteristics – his deep voice, his body and facial hair, his stronger muscles and the more rugged form of his bones.

THE OVARIES

The ovaries secrete a number of female sex hormones which appear in the reproductive years of the woman. They are responsible for the female type of hair, for the development of the breasts and the typical fat distribution. Each month they also prepare the uterus for the possible embedding of a fertilized ovum.

The follicle which a discharged ovum leaves behind in the ovary converts itself into an endocrine centre secreting another hormone which, if fertilization has taken place, further influences the uterus for the maintenance of pregnancy. However, if fertilization does not occur then the secretion of that hormone ceases after a fortnight.

THE PLACENTA

This is the 'afterbirth' which is formed within the pregnant uterus to let nourishment pass from the mother's blood to that of the foetus. It too acts as an endocrine organ, secreting hormones to help develop the breasts to give milk and also taking over from the follicle in the ovary the main production of the pregnancy maintenance hormone. In addition (a nice example of hormonal interdependence) it secretes yet another hormone one of whose effects

is to keep up the follicle's endocrine activity.

All these various sex hormones are not uniquely male or female. They are found in all men and in all women but their relative proportions vary greatly.

THE ADRENALS

Sitting on top of each kidney, like a cap set at a jaunty angle, is the adrenal gland. It is in fact a double gland, the outer layer (cortex) and the inner mass (medulla) each having quite different roles. The **cortex** produces three types of secretion. Corticosteroids is the name for a group of chemicals which includes hydrocortisone. Their actions cover some control of the body's use of proteins (forming them into sugar) and of fats; they reduce inflammation; they combat allergic reactions and they play an important part in the body's response to stress. Another hormone from the

cortex controls the balance in the body of elements like sodium by altering the filtering effects of the kidney. The cortex also produces some forms of male sex hormones but the power of these is relatively weak compared to that from other sources. They may initiate the male changes at puberty. The **medulla** of the adrenal has a very different set of hormones which includes **adrenaline**, whose actions arise in emergency and emotional excitement. Associated with the sympathetic nervous system, they have been described as tuning the body to 'fright, flight or fight'. In sudden crises they reduce the blood supply to less urgently needed areas of the body such as the skin or the intestines but augment it to muscles. From its store in the liver they extract sugar for immediate energy and they increase the force of the heart beat.

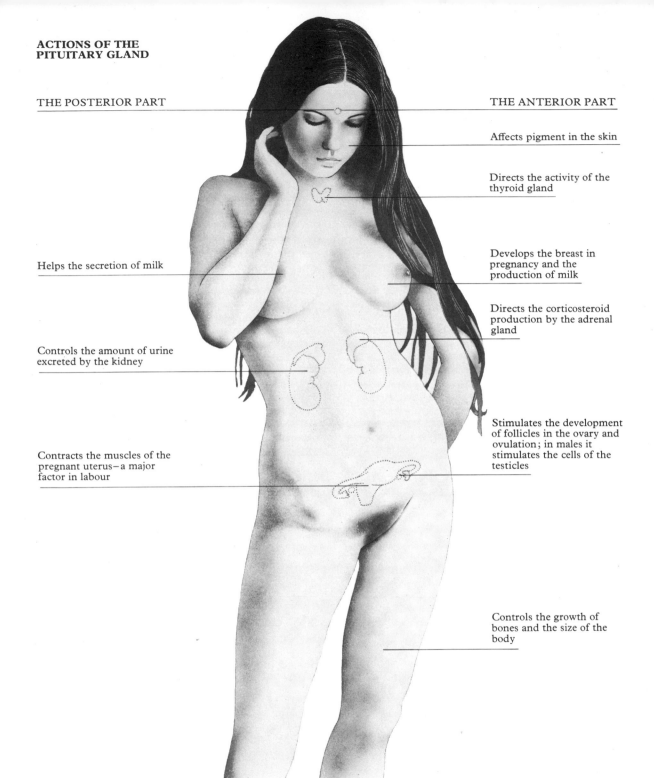

THE POSTERIOR PART

THE ANTERIOR PART

Affects pigment in the skin

Directs the activity of the thyroid gland

Helps the secretion of milk

Develops the breast in pregnancy and the production of milk

Directs the corticosteroid production by the adrenal gland

Controls the amount of urine excreted by the kidney

Stimulates the development of follicles in the ovary and ovulation; in males it stimulates the cells of the testicles

Contracts the muscles of the pregnant uterus—a major factor in labour

Controls the growth of bones and the size of the body

THE PITUITARY

So far we have seen all these endocrine glands playing different parts in the concerted programme of keeping the body in tune, coordinating and correlating with each other rather like members of an orchestra. The pituitary has been compared to the conductor of this orchestra for it directly commands and influences a great many of the other endocrines. Quite small, about the size of a pea, it consists of two parts, an anterior and a posterior. The different sets of action of each are summarized in the diagram. The gland lies beneath the hypothalamus of the brain (see page 30) to which it is connected. In fact it is very closely influenced by the subtle reactions of the hypothalamus.

THE KIDNEYS

As seen on page 27, the kidneys can under certain circumstances act as endocrine glands by producing hormones affecting blood pressure and also the formation of red blood cells.

THE PANCREAS

Here is another organ with an endocrine role in addition to its other function (see page 24). Of immense importance is its production of **insulin** into the blood stream. Insulin enables the sugar in the blood and tissues to be 'burnt up' for energy and also to be stored in muscles and in the liver. It also helps the conversion of sugars into body fats.

Its adequate secretion keeps the amount of sugar in the blood within normal levels. Insulin lack or malfunction (as in sugar diabetes) makes the sugar level in the blood rise abnormally high without being available as a body fuel or body builder.

THE STOMACH AND INTESTINES

These are further examples of organs with a secondary endocrine action. Under the effect of food passing into them the intestines produce hormones which stimulate the flow of bile from the gall bladder and of digestive juices from the pancreas. As for the stomach it has the faculty of creating a hormone which acts not on a distant organ but actually on itself. Entry of food into the stomach makes it secrete this hormone into the blood; the hormone then circulates with the blood back to the stomach to incite it to pour out juices to digest what lies within it.

THE THYMUS

This gland appears to have the task of championing the body in youth in its fights against newly met infectious microbes and foreign substances. Tucked behind the breastbone, the thymus is of prominent size in the baby, reaches its maximum in the toddler and then, after puberty, shrinks into almost nothingness. Its hormones increase the number and potency of the special white blood cells which protect the body against infection and help it develop its immunities.

THE THYROID

Lying in the front of the neck the extremely important **thyroid gland** regulates the pace of life and the heat production in the body. Its hormones speed up activity of both mind and body and determine the rate at which energy can be created. Also by means of a quite different hormone it plays a balancing part with the parathyroids in adjusting the level of calcium in the blood.

THE PARATHYROIDS

The four smaller parathyroids are embedded within the thyroid gland. They regulate the amount of phosphorus and of calcium in the blood. Bone substance, containing these two elements, is constantly breaking down and being reformed and the maintenance of the right calcium and phosphorus levels is an essential part of the process of keeping bone density correct.

THE PINEAL

The pineal gland remains much of a mystery. Set as a small projection from the brain, it is believed to react to light and dark impressions within the eyes and that its hormone is related to the body's circadian rhythm—that is, its sense of and reaction to the regular successions of day and night. It also certainly plays some part in sexual development, for an excess of its hormone in childhood can result in precocious puberty.

FINALLY . . .

There is no 'finally' in any account of the body. There is no conclusion as discovery after discovery keeps on being made.

In another sense it is impossible to be complete, especially in such a brief survey as this. But surely one point comes out clearly. The body is not a collection of separately working units. It is an extremely complex coordination of interdependent chemicals and tissues. No single cell, no single organ has its free autonomy. They are all in collaboration.

PART 2

STAY
HEALTHY

SIX ASPECTS OF BODY MAINTENANCE. INDIVIDUAL SECTIONS ON:

EATING WELL

Why do you eat?

Eating is so much a part of everyday life that few people think much about it. And if they do, thoughts generally revolve around the housewife's nightmare of what to eat that's not going to break the bank, can be prepared in the time available, is different from yesterday's and – above all – is something the family will eat.

With all those things to consider, it's perhaps not surprising that the nutritional value of the food is usually forgotten. But if you stop for a minute and wonder why you eat at all, there may be a few surprises. The fatalists would probably say that without food you'd die! True, of course, but such extremes of deprivation are not likely to happen to anyone in this country, or in any other 'developed' nation.

The real motivation to eat should be hunger, the feeling in your stomach that it's time to replenish the nutrients and energy expended during the previous six to 12 hours. But how many people ever feel really hungry? Certainly some do. There are even a few normal, healthy people who are positively faint if a meal is delayed by just one hour. The vast majority, however, can't remember what it's like to feel hungry. We tend to eat before hunger sets in. Why? Because the clock says it's breakfast time or lunch time, or time for tea break or the evening meal.

There's little doubt that for most people eating is an act of habit. It's not surprising. There's a lot to think about during our waking hours and any habit that can be formed to make an activity a 'mindless' process will be a help. To a large extent that's what has happened to food and eating. Once you've discovered the family's likes and dislikes and you know you get through five loaves of bread, 12 eggs, three pounds of meat, etc., in a week, shopping becomes so much easier and quicker if you can buy much the same food every week.

That's a slight exaggeration, of course. We do try new foods if the packaging is eyecatching or the advertisement memorable or our lifestyle changes and we need to seek out different foods. For the most part, however, man is a creature of habit. As long as the habits are good ones it is to his advantage that he should be. But when people get into the habit of eating less than perfectly there are problems. It isn't all that easy to exchange a bad eating habit for a good one.

Eating too much is one of our most common failings. The habit is established early in life, but may not be recognized as a problem until adulthood. This is where the great army of slimmers comes from – the biggest diet-conscious group in the UK.

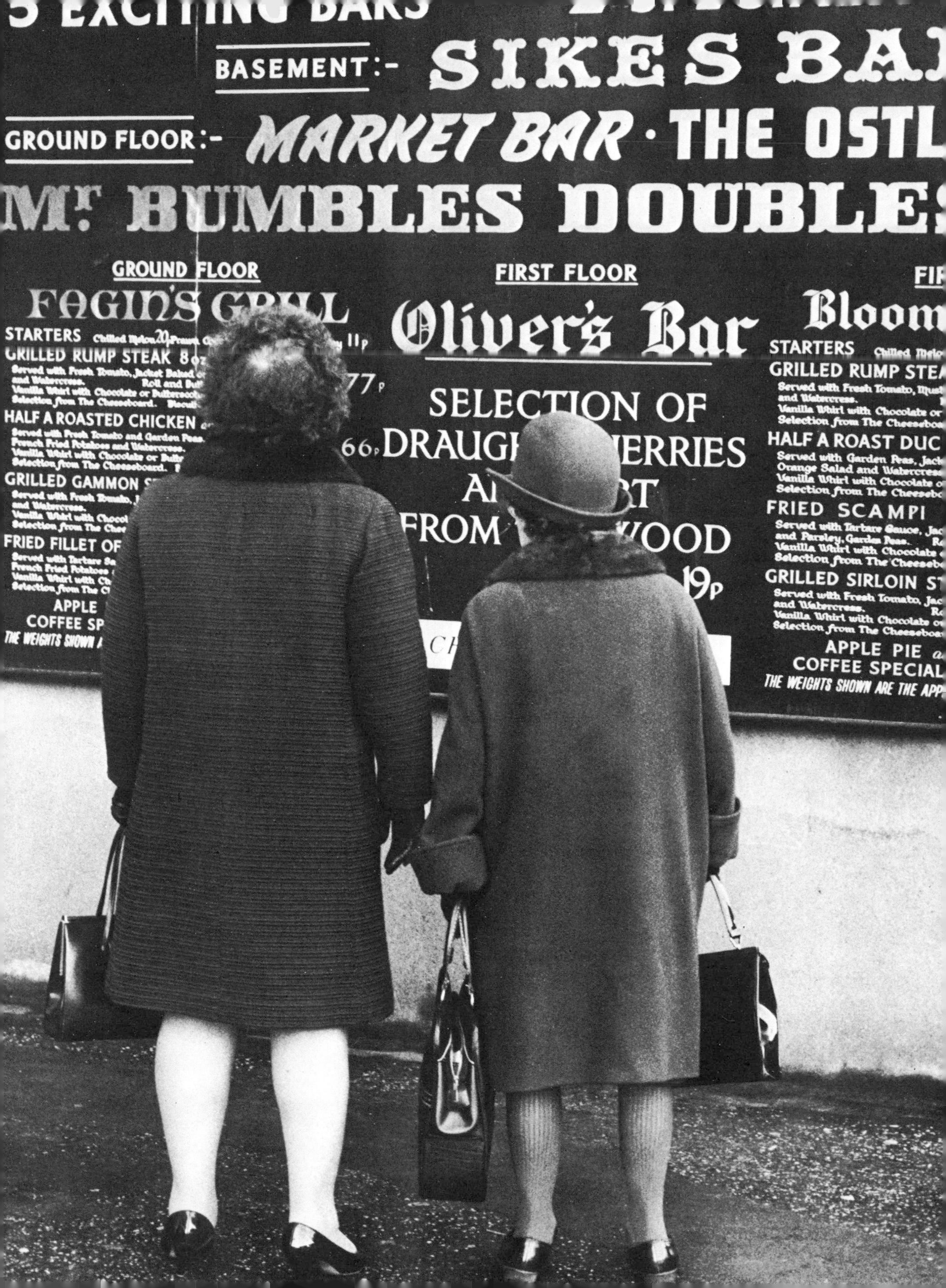

5 EXCITING BARS

BASEMENT :- SIKES BA

GROUND FLOOR :- MARKET BAR · THE OSTL

M? BUMBLES DOUBLE

GROUND FLOOR
FAGIN'S GRILL
STARTERS   Chilled Melon 20 Prawn Co...   11p

GRILLED RUMP STEAK 8oz
Served with Fresh Tomato, Jacket Baked or ...
and Watercress.   Roll and But...
Vanilla Whirl with Chocolate or Butterscot...
Selection from The Cheeseboard.   Biscuit...

HALF A ROASTED CHICKEN a...
Served with Fresh Tomato and Garden Peas.
French Fried Potatoes and Watercress.
Vanilla Whirl with Chocolate or Butt...
Selection from The Cheeseboard.   F...

GRILLED GAMMON S...
Served with Fresh Tomato, ...
and Watercress.
Vanilla Whirl with Chocolate ...
Selection from The Chee...

FRIED FILLET OF ...
Served with Tartare Sa...
French Fried Potatoes a...
Vanilla Whirl with Ch...
Selection from The Ch...

APPLE
COFFEE SP...
THE WEIGHTS SHOWN A...

FIRST FLOOR
Oliver's Bar

SELECTION OF
66p DRAUGH... ...ERRIES
A... ...T
FROM ...WOOD
19p

C...

FIF
Bloom
STARTERS   Chilled Melo...

GRILLED RUMP STEA...
Served with Fresh Tomato, Must...
and Watercress.
Vanilla Whirl with Chocolate or ...
Selection from The Cheeseboar...

HALF A ROAST DUC...
Served with Garden Peas, Jack...
Orange Salad and Watercress.
Vanilla Whirl with Chocolate or ...
Selection from The Cheesebo...

FRIED SCAMPI
Served with Tartare Sauce, Jac...
and Parsley, Garden Peas.   R...
Vanilla Whirl with Chocolate ...
Selection from The Cheesebo...

GRILLED SIRLOIN ST...
Served with Fresh Tomato, Jac...
and Watercress.   R...
Vanilla Whirl with Chocolate or ...
Selection from The Cheesebo...

APPLE PIE a...
COFFEE SPECIAL
THE WEIGHTS SHOWN ARE THE APP...

Something like 11 million people in Britain try to lose weight each year. Many of them really want to be slim. But to achieve their ambition they have to 'unlearn' the habits of a lifetime and adopt new ones. That isn't easy. Forty per cent of adults are too fat. In 1978 the figure was 40 per cent and it was the same the year before—evidence enough of how difficult it is to achieve long-term success in changing food patterns significantly.

Some people do manage to change their habits permanently. It could be because they simply want to look more attractive or because they have developed diabetes and their life depends on eating in a certain way. But for the majority the best hope of eating in a well-balanced way at the age of 30, 40 or 50 and beyond is to start young, to teach your children the kind of eating patterns you'd like them to have for the rest of their lives.

Because many of today's nutrition-related disorders don't appear until middle age, many people think that what children eat doesn't matter much. Not true. The foundations of several of these diseases are laid in childhood. That may sound ridiculous when you look around and see apparently healthy, energetic children, when you know that they are most unlikely to lose their teeth through scurvy and lack of vitamin C, and when every supermarket is bulging with an enormous variety of appetizing foods that children love to eat. But therein lies part of the problem.

There was a time, before man learned how to extract and concentrate sugar and fats and make them into a thousand different confections, when the foods that tasted best were the best nutritionally. Admittedly it was a long time ago—thousands of years—but how things have changed. Now if children were allowed to eat only the foods they thought tasted best many would live on sweets, biscuits, crisps and sugary drinks. And not only children . . .

All these foods have a role to play in the well-balanced diet. The trouble comes when they are eaten on top of adequate meals or in place of them. We don't need sugar and fat-rich foods; we don't feel hungry but we have an appetite for them.

Appetite—the desire to eat specific foods because they taste good—has to a large extent overridden the normal sensations of hunger. How many times have you seen small children refuse to eat meat or fish and vegetables because they're 'not hungry' and devour biscuits, trifle or chocolate pudding as though they hadn't seen food for a week?

There's no doubt that the so-called sophisticated diet of today is very different from the kind of food our ancient ancestors ate. It's even different from the food we or our parents ate 25 or 30 years ago! True, that was not long after the end of the war, but times have changed a great deal since.

What do we eat?

Long before the development of the food industry, in the days when man obtained his food as the wild animals still do, he relied on carcase meat and offal, fish, fruits, berries and some vegetables and nuts. Cereals were coarsely ground and made into a kind of rough bread. Foods like sugar, biscuits, chocolate, butter, cakes and ice cream, fish fingers and yeast-raised bread, jams and breakfast cereals are all inventions of very recent times—recent, that is, in terms of man's evolution.

Of course, if we had to rely on the food we grew and gathered ourselves, we would very soon starve. The lifestyle we have chosen is totally dependent on the food industry. But many people argue that modern man has not had time to adjust to the changes, to the high-sugar, high-fat, low-starch and dietary-fibre diet of today, nor to the sedentary lifestyle. In a few thousand years from now he might. Until then, they argue, many of today's diet-related disorders could be prevented by a return to the kind of diet man ate thousands of years ago.

Whether the full-scale 'back-to-nature' message has any more than emotional appeal is doubtful. But there is evidence based on modern research that health could be improved if we made changes in the balance of nutrients and therefore in the kinds of foods we eat. That doesn't mean foregoing all the time-saving, appetizing foods modern food technology has given us. It means being selective and knowing the best combinations of foods to choose. The foods available in every supermarket enable everyone to choose a nutritionally well-balanced diet—provided that people do select sensibly.

Many of the suggestions for a healthy way of eating mean adopting the diet patterns which were common some 25 years ago—when foods were rationed! How far have we come since 1953? What's different about the food and the nutritional value of our diets?

Whether you remember food 25 years ago or not, it's not difficult to accept that food in 1953 was somewhat less processed and more readily recognizable as meat, fish or cereal, sugar and fat than it is today. Since 1952 total bread consumption has fallen by 50 per cent, that of potatoes by one-third and of fish by almost half. Meat consumption rose dramatically as soon as rationing finished and thereafter remained fairly steady.

The effect of these and other changes has been to decrease the average amount of dietary fibre and starch we eat. The protein and fat intake per head have remained fairly constant.

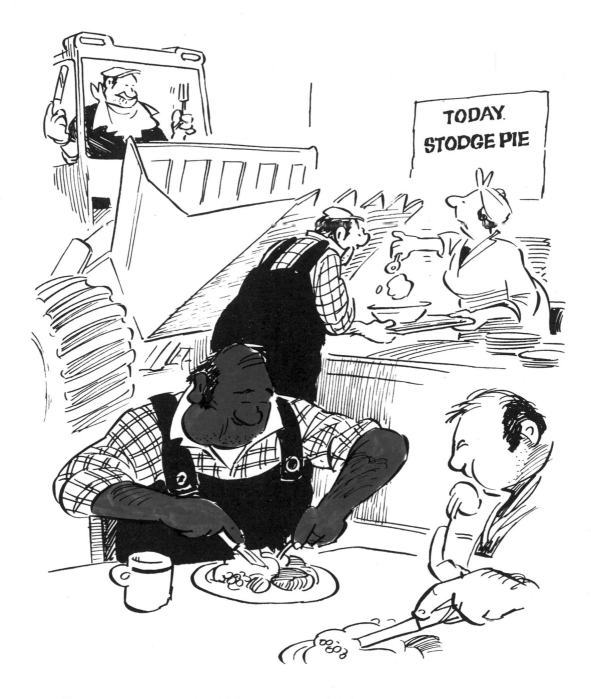

We now eat more meals which are prepared outside the home than we used to—not only in work canteens, in schools and restaurants but also as take-away Chinese or American food and quick snacks like pizzas, fried chicken and hot pies. When food is so highly prepared before we even buy it, it can be difficult to know what's in it in terms of proteins, fats, carbohydrates, vitamins and minerals. But choosing foods for a healthy diet needn't be a computer exercise nor an expensive pastime as long as you know something about the nutrients you need and where you're likely to find them. Armed with this knowledge you are also in a better position to judge for yourself the claims made for certain foods. Above all, healthy meals can be just as varied and interesting as unhealthy ones. They needn't be boring or dull if you use a little imagination in preparing them.

NUTRIENTS – WHAT THEY ARE, WHAT THEY DO

Most people have heard of protein, vitamins, fat, starch, sugar and calcium, but not of many more nutrients than that. So it would probably come as a surprise to know that there are about 50 different nutrients in foods, as well as water and dietary fibre.

WATER This is something we take for granted, rarely seeing how important it is to life. About 80 per cent of the weight of a baby is water. As he gets older he dries out a bit so that by adulthood only two-thirds of his weight is water. This abundance of water in our bodies is crucial to good health. Nutrients are carried around the body in water, waste materials are removed from tissues in it and all the chemical reactions which constitute life cannot continue unless an adequate amount of water is in the body.

A healthy person of normal weight can live for several weeks without any proteins, fats, vitamins or minerals. But he can survive for only two or three days without water. Each day the body has to lose about 850 ml water in urine. Normally it is more than that because we lose all the excess we take in, but 850 ml is the irreducible minimum which must be lost irrespective of the amount taken in. The water lost in faeces is quite small–about 60–100 ml a day–and the amount lost in sweat is very variable. It could be almost none if the climate is cool and physical activity very low. So about 1 litre of water is the minimum we need each day.

In most diets of sedentary people about half the water comes from solid foods and half from liquids. It is often surprising how large a proportion of apparently solid foods is, in fact, water. Our table shows that it is not uncommon to find a water content of 60 per cent in many of the foods we eat. In contrast, some foods like butter, biscuits and sugar contain very little water.

There is a theory that eating many foods with very low water contents is one of the factors responsible for the high incidence of overweight in this country. Water provides no energy (Calories or joules) but it is bulky. Most foods which are high in water are low in energy. The exceptions are the foods which are rich in fat as well as water; examples of such foods are cream and milk.

In general, thirst is a good guide to the fluid intake needed. It is particularly important for babies and people eating large amounts of dietary fibre to take enough water, but more will be said about these two later. Athletes may lose large volumes of water, which

Water content of foods

	% water
Cornflakes	3
Biscuits	4
Chocolate	4
Peanuts	4
Butter, margarine	15
Cheddar cheese	37
Bread	40
Fried sausages	46
Apple	65
Avocado pear	65
Lean meat, cooked	65
Roast chicken	68
Salmon	69
Egg	75
Grilled cod	78
Broad beans	84
Orange flesh	86
Milk	87
Tomatoes	93

It is surprising how much water apparently solid foods contain; even meats are two-thirds water.

contains salt, in sweat and it is especially important that this is replaced as soon as possible–even during the event if it is a long one. A loss of one-tenth of the total body water can result in severe symptoms of dehydration and muscle inefficiency.

PROTEINS If there's one nutrient everyone has heard about it's protein. Over the years many myths have developed around this nutrient and the sooner they are laid to rest the better–both for health and the housekeeping budget. It isn't true that the more protein you eat the better your health. It isn't true that protein is not fattening and it isn't true that vegetable proteins are inferior to animal proteins.

But first, what are proteins? The plural is deliberate. Both foods and the human body contain many different kinds of proteins. All of them are made from **amino acids**. It's not difficult to see an analogy in houses. All houses are built of the same basic materials– bricks, wood, glass, plastics, metals. But these can be used in different proportions to produce a huge variety of end products: small houses and large ones, houses with many windows or a few windows, houses with wood or metal window frames. So amino acids are put together in different combinations to form very different proteins. Liver proteins, for example, are different from muscle or bone proteins.

Twenty amino acids are used to make the proteins of the human body. Twelve of them can be made by the body itself if foods contain enough of the other eight. But these eight can't be made, they have to be eaten in foods and are called the 'essential' amino acids. (The other 12 are just as necessary for protein formation, but because they don't have to be eaten as such they don't qualify for the title 'essential'.)

If these eight essential amino acids are present in food in roughly the same proportions as the body needs to build its tissues then the protein is said to be of good quality. If one of these eight amino acids is absent or poorly represented in a food, then that food's protein quality is low. It was this reasoning which gave rise to the artificial and wrong distinction between animal and plant proteins. Most animal proteins are very similar in structure to man's, which is not really surprising. Many plant proteins–wheat, rice, peas, beans, oats–are short of one or more of the essential amino acids.

Protein content of food portions

	Weight of food in grammes	Proteins in grammes
2 slices lean meat	100	30
1 chicken joint	250	30
1 cod steak	120	19
Small piece Cheddar cheese	50	13
2 tbsp peanuts	50	12
Small can baked beans	150	8
Glass of milk	200	7
1 egg	50	6
2 slices bread	80	6
1 medium potato	150	4
2 tbsp peas	50	3
1 medium banana	150	2
2 tbsp cooked rice	50	1
1 tbsp butter, margarine	20	0

Although plant foods contain smaller amounts of protein than animal foods, they are still important sources of proteins because we tend to eat a lot of them.

However, the reason the distinction between plant and animal proteins is misleading is that almost no one eats just one protein-containing food; we eat several at the same meal. And one protein 'helps out' another. In cereals an amino acid called lysine is deficient. But there's plenty of lysine in peas, beans and other pulse vegetables. So, by eating spaghetti or bread with pulse vegetables, the protein quality of the meal is every bit as good as one containing animal protein.

Proteins are a fundamental part of every body cell. They form part of the structure of bones, teeth, muscle, liver, brain, blood and hair. Many enzymes, the organic substances which help in all the chemical processes and digest food, are also based on proteins. So proteins are important in forming body tissues and enabling the functions of the body to continue.

But proteins don't just go to the liver or other tissue and stay there for ever. There is a constant turnover in all tissues. Old proteins are broken down and replaced by new ones. When the old proteins are dismantled they liberate their constituent amino acids and these are further broken down in order to release energy.

FATS Not so long ago most people believed that one kind of fat was much the same as another and that all fats really did was to provide energy for the body. Indeed, the general opinion was that it didn't matter how much of our food energy came from fats and how much came from carbohydrates. Things are different now.

Each fat is made of two components– fatty acids and glycerol. All the common fats contain three fatty acids, hence the name triglycerides. They are joined to a glycerol molecule, as shown below:

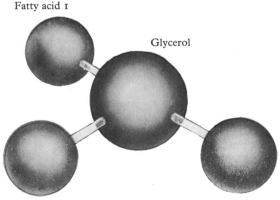

Fatty acid 1

Glycerol

Fatty acid 2

Fatty acid 3

In any one triglyceride the three fatty acids don't have to be all different; sometimes they are, sometimes two are the same. It is the structure of the fatty acids which gives the fat its characteristic properties and determines whether it is liquid or solid at room temperature.

Just as there are 20 different amino acids in proteins so there are about 40 different fatty acids in foods, but some are much more common than others and about 16 make up the bulk of the fatty acids in our food.

There has been a great deal of discussion about saturated and polyunsaturated fats and their relationship to heart disease (see also page 57). These two terms are sometimes used incorrectly in an effort to simplify explanations.

A fatty acid consists of a carbon chain:

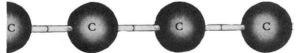

We can think of each carbon as having four hands:

If carbons link hands in a chain, each one uses two of its four hands leaving two free. If both of these link with a hydrogen on the following pattern:

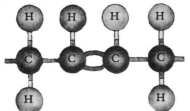

the fatty acid is saturated, i.e. it has no free hands to hold anything else.

If, somewhere along the chain, two carbons next to each other have one free hand each, they may link together in the double bond illustrated below:

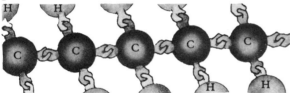

A fatty acid with just one such linkage is monounsaturated, i.e. it could accept a pair of hydrogens. A fatty acid with two or more such linkages is polyunsaturated. In other words it could accept many hydrogens, as below:

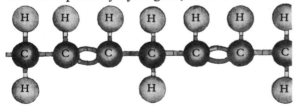

Many naturally occurring vegetable fats are polyunsaturated, e.g. corn oil, soya bean oil, sunflower seed and safflower seed. Some are monounsaturated, e.g. olive oil. But palm and coconut oil are saturated.

In general the more unsaturated a fat the more likely it is to be liquid at room temperature. Sometimes this is undesirable and a hard fat would be preferable. To make unsaturated, liquid fats hard, food manufacturers can add hydrogen. But in so doing they are likely to add so much that what started off as a polyunsaturated oil finishes up saturated.

Today there are special techniques which can be used in making margarine so that a part of the oil has hydrogen added, which makes it very hard, and this is mixed with polyunsaturated fats which are very soft. The result is a soft polyunsaturated margarine. By no means all the soft margarines on the market are polyunsaturated and certainly not all vegetable oils are polyunsaturated. Fish oils are among those that contain a high proportion of polyunsaturates.

Fat content of food portions

	Weight of food in grammes	Fats in grammes
1 pork chop, lean and fat	150	27
2 tbsp peanuts	50	25
Small packet crisps	25	18
Small piece Cheddar cheese	50	17
1 tbsp butter, margarine	20	17
Small bar chocolate	50	15
Small piece pastry	50	15
Glass milk	200	8
Individual tub yogurt, low fat	150	7
1 chicken joint	250	7
2 small biscuits	50	6
1 egg	50	5
2 slices lean meat	100	4
Custard (made with powder)	100	4
2 slices bread	80	2
Small can baked beans	150	1
1 cod steak	120	1
1 medium baked potato	120	Trace, i.e. negligible
2 tbsp peas	50	Trace
2 tbsp cooked rice	50	Trace
1 medium banana	150	Trace

Some foods like butter are obviously fatty, but many contain large amounts of 'hidden' fat, e.g. pastry, biscuits, chocolate.

Apart from their energy, we also need a small amount of fat to help make some hormones–prostaglandins–and the polyunsaturated fatty acids form part of the structure of cells. We certainly need some fats in food to give enough energy and to make food taste good. But everyone in Britain eats far more fat than he needs. Indeed, the amount we eat is so large that it could positively damage health. More will be said about this later.

CARBOHYDRATES If ever a group of nutrients was misunderstood it's the carbohydrates, or more specifically the starches. There are many different kinds of carbohydrates but basically they fall into two groups–the **sugars** and the **starches**. And the two groups are viewed very differently by nutritionists in terms of their health-promoting or health-inhibiting properties.

Starches are long chains of glucose units. Sugars are much smaller and consist of one or two units. Glucose is one sugar unit, and sucrose or common table sugar consists of two units, one glucose and the other fructose. Milk sugar consists of two units also, one of glucose and one of galactose.

Current nutrition research suggests that most people ought to be eating more starch and less sugar. Dietary change is difficult at the best of times, but particularly so when a nutrient has such a bad 'image' as starch. For decades starch and sugar have been almost

Starch content of food portions

	Weight of food in grammes	Starches in grammes
1 medium baked potato	150	37
2 slices bread	80	34
2 tbsp cooked rice	50	15
Small can baked beans	150	8
1 medium banana	150	3
2 tbsp peanuts	50	3
2 tbsp peas	50	2
2 slices lean meat	100	0
1 chicken joint	250	0
1 cod steak	120	0
Small piece Cheddar cheese	50	0
Glass milk	200	0
Butter, margarine	20	0

Nutritionists recommend that we eat more starch, and that means more potatoes, bread, rice and pasta. These foods also contain useful amounts of proteins, vitamins and minerals.

synonymous with 'stodge' (whatever that means) and with 'fattening'. People have thought they should try to cut down on the amount of starch they eat, probably because the advocates of the low carbohydrate reducing diet gave the impression that carbohydrates, and carbohydrates alone, were responsible for the excess weight. They aren't. An excessive intake of energy from whatever source is responsible for overweight. And it isn't possible to talk about starches and sugars in the same breath. They are different and behave differently in the body.

Sugar content of food portions

	Weight of food in grammes	Sugars in grammes
1 small bar chocolate	50	30
Small slice fruit cake	50	23
1 individual tub fruit yogurt	150	22
1 level tbsp sugar	15	15
1 medium banana	150	15
1 level tbsp honey	15	12
1 glass milk	200	9
Small can baked beans	150	8
2 slices bread	80	2
1 medium baked potato	150	1
2 tbsp peas	50	1
2 tbsp peanuts	50	1
2 slices lean meat	100	0
1 cod steak	120	0
1 chicken joint	250	0
1 egg	50	0

There are several different sugars in foods. The most common is sucrose–table sugar. Only milk contains significant amounts of lactose, which does not decay teeth. Honey contains some fructose.

Once digested, all starches and a large part of the sugars are converted into glucose, and ultimately into fat. An adequate level of glucose in the blood is necessary for the proper functioning of the brain and nerves. But we don't need to eat glucose as such. It can be produced in the body from dietary starches and from amino acids.

ALCOHOL When people think of food and its nutrients alcohol is very often–perhaps conveniently–forgotten. But it is a nutrient and in small quantities harmless. Unlike proteins, fats and carbohydrates, alcohol is a single substance. It can be used to provide energy, but otherwise has no nutritional value. So an excessive alcohol consumption may well lead to overweight. More seriously, gross overconsumption of alcohol to the exclusion of other foods can lead to liver damage and to deficiencies of B group vitamins and other nutrients. The hazards of sustained overconsumption, allied to a growing dependence, are explained on page 114.

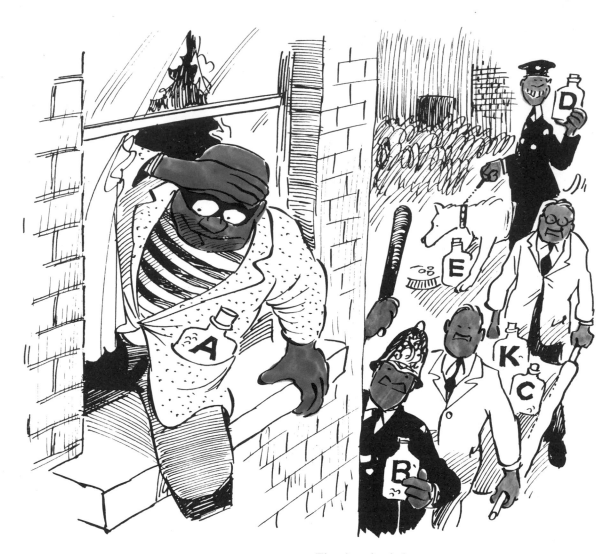

The vitamin chain

VITAMINS There have been more claims for the miraculous cures wrought by doses of vitamins than there are pages in this book. The imaginations of those who propound these works of fiction seem boundless. Even today, when vitamins have become as well known to nutritionists as water or proteins, we still have to endure ridiculous stories from the fanatical few who claim that food today is so devitalized that there's no alternative to resorting to vitamin tablets. What nonsense.

Of course vitamins are important in everyone's diet: the very name was originally derived from the word 'vital' because animals fed diets devoid of vitamins became very ill and even died. But they would have died if they had been deprived of protein or energy.

A vitamin is a substance which is essential to life and tiny amounts must be supplied by food. There are 13 vitamins which have almost nothing in common as far as their structure is concerned. In a way they are a motley collection of chemicals whose functions are as diverse as their structures.

The best-known is probably vitamin C, and most people have probably been told that it prevents scurvy—though the usefulness of that bit of information is doubtful in any of the developed nations. Recently much research effort has been put into the task of proving or disproving the theory that huge doses of vitamin C help to reduce the number of winter colds we get. For every piece of work which suggests that it is true, another investigation shows that vitamin C has no effect on the number, severity or duration of colds.

Next to vitamin C, the best-known of the vitamins is A, associated with good night vision, then B vitamins which are commonly thought to give healthy nerves. Many vitamins help the body's enzymes to work properly so that the thousands of chemical reactions which sustain life and the functioning of muscles, bone, brain and nerves can continue. The main functions are summarized in the table below.

Main functions of some vitamins

Vitamin A (retinol)	Good condition of body surface tissues, e.g. skin, respiratory tract. A tiny amount is needed in the eye to give good vision in dim light.
Vitamin B group (there are 8 vitamins in the group)	Converts one amino acid into another. Breakdown of carbohydrates to release energy. Indirectly concerned with functioning of nerves and brain. Prevents some kinds of anaemia.
Vitamin C (ascorbic acid)	Repair of skin wounds and broken bones. Holds adjacent cells together.
Vitamin D (calciferol)	Helps body to absorb calcium and phosphorus and deposit them in bones and teeth.
Vitamin E (tochopherol)	Involved in normal reproduction in animals— function in man not certain!
Vitamin K	Helps normal blood clotting after injury.

MINERALS The vitamins are a diverse group of chemicals with many unrelated functions, but the minerals are even more complex, not in structure but in number and function. There are far more minerals than vitamins—and we're not yet sure we have identified all those that are essential to health because some are needed in such small amounts. But a mixed diet is so unlikely to be short of any of the 'trace' elements that it is necessary to consider only a few of the more established minerals.

Calcium is well known as a constituent of bones and teeth, but a small and constant amount is needed in the blood to make sure blood clots quickly over a wound. Tiny amounts of calcium are also needed to enable muscles to contract properly.

Iron is probably as well known as calcium but its precise function is less well known. Iron is the part of the red blood cells which takes oxygen from the lungs to muscles where it is needed to break down fats and glucose to release their energy. This means that muscles can contract and move the body. It's not surprising that frequent symptoms of iron deficiency are breathlessness and tiredness. A shortage of iron in the blood means that insufficient oxygen gets to muscles. More rapid breathing and beating of the heart are attempts to overcome the deficit.

Many people, especially women, believe they have iron deficiency anaemia, but there is very little evidence that giving the majority of people iron supplements, or adding iron to foods, does any good. There certainly are cases of iron deficiency anaemia in many countries and probably some in a developed country like Britain, but not nearly as many as one might think from the sales of iron tonics and tablets. That isn't to say we should be complacent about the iron content of the diet.

For most nutrients the total amount of the nutrient in a food is a good guide to the value of the food in supplying that nutrient. If that sounds ridiculously obvious—read on, because the same is not true of iron. There are two kinds of iron in food, and one is much more readily absorbed by the body than the other. Iron in meat and offal is much better absorbed than iron in vegetables, eggs or cereals. Even so, the amount absorbed is only about 15 per cent. But the very poor absorption from plant foods—about 4 or 5 per cent—can be improved by taking a source of vitamin C at the same meal. So orange juice with the breakfast egg and toast makes more sense than you might have thought. Vitamin C has no effect on the proportion of iron absorbed from meats.

Other substances of importance are **fluoride** and **iodide**, both of which may be in short supply in some areas.

There has been considerable debate about the addition of fluoride to the water supply in some parts of the country. It's difficult to see why when all that is proposed is to raise the amount of fluoride in these parts to the level that exists naturally in others. There is no doubt that 1 part per million of fluoride in the drinking water, whether present naturally or added, does reduce the amount of tooth decay in young children. If the water supply in a particular area does not contain this level of fluoride, tablets are available but—as with anything else—enough is enough. There is no benefit from taking more than the recommended dose and large excesses may produce mottling of the teeth.

Iodide deficiency used to be much more of a problem than it is now. 'Derbyshire neck' or goitre was common among people living in certain inland districts where the soil was deficient in iodide. But much of the salt on sale now is fortified with iodide and cases of goitre from this cause are rare.

Sodium is a mineral no one is normally short of but it's important nevertheless to the normal functioning of nerves and muscles. Only people who are in very active occupations, athletes or those living or working in hot climates are likely to lose so much sodium in sweat that they need contemplate taking salt supplements. For the rest of us, cutting down on salt is more the order of the day as there is some evidence that an excessive intake in the form of added table salt may help to cause high blood pressure.

DIETARY FIBRE This is the new name for roughage. For years even the most esteemed authorities thought roughage was only important because it obviated the necessity to take laxative drugs. Many nutritionists believed fibre didn't really serve a useful purpose because, they thought, it went straight through the body unchanged.

Research on dietary fibre has accelerated in the past five years or so and we are beginning to learn what a complex and valuable substance it is. In fact, dietary fibre is not one substance, it is a mixture of chemically unrelated compounds–much the same as the vitamins. There are three groups of compounds in dietary fibre–**cellulose, non-cellulosic polysaccharides** (in other words long sugar-based units other than cellulose!) and **lignin**. Cellulose is the sole ingredient of cotton and is the basis of every plant cell wall. Lignin is the material deposited on the cellulose walls as plants age and become woody. Generally we make a particular effort to remove such parts of plants before we eat them and lignin is not a large part of the fibre we eat. One of the non-cellulosic polysaccharides familiar to most people is pectin–the substance responsible for the setting of jams and jellies.

From this description of dietary fibre, it must be clear that it occurs only in plant foods. Animal foods like cheese, meat, fish and eggs contain none. By definition, none of the components of dietary fibre is digested by the normal enzymes which digest proteins, fats and carbohydrates. It used to be thought that because fibre wasn't digested and absorbed into the body it couldn't be classed as a nutrient.

It may not be digested, but it is far from an inert lump moving along the intestines. One of the better known functions of dietary fibre is that it forms a large bulky soft mass in the intestines. This is much easier to expel from the body than small, hard stools. The muscle pressure needed to propel the large mass along the intestine is very much reduced. There are

two major consequences. Firstly, for nearly everyone in otherwise good health, the need for laxative drugs is eliminated. Long-term laxative use can be addictive which means that the longer the drug is taken, the greater is the dose needed to obtain the desired effect.

The second benefit is that a reduced pressure in the intestines is very likely to reduce the incidence of diverticular disease of the colon. This occurs when the inner layer of tissue in the large intestine bulges through the outer two muscle layers to form small pouches, known as diverticula. These pouches may cause no problem at all until they become infected and the condition becomes diverticulitis. This can be very painful.

Dietary fibre content of food portions

	Weight of food in grammes	Dietary fibre in grammes
4 tbsp All bran	50	13
2 slices wholemeal bread	80	7
2 tbsp peas	50	5
2 Weetabix	35	4.5
1 medium banana	150	3
4 tbsp cornflakes	25	3
2 slices white bread	80	2
1 medium potato	150	2
1 medium apple	120	2
2 tbsp cabbage	50	1.5
2 tbsp carrots	50	1.5
10 lettuce leaves	20	0.3
Small piece Cheddar cheese	50	0
2 slices lean meat	100	0
1 cod steak	120	0
Glass milk	200	0
1 egg	50	0

The texture of foods isn't a good guide to their dietary fibre content. Some smooth foods like banana or peas contain more fibre than rough foods like apple or lettuce. Both fruit and vegetables and cereal sources of fibre should be eaten.

A high-fibre diet is now the standard treatment for diverticulitis. The pouches won't go back to their normal state, but the symptoms are alleviated.

As if that were not enough to commend dietary fibre, there is some evidence that dietary fibre's components alter the 'environment' in the large intestine so that toxic materials are held by the fibre and prevented from coming into close contact with the wall of the gut. In addition, any toxins are removed from the intestine more quickly when the diet contains adequate amounts of fibre. The net result could be that cancer of the colon is less likely to occur. At present this is no more than plausible speculation, and like many of the other claims for the health benefits of dietary fibre has yet to be proved conclusively or refuted.

So much for the major nutrients in foods, what they are and what they do. Perhaps it is surprising that scant mention has been made of calories, kilojoules or energy. But energy is not a nutrient, it can't exist on its own.

WHERE'S THE ENERGY IN FOOD?

Energy in food and drink is contained in proteins, fats, sugars, starches and alcohol. For some years now there has been such interest in slimming that 'calories' have become rather undesirable in many people's eyes. But even slimmers need some energy from food each day. Total starvation may be alright under the strict supervision of a hospital ward, but for everyone else a minimum of about 800 Calories a day is needed for healthy slimming. Eat fewer than that and body protein is lost at a greater rate than normal and much of the weight loss is muscle rather than body fat. And that's not the object of the exercise at all.

Food energy has, for decades, been measured in calories because it was assessed by burning the food and measuring the heat given off—so many calories. In fact the calorie (with a small c) is very small indeed—so small that a woman might need 1,500,000 a day. Measured by this system an apple, for example, contains 50,000 calories. Such figures are too large to handle easily and we divide them by 1,000 and use the kilocalorie or Calorie (with a capital C). Then the apple contains a respectable 50 Calories and the woman needs a mere 1,500 Calories a day. Unfortunately people often become lazy and use a small c when they should use a capital C.

As if that were not complicated enough, it seems possible that, in the interests of standardized measurement in different sciences, we may one day have to change from kilocalories to kilojoules. The approximate relationship between the two units is: 1 kilocalorie (Calorie) = 4.2 kilojoules (kJ). So a 1,000 Calorie diet becomes a 4,200 kJ diet. When such a change will be imposed is not certain, but some people, notably dietitians in hospitals are already using kilojoules. But for the present it seems sensible to use both units.

Whatever measurement one uses, a Calorie or kilojoule in proteins is no different from a Calorie or kilojoule in fats, starches or sugars, or alcohol. But these nutrients contain different amounts of energy:

1 g of fat	9	Calories or 37 kJ
1 g alcohol	7	Calories or 29 kJ
1 g proteins	4	Calories or 17 kJ
1 g starches or sugars	3.75	Calories or 16 kJ

That should make it pretty clear that there's nothing inherent in starches or sugars that makes them more 'fattening' than proteins, fats or alcohol. Indeed, the high energy value of fats makes it more likely that high-fat foods play a major role in causing obesity.

WHEN YOU EAT TOO MUCH

It must seem amazing that, with all the complexity of the human body's nutritional needs, we don't suffer more than we do from excesses or deficiencies of one or more nutrients. Is it because people are such amazingly good judges of their needs, or does the body adjust despite efforts to over- or underfeed it?

Not surprisingly, the latter is usually the case! The safe rule is to eat a bit more than the body needs of proteins, minerals and most vitamins and the excesses will automatically be eliminated. Unfortunately, the rule doesn't apply to energy intake for most of us. Eating a bit more is precisely what happens in countries where food supplies are plentiful. A small or large excess of vitamins B and C and of many minerals is simply excreted by the kidneys. It's a bit more complex than 'in one end and out the other', but not much.

To some extent the body can store all nutrients. When the stores are full there is enough vitamin C to keep a person supplied with the vitamin for at least four weeks, even if he ate none at all. And there's enough of all the B group of vitamins to last for at least two weeks.

In the case of calcium and iron, when the body has as much as it can store the intestine adapts and simply refuses to absorb the normal proportion of these minerals; they really do go straight through the body. Only in conditions of extreme over-nutrition does the body become so overloaded with iron that a person becomes ill. The situation is most unlikely to occur in a country such as Britain by eating normal foods.

Very large stores of vitamin A can be built up in the liver. The same is true of fish and animals, which is why liver and liver oils are such good sources of this vitamin. When the human liver is full, it contains enough vitamin A to last for many months or years. But there isn't a very good regulatory mechanism which limits absorption of vitamin A or D and it is occasionally possible that too much of these vitamins can be taken. This is especially true if halibut liver oil is mistaken for cod liver oil. The former is much richer in vitamin D and care should be taken to use only the recommended dose.

The only food which contains toxic amounts of vitamin A is polar bear liver. Hardly a main item of diet for most of us, but early explorers in the Arctic soon learned not to eat polar bear liver, even in times of severe food shortage.

The body has very small reserves of carbohydrates and proteins but an excess of these in the food you eat, together with any excess of fat, is converted into body fat in most people. Most of the store is just beneath the skin, but some fat is around internal organs, where it protects them from impact damage.

There are some people who really can eat vast amounts of energy and never accumulate a store of fat. Quite how they manage it isn't known, but therein could lie the salvation of every slimmer, if only the scientists could discover what the secret is. Eating too much fat and sugar have other undesirable consequences for the heart and teeth respectively, and more will be said about them later.

Eating too little of anything isn't something most of us experience very often. But it should be clear that the body has enough of every nutrient to last it for at least two weeks of total starvation, provided enough water is taken. Many people have survived much longer periods without food. Over the course of a week or so, excesses and deficits tend to balance out. The well-known consequence of eating too little food-energy is that body fat is mobilized and its energy released to make up the deficit—and weight is lost.

HOW MUCH IS ENOUGH?

People vary enormously in height, hair colour, the length of their fingers, their pulse rate and stamina. So it's not surprising that they need very different amounts of nutrients and energy. Indeed it is not uncommon to find two apparently similar people of the same age, sex, weight, height and activity, one of whom needs twice as much energy and nutrients as the other. So it is impossible to make precise statements about the amounts of any nutrient or energy one person needs. But some guide is better than none. The best yardstick at present available is a set of figures from the Department of Health and Social Security called 'Recommended Daily

Amounts of Food Energy and Nutrients for Groups of People in the UK (1979)'. The figures for nutrients are set higher than the average requirement so that they cover the needs of most people. They therefore represent more than most people actually require, but that doesn't matter. The recommended amounts of energy are based on average requirements of people of different age and sex and activity. Some will need more, some less than the average to maintain weight.

Clearly the amount of energy the body needs depends on activity. Someone who leaps about a squash court for 30 minutes every day, cycles to work and spends eight hours digging ditches is going to need more energy than his neighbour who may travel to work by car, sit at a desk all day and do nothing more energetic than watch television in the evening. But apart from obvious physical activity, the amount of energy we need depends on body size. During sleep a small child needs much less energy than an adult. His smaller body needs less energy to keep it ticking over.

For adults about 1,100 to 1,600 Calories (4,500 to 6,700 kJ), depending on body size, are needed every 24 hours to keep the heart beating and the chest wall moving to allow breathing, to maintain a constant body temperature, and keep all the other life processes going. Physical activity needs extra energy. Despite popular ideas to the contrary, mental activity in terms of creative thought and

Energy expenditure of different activities for a person of normal weight

	Calories/ minute	kJ/ minute
Sleeping	0.7–1.4	3–6 depending on weight of bones and muscle
Sitting	1–2	4–8
Standing	1.2–2.4	5–10
Walking, moderate pace	3.5	15
Golf	3.5	15
Light domestic work	3.5	15
Cycling	6	25
Tennis	6	25
Swimming	12	50
Running, sprinting	15	65

Different people can use very different amounts of energy even when they are apparently performing the same activities. These figures are averages. Contrary to popular opinion, golf is hardly a strenuous activity, unless the course is on a 20° slope! All figures for energy expenditure during activity are higher in heavy people than in light ones.

mental arithmetic uses up no more energy than 'thinking' about nothing.

It is surprising how little energy apparently demanding physical tasks use. Housework is, frankly, physically light work. Let's face it, it doesn't demand much effort to push the buttons on the automatic washing machine, to walk around with the vacuum cleaner and lift the freezer lid to get the evening meal.

To be significant in terms of energy expenditure it is far more important that an activity is taken regularly, i.e. daily than that it is cripplingly exhausting for 10 minutes a week. The former will do you good. The latter may well knock you out.

Not only does exercise help to burn up any excess energy that your food may have supplied, and keep your heart and lungs in good condition, but there is an additional benefit. It seems that we need to take a small amount of exercise regularly for the body's normal hunger control mechanism to work. An extremely active person is almost certainly going to have a good appetite but he is equally certainly going to know when he's eaten enough and so maintain the correct body weight. On the other hand it is

quite likely that a totally inactive person will never feel really hungry and never feel full. The result is that he is liable to go on eating until he has consumed far more calories than he needs: and he'll get fat. In other words, his 'appestat' or control mechanism in the brain, which tells the body when to start and when to stop eating, just doesn't work.

A moderate amount of exercise daily is enough to get the "appestat" working so that the amount of food eaten can be controlled. Something like jogging for 20 to 30 minutes, walking for a mile or two or, if you're fit, a game of squash each day is all most people need.

At present there are no official recommendations for the amount of fat and carbohydrate we should be eating. But most authorities think that fat should account for about 30 to 35 per cent of the total energy of the diet. So the figures in our table of daily intakes are a guide to the amounts of proteins, fats, and carbohydrates (starches and sugars) which make up a healthy eating plan.

If we eat more protein than we need the body simply breaks it down, turns the amino acids into fat and either stores it or uses it as a

A guide to daily intakes of some nutrients and energy

	Proteins Grammes	Fats Grammes	Carbohydrates Grammes	Energy Calories	kJ
Boys aged 3–4	25–40	55–65	240–270	1,650	6,900
5–6	30–45	60–70	260–300	1,750	7,300
7–8	30–50	65–75	290–340	2,000	8,370
9–11	35–55	75–90	340–390	2,300	9,620
12–14	50–65	90–105	390–440	2,650	14,100
15–17	50–70	100–115	430–480	2,900	12,100
Girls aged 3–4	25–35	50–60	220–250	1,500	6,280
5–6	30–45	55–65	250–290	1,700	7,100
7–8	30–45	65–75	280–320	1,900	7,950
9–11	35–50	70–80	300–340	2,050	8,580
12–17	45–55	70–85	320–360	2,150	9,000
Men aged 18–34 (moderately active)	45–70	100–115	430–480	2,900	12,100
35–64 (moderately active)	45–70	90–105	400–460	2,750	11,500
65–74 (sedentary)	40–60	80–95	350–400	2,400	10,000
75 and over (sedentary)	40–55	70–85	320–360	2,150	9,000
Women aged 18–54 (moderately active)	40–55	70–85	320–360	2,150	9,000
55–74 (sedentary)	35–45	65–75	280–320	1,900	7,950
75 and over (sedentary)	35–45	55–65	250–280	1,680	7,030
Pregnant women (after 3rd month)	45–60	80–95	350–400	2,400	10,000
Breast-feeding women	55–70	90–105	400–460	2,750	11,500

These figures are only a guide. Some people will need more energy, some will need less to maintain weight, and nutrient needs will also vary within groups.

source of immediate energy. So it's pointless eating more and more protein. It won't do a scrap of good, and many protein-rich foods are expensive so it's also a waste of money.

The effect of eating more fat and carbohydrate than we need is too obvious to need restating.

Recommendations do exist for the amounts of certain vitamins and minerals that people should be eating, but there's not much point in delving into them. A good mixed diet which supplies the right proportions of proteins, fats and carbohydrates (with far more starch than sugar) is almost certainly going to contain enough of those nutrients.

ARE WE EATING ENOUGH?

A more appropriate question for most people would be: are we eating too much? All the evidence suggests that most people are eating enough of all the vitamins and minerals. They are certainly getting enough energy from food and drink, and enough protein.

Each year some 7,000 households throughout Britain complete an inventory for one week of the food already in the home, the food brought into the home during that week and the food remaining at the end. So we have a measure of the amount of different foods eaten by households of different composition. By using food composition tables the nutrients and energy this food contains can be calculated.

The survey is the Household Food Consumption and Expenditure Survey, better known as the National Food Survey. It measures only the foods brought into the home and takes no account of sweets, chocolates, soft drinks and meals eaten outside the home. But even without these foods, there is no general nutritional deficiency in Britain. The survey monitors groups of people so it doesn't pick up individual cases of undernutrition which may exist. But these are in any case very few and far between.

The only nutrient which may be poorly represented in some diets is vitamin D. But for the vast majority of people that doesn't matter at all. Sunlight falling on the skin enables the body to make its own vitamin D. If exposure to the sun is adequate a dietary source of vitamin D is unnecessary. 'Adequate' doesn't mean lying in the sun all day during the summer or under an ultra-violet lamp for hours in the winter. Just a few hours a day during which the face and legs are in sunlight is enough for everyone except young children and pregnant women, and women who are breast-feeding.

The National Food Survey shows that, on average, we eat at least 20 per cent more of most nutrients than the recommended intakes.

SO WHO NEEDS HEALTH FOODS?

In the past decade health food stores have sprung up in almost every high street in town and country. Health food magazines and health food fanatics try to persuade people that the 'normal' food of the masses is so devitalized and artificial that responsible people who care about their health should shun the supermarket's offerings and eat only foods from health stores.

It is difficult to see how some of the claims made for various foods like honey, organically grown vegetables and herbs like ginseng can be substantiated. Indeed, the only sensible definition of a health food seems to be 'one that is sold in a health food store'. Organically grown foods contain the same nutrients as equivalent foods grown normally, no one needs extra vitamins in tablet form. Health food stores offer some unusual foods you may not be able to buy elsewhere and you can be pretty certain that the brown bread you buy in a whole food shop is 100 per cent wholemeal, whereas in some other shops it is unclear which bread is wholemeal and which is just brown.

Eating enough of all nutrients and energy is extremely important. Eating more than you need is at best a waste of money, at worst damaging to health.

WHAT IS A BALANCED DIET?

Maybe you think that if we're all eating enough protein, energy, vitamins and minerals there is not much point in saying any more about nutrition. But there is plenty of evidence that all is not quite perfection in terms of the balance of nutrients we eat. It used to be thought that the relative amounts of fats and carbohydrates had no effect on health. This is now less certain as research indicates that too high a proportion of fats may be one of the factors associated with several of today's major diseases. Nonetheless the basic rules of general healthy eating can be summarized very simply.

Many sciences have a multitude of laws which students learn. Nutrition has one that is simple enough to remember: eat a wide variety of foods—a little of each and not too much of any.

Because nutrients are distributed in a somewhat random fashion among foods, and almost every food contains a great many different nutrients, a varied diet is almost bound to give you enough of every one of them. There are some people, however, especially children, who think a varied diet involves eating different flavoured crisps every day. That's not quite the interpretation nutritionists put on the term. But eating some foods from each of the following five groups every day is the basis of healthy meals for everyone.

Foods and some of their nutrients

Foods	Main nutrients
1 Meat, offal, fish, eggs, poultry	Proteins, fats, iron, B vitamins
2 Milk, cheese, yogurt	Calcium, proteins, fats, vitamins A and D
3 Fruits, vegetables	Vitamin C, dietary fibre, starches, proteins
4 Bread, pasta, rice, other cereals	Starches, proteins, iron, B group vitamins, dietary fibre
5 Margarine, butter	Vitamins A and D, fats

Eating some foods from each group daily ensures that all nutrients are obtained.

If you analyse the meals you eat now, it is likely that you'd find your diet contains two or three portions of food from each of these groups. So what's wrong with that? Recent research has revealed that further modifications to the kinds of foods within each group could make the diet even healthier and could help to reduce the incidence of several diseases which are common today.

DIET AND HEART DISEASE

Heart disease in every Western country is no longer a disorder which affects a few wealthy businessmen eating expense account lunches and doing 'stressful' jobs. An unskilled or skilled worker is even more likely to have a heart attack. Very many factors seem to be associated with the disease and the real causes are not yet clear. It is likely that heredity, smoking, blood pressure and inactivity are just as important as diet, or more so, in determining susceptibility to heart disease.

In their research, some scientists study the diets of people in different countries and look at the diseases they get. It may be possible to draw some conclusions about the eating habits which are often associated with a particular disease. This method of investigation is epidemiology. It doesn't prove that a particular eating pattern definitely causes the disease; it might be pure coincidence that, for example, a high intake of fats is found in communities that have a high rate of heart disease. But by using other bits of information it is possible to get a little closer to finding the causes of certain diseases.

Various studies have indicated that a high level of blood cholesterol is associated with a high incidence of heart disease. The amount of cholesterol in the blood is affected by two main elements of diet—the amount of cholesterol in food and the amount and kind of fat in food. In fact, the amount of ready-made cholesterol you eat in foods like liver, kidney, brain and eggs doesn't affect the blood cholesterol very much. Of greater significance is the amount and kind of fat. The different types of fatty acids were discussed earlier, and the table below shows the foods which contain predominantly one of these types.

Fatty acid contents of different foods

Mainly saturated fatty acids (increase the blood cholesterol)	Coconut oil, palm oil, hard margarines, dripping, suet, white cooking fats, beef and mutton fats, butter, cream, hard cheeses, cream cheeses
Mainly monounsaturated fatty acids (no effect on blood cholesterol)	Olive oil, lard, poultry
Mainly polyunsaturated fatty acids (reduce blood cholesterol)	Corn oil, soya bean oil, sunflower seed oil, safflower seed oil, fatty fish, margarines labelled 'high in polyunsaturates'

Eating saturated fats tends to increase the amount of cholesterol in the blood; monounsaturated fats don't have any effect and eating polyunsaturated fats often reduces blood cholesterol levels a bit. Although high blood cholesterol levels indicate a high risk of a heart attack, there is no conclusive proof that changing the levels by altering diet will reduce the risk of a heart attack. But it might help and it won't do any harm.

Whether lowering high blood cholesterol levels will prevent someone having a heart attack is not absolutely clear, but most authorities in many countries think the lowering of blood cholesterol by dietary change is worthwhile. There is general agreement that eating fewer fats in total and eating less saturated fat in particular is sensible.

Eating less fat clearly means eating less food energy. If you're overweight this is a good thing. But if you don't want to lose weight, replacement of the fat by starch is recommended, and that means eating more bread, rice, potato, and pasta.

The only point on which there is disagreement concerns the role of polyunsaturates. Some actually lower the amount of cholesterol in blood and for that reason some countries advocate an increase in the amount of polyunsaturates in the diet. Others believe that research does not show any reduction in heart disease if polyunsaturates are increased.

The best policy at the moment seems to be to cut down on all fats, including those used for cooking food. If you want to go on eating a small amount of butter or cream *within a low fat diet*, do. If you want to change to a polyunsaturated margarine *within a low fat diet*, do so, it may do some good. The obvious advantage of using a polyunsaturated margarine is that it can be spread thinly straight from the fridge, so enabling you to eat less total fat.

The other diet-related factor which may play a part in protecting people against heart disease is dietary fibre—especially the components of fibre found in cereals. Recent research showed that men who ate relatively large amounts of cereal fibre in the form of wholemeal bread, bran and other bran-containing foods and who also took more exercise than the average had fewer heart attacks. Whether or not additional dietary fibre does help in reducing this ailment has yet to be decided, but it could be another reason for making sure that everyone in your family eats enough fibre now.

This piece of research also highlights the importance of regular activity. It is important to remember that diet is probably not the major determinant of whether a person gets heart disease or not. A family history of the disease is relevant, and factors like smoking and physical inactivity are likely to be as important as diet, if not more so. But because smoking and inactivity are relatively more difficult to change than diet, the food we eat and its relation to heart disease has received more than its due share of attention.

It seems that the more of these aspects of lifestyle that can be changed the better are the chances of avoiding heart disease. And the sooner the healthy pattern is adopted the better the chances of success.

Heart disease occurs in the arteries taking blood to the heart muscle. And the beginnings of the problem occur in early adolescence. Somehow fatty substances are deposited in the artery walls and reduce the size of the channel through which blood flows. If an extra demand is made on the heart—as, for example, when someone exercises violently when he is unaccustomed to exertion—the artery channel isn't wide enough to allow the extra blood needed to reach the heart quickly. The result is either a pain in the chest—angina—or, in very severe cases, collapse as a heart attack occurs.

Complete blockage of an artery can be caused in two ways. Either so much fatty material is deposited in the wall that the channel becomes completely closed or a blood clot forms—a thrombosis. When a portion of heart muscle is deprived of oxygen and food it dies. Clearly the damage will be much more extensive if an artery supplying a large area of muscle is affected than if a tiny artery is blocked. There is not much evidence that thickening of the arteries can be reversed, although it can be slowed by appropriate measures, so it makes sense for people to take preventive measures at an early age.

DIET AND BLOOD PRESSURE

Many people suffer from high blood pressure, especially with advancing years, and it is one of the factors closely associated with heart disease. Some doctors believe that modern drugs are so effective in reducing high blood pressure that they alone should be used to control the condition and diet has no role to play. Other doctors believe that being the correct body weight is very important and that many cases of high blood pressure can be cured simply by slimming overweight people to their ideal weight.

It is much less clear whether the amount of sodium eaten is important in causing or curing high blood pressure. Certainly, people eating very low sodium diets have a very low incidence of high blood pressure. But the food they eat is very different from ours. They don't use salt (sodium chloride) and eat very little meat, which contains relatively large amounts of sodium. The diets consist mainly of cereals, fruits and vegetables which are naturally low in sodium. Such a diet would not be acceptable to most of us, but there is some evidence that keeping blood pressure low in childhood may be helpful in middle age. So keeping the sodium content of babies' and toddlers' foods down makes sense, and they don't seem to mind the taste. The rule is not to add salt to children's food and to avoid giving large amounts of very salty foods like cured meats, cheese, meat extracts, bacon and crisps, salted nuts and salt at table.

DIET AND CONSTIPATION

Constipation may be an embarrassing joke to some people, but it is a very real affliction for many others. It's as bad to think you are constipated even if you're not, and to self-medicate with laxative drugs.

Of all the aspects of diet and health which are being scrutinized now, few are as uncontroversial as the role of dietary fibre in preventing or curing constipation. Not only are laxatives addictive, but some, like liquid paraffin, may well prevent absorption of adequate amounts of vitamins A and D. So they are definitely not a good idea, especially for the elderly.

Dietary fibre will only exert its effect as a bulking agent if the diet also contains enough fluid to allow it to swell to its maximum extent. Taking breakfast cereal containing bran, wholemeal bread as well as fruits and vegetables is obviously sensible, together with an additional 500 ml of fluid a day.

Many claims have been made for the benefits of dietary fibre, most of them based on epidemiological studies. Groups of people eating more dietary fibre than we do in Britain don't get as much appendicitis, gallstones, hiatus hernia, heart disease, cancer of the colon or varicose veins. That doesn't mean eating enough fibre surely prevents all these disorders but it indicates that it might.

At present there is no official recommendation about the amount of dietary fibre we ought to be eating. The average daily intake at the moment is 20 g each a day. Many authorities think it would be much better if this average were nearer 30 or 40 g a day.

The different components of dietary fibre have different properties and different functions. Until we know more about the precise roles of each, it is sensible to eat a good mixture of cereals and fruits and vegetables to obtain all the components.

DIET AND TEETH

Only nine per cent of children in this country have a full set of perfect teeth by the time they are eight years old. Adequate brushing of course is important. Indeed, if everyone cleaned his teeth well enough after every bout of eating there probably wouldn't be any need for dentists. But it's not always convenient to use a toothbrush in the middle of the high street, the car or the cinema–the very places where sweet consumption is likely to be highest.

The alternative is to restrict sweet eating to the times and places it is possible to remove the sticky remains immediately. It may seem surprising, but the amount of tooth decay is not very closely related to the total amount of sugar eaten. It is much more dependent on the form of sugar. Maximum tooth decay results from eating sticky forms of sugar frequently– toffees, boiled sweets, biscuits, treacle tart, etc., which adhere to teeth for a long time and effectively give a constant supply of ammunition to the bacteria which eat into the tooth enamel. The least harmful forms of sugar are those which dissolve quickly like ice cream and jelly. And sugar as part of a meal is preferable to sugar between meals. Less sugar all round is better still.

If it is impossible to clean your teeth after eating sweet foods, a small piece of cheese or a few nuts will be a reasonable substitute. These foods reduce the acidity in the mouth and effectively neutralize the acid produced by the bacteria.

TODAY'S IDEAL EATING PLAN

The five food groups shown on page 57 enable you to eat the variety of foods necessary to obtain proteins, starches, vitamins and minerals. But clearly some modification is needed within the groups to reflect present-day thinking about what makes a healthy diet. The plan then becomes something like the one below.

The master plan	
1 Lean meat, fish, poultry, eggs	Eat 2 or 3 portions a day
2 Skimmed milk, cottage cheese, yogurt	Two portions a day
3 Fruits and vegetables including potatoes	At least 3 good portions a day
4 Cereals, e.g. bread, pasta and breakfast cereals, especially wholemeal varieties	At least 3 good portions a day
5 Margarine, butter	Small amounts

Cut down on sugar, especially between meals, cream, hard cheese, oils and whole milk. Use the grill rather than the frying pan, but don't smother food in oil before grilling.

Just eating the number of portions indicated may not provide enough energy for very active people. Additional foods can come from any of the five groups or from other foods like nuts, biscuits and snacks.

It may seem surprising that you are now being asked to eat more potatoes and bread, rice and spaghetti in the interest of better health. These foods are not only good sources of starch and low in fat, they also contain significant amounts of proteins, vitamins of the B group, and iron. And they don't contain all that much energy.

SPECIAL EATING PATTERNS

No matter what the size of a child or adult our ideal eating plan, above, is the basis of good meals for all the family. But there are some states where special nutritional needs have to be met, and some people choose to eat rather differently from the rest of us.

DIET IN PREGNANCY The additional nutritional needs of the pregnant woman are remarkably small. Although the foetus grows considerably after the third month, its growth is very small before then, and there is no reason why a woman should eat any more food, or eat any differently from normal at this time, provided she was eating a well-balanced diet to begin with. Even during the fourth to ninth months of pregnancy the daily increases in nutritional needs are quite small.

Early morning sickness during the initial weeks of pregnancy can be a problem. Different solutions seem to suit different women. Some find it helpful to eat a few dry biscuits before getting up, others are best helped by taking many small meals throughout the day. Yet others just have to wait for a few weeks to pass and for the condition to clear itself.

During the fourth to ninth months the additional energy needs are real but small— about 200 Calories (840 kJ) a day. In food terms that is about 2 slices of bread or 2 eggs or 250 ml milk or 40 g cheese. In fact the additions of milk or cheese to the normal diet make a great deal of sense because these foods also help supply the extra calcium needed.

Many pregnant women do become anaemic due to iron deficiency and are prescribed iron tablets. These may also contain folic acid—one of the B group of vitamins—and vitamin C. The folic acid helps to prevent a second type of anaemia, and the vitamin C promotes absorption of the iron. Even if tablets are prescribed it is wise to eat beef, lamb and particularly liver and kidney regularly, as well as fruits and vegetables.

Excessive weight gain in pregnancy may lead to difficulties during birth. It is certainly not easy to remove that extra weight afterwards. But equally it is not sensible to try to cut down on food intake during pregnancy so that weight is actually lost. Insufficient food can damage the developing foetus, especially the brain. The accumulation of some additional fat in the mother's body is desirable because this will be needed to provide some of the energy for lactation. Indeed, breast-feeding a baby is a very effective way of regaining your pre-pregnancy weight and shape.

LACTATION The energy needed to produce breast milk comes partly from the fat stores of the mother and partly from the food eaten during lactation itself. An additional 500 Calories (2,100 kJ) a day compared with the normal diet is the average requirement for successful lactation. Needs for all nutrients are increased slightly during lactation but particularly so for calcium and vitamin A. Again, taking an extra 250 ml of milk or 30–50 g cheese a day as well as the balanced diet is all that is needed. It is also important to drink enough fluid because about 800 ml of breast milk are produced every day.

FEEDING BABIES Very young babies don't eat, they drink, so why bother to mention them? Simply because the kind of food the baby receives during the first four months, and especially during the first two weeks of life, may affect his health for the rest of his life.

More women these days are deciding to breast-feed, and there is no doubt that this is the best start any mother could give her baby. It is not only nutritionally best, it is hygienic, convenient and satisfying for both mother and baby. Apart from the suitability of the nutrients in breast milk, there are also other components which mean the child is less likely to develop allergies later in life. Even if breast-feeding is continued for only two weeks it is better than nothing, but the ideal is four to six months.

No matter what the benefits of breast-feeding, there are some mothers who can't or won't breast-feed. The health of thousands of bottle-fed babies testifies to the effectiveness of artificial formulae. But it is important to choose a feed which has been modified to make it as similar to human milk as possible. Cow's milk contains too much protein, sodium and calcium for the human baby. Young kidneys can't excrete a very concentrated urine and it is important that all babies are given enough water.

Using more milk powder than is recommended on the label is positively dangerous. It effectively reduces the amount of water available to the baby and, far from making the baby healthier, it can harm him. Don't pack the scoops with powder, and don't use heaped scoops. In hot weather, or if the baby has diarrhoea, he will need extra water, not extra feed.

WEANING There is some evidence that the early introduction of cereals—at four to 12 weeks—may increase the risk of a child developing coeliac disease. This means that, for the rest of his life, he will not be able to eat anything which contains wheat flour or other wheat products, and maybe not oats, barley or rye either. Of course it is possible to live and eat happily without these foods, and many people do, but it's inconvenient. By no means all cases of coeliac disease can be eliminated simply by delaying the introduction of cereal foods, but some probably can.

Moreover, early weaning may lead to obesity in the infant. The ideal time to begin solids is four to six months. And it is sensible to take it slowly. The first week or so is a time when the baby gets used to a range of tastes and textures and the more he will accept at this stage the better are the chances of him not being a 'fussy eater' later.

It is wise not to add salt and sugar to the baby's foods to suit your own tastes. They are not necessary and the former may lead to high blood pressure later on. Sugar is better avoided for as long as possible, especially sugar in comforters. These are very damaging to teeth as a concentrated sugar solution may be in contact with teeth for hours on end.

VEGETARIAN DIETS

For some reason many people who eat meat can't imagine how vegetarians manage to keep body and soul together. The truth of the matter is that the only food most vegetarians deny themselves is meat, and maybe fish. Nutritionally valuable though these foods are in most people's diets, they are not indispensable. The protein, iron and B group vitamins they supply can very well be obtained from cereals, fruits and vegetables, eggs, milk and cheese. A new vegetarian in the family should cause no mother, husband or wife to worry one scrap about the health and fitness of the non-meat eater.

A bit more restrictive is the vegan diet which doesn't include any meat, fish, eggs, milk, cheese or any animal product like gelatine. But even vegans with a little guidance from the Vegan Society or other vegans can eat nutritionally adequate meals—provided they keep up the iron content in their diet. Nuts, pulses and other vegetables, cereals and vegetable fats, if eaten in sufficient amounts to maintain weight, are nutritionally satisfactory.

But it is likely that some help will be needed in finding interesting ways of presenting these foods.

Rather than being poorly fed, if the current thinking about a healthy diet is right, vegans should be even healthier than most of the rest of us. They certainly eat enough dietary fibre and their fat intakes are usually low.

MACROBIOTIC DIETS Any eating programme which is even more restricted than the vegan's is very likely to be nutritionally inadequate. The most widely publicized of these regimes is the macrobiotic diet in which more and more foods are eliminated from the diet until only rice remains. Valuable as this food is as part of a mixed diet, alone it is not adequate to sustain health, especially for children. Neither is a diet composed entirely of fruits.

SLIMMING

So much has been written about ways to lose weight that you'd think there was no more to say. But it seems there are still some people who believe the extravagant claims made by some food manufacturers. Despite what anyone may try to tell you, the only way to lose weight is to eat less energy than you need. This can be achieved either by reducing food intake or by increasing energy output, or, ideally, by doing both these things.

There are several popular methods of slimming, but if the diet works it will have reduced the amount of energy eaten. The most certain method is simply to count calories (or kilojoules). If you don't cheat, it must work. Cut back to:
    1,000–1,200 Calories a day for women (4,200–5,000 kJ)
    1,200–1,500 Calories a day for men and children (5,000–6,300 kJ).

Another healthy way of slimming is to concentrate on reducing the amount of fat. Cut back to:
    35–45 g daily for women
    40–55 g daily for men and children.
As long as you don't eat loaves of bread, plates of plain spaghetti or boiled rice, which are fat free and therefore theoretically 'free' on this diet, it should work.

And the final nutrient you can restrict is carbohydrate. Cut back to:
    60–100 g daily for women
    120–150 g daily for men and children.
Again, as long as you don't drink double cream neat or eat butter with a teaspoon (they are both carbohydrate free) the total energy intake should be reduced and the net result will be on the side of success: you will lose weight.

There is no food which actually

Energy values of some foods

	Amount	Calories	Kilo-joules
Cereals			
All bran	4 tbsp/50 g	140	580
Biscuits, plain	2 small/50 g	200	840
Bread	1 medium cut slice/40 g	90	390
Cornflakes	4 tbsp/25 g	90	390
Flour	1 rounded tbsp/ 25 g	80	330
Pasta, cooked	2 tbsp/50 g	60	260
Rice, cooked	2 tbsp/50 g	60	260
Weetabix	1/20 g	70	290
Milk, milk products, eggs			
Milk, whole	200 ml	130	540
skimmed	200 ml	70	290
Cream, single	1 tbsp/15ml	30	130
double	1 tbsp/15 ml	65	280
Yogurt,			
natural	indiv. tub/150 ml	80	330
fruit	indiv. tub/150 ml	140	580
Cheese,			
Cheddar	small piece/50 g	200	840
cottage	indiv. tub/110 g	100	420
Egg, boiled			
poached	size 3 or 4	90	390
fried	size 3 or 4	140	580
Fruits			
Apple, pear, orange	1/150 g	50	210
Avocado pear	½/100 g	220	920
Banana	1/150 g	120	500
Dried fruit	1 tbsp/25 g	60	260
Grapefruit	½/100 g	10	40
Fish			
White fish – cod, haddock, plaice poached or baked	100 g	70	290
fried in batter	100 g	200	840
Oily fish – salmon	50 g	80	330
Sardines, drained	1/25 g	50	210
Trout, grilled	1/200 g	190	800
Shell fish	50 g	50	210
Fish fingers, grilled	1	55	230

Vegetables

Beans, baked	1 small can/150 g	100	420
green	1 tbsp/25 g	5	20
Cabbage, cooked	1 tbsp/25 g	3	15
Cauliflower, cooked	25 g	3	15
Carrots	25 g	5	20
Parsnip, boiled	25 g	15	60
Peas	1 tbsp/25 g	15	60
Potato, boiled	1/150 g	120	500
roast	1/120 g	200	840
chips	120 g	320	1,340

Meats

Beef, lean, roast	2 slices/50 g	80	330
Lamb, lean, roast	2 slices/50 g	95	400
Pork, lean, roast	2 slices/50 g	90	390
Lamb chop, lean only	1/150 g raw	180	750
lean and fat	1/150 g raw	410	1,720
Chicken joint	1/250 g w. bone	200	840
Liver, fried	100 g	230	960
Sausage, cooked	1 large/55 g raw weight	130	540

Fats/oils

Butter, margarine	25 g	185	760
Oil	1 tbsp/15 ml	130	540
Lard	25 g	220	920

Nuts

Hazelnuts	1 tbsp/25 g	100	420
Peanuts	1 tbsp/25 g	140	580
Walnuts	1 tbsp/25 g	130	550

Others

Chocolate	1 small bar/50 g	260	1,090
Crisps	1 small pkt/25 g	130	550
Jam/honey	1 tsp/5 g	15	60
Sugar	1 tsp/5 g	20	80

makes you slim. There is no food which is inherently fattening. Certainly some foods contain more energy than others, but it is the sum total of the day's or week's diet that decides whether you gain or lose weight or stay the same. Slimming biscuits, meals in a glass and the like are effective in making you lose weight in the short term, but they are unlikely to help much in the longer term because they don't help you to learn the energy or fat contents of normal foods. The minute you stop the biscuit eating diet and return to normal foods, there is every chance you will go back to the eating pattern which made you fat in the first place.

Both slimming and general healthy eating are not achieved overnight. The benefits take a long time to be evident, but it does make a lot of sense to think about your family's diet and see if there are some changes you can make to improve it.

TAKE EXERCISE

Do you hate exercise? Or do you, perhaps, love the thought of it, but somehow never quite get round to it? If so, take heart. You are no different from millions of others.

What is more important, thousands who hate the thought of exercise just as much as you do have found ways to keep their bodies in good shape without making a part of each working day into a time of misery.

Remember, almost everyone has been fit and healthy at some time during their lives. Do you recall a time, perhaps as a child or teenager, when a game, a walk, hard physical work, a swim, would leave you tired–but glowing? The memory, like your legs, might well be a little rusty now. But the truth is that your body and mind have a memory of fitness that is invaluable to you.

It is this feeling that we shall try to help you recapture– however old and out of shape you may be at present. One of the lessons to be learned from remembering how you used to feel is that it was as a child you felt that way. Be like a child. . .and you will feel that way again. Approach your exercise with the thought that it is play, not hard work. You will find eventually that it's fun to be fit.

It won't happen overnight. But if you start gently, and progress gradually, you will begin to feel alert and alive, perhaps for the first time in years, and you'll be moving with the relaxed ease that you once had as a child.

WHAT IS FITNESS?

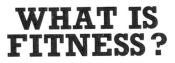

A lot of people make the mistake of believing that there is some mysterious state of 'absolute fitness'–like a sort of Everest peak of physical conditioning that you can clamber your way towards but which is way out of reach for most mortals like you and me.

There's no such thing. Fitness is very specific–it means different things to different people. The woman who is fit as a tennis player will not necessarily be fit as a swimmer. The man who can run for an hour every day is unlikely to shine as a weightlifter. What is fitness for the office worker is not going to be enough for the athlete.

There are inevitable differences between young and old, men and women, athletes and spectators. Yet all, in their own way, can enjoy the wonderful feeling of being fit. Probably, like most people, you have a vague feeling that you want to be more fit. But you must learn to be specific about *why* you want to be fit. You don't need the fitness of an astronaut bound for the moon to get you round

the supermarket feeling fresh and full of energy. You don't need the sharpness of a four-minute miler to take the dog out for a jog.

Fitness is a blend of a number of qualities, and the truth is that almost everyone– no matter how old, how young, how fat or how thin–can experience the benefits of increased fitness by taking the sort of exercise that they and their body will enjoy taking. You possibly have no great aspirations to shine in sports and games. You probably have no wish to amuse your neighbours by running the roads like mutton tracksuited as lamb. And you almost certainly have no wish to spend endless hours in some gymnasium aping the workouts of athletes.

But if you never experience the joy of mere existence that comes from being fit and healthy, then you're being robbed. It's the joy in movement that you can see in the playing of the child, in the running of the deer or the leaping of the horse. It's something that the rich would pay a fortune for–if it were for sale. And it's something that you can have for almost nothing. The price is just a little regular effort.

In the following pages we analyse the factors that contribute to fitness and suggest a variety of exercise programmes.

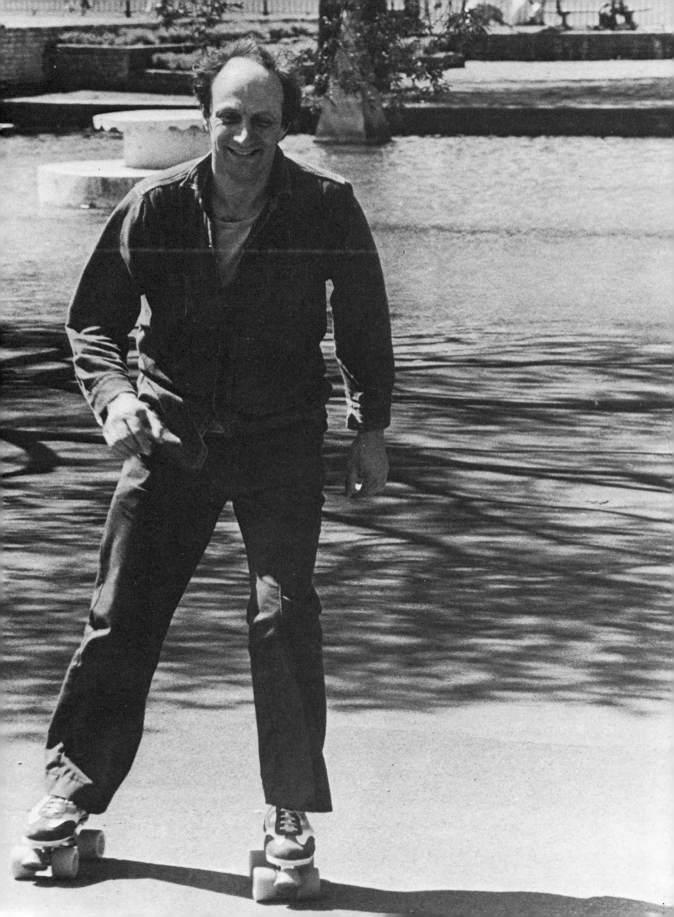

THE INGREDIENTS OF FITNESS

Fitness and exercise go together. There are various ingredients that you can choose from to mix your own blend. The secret is to find out what you need, and then choose the kinds of exercise that you will enjoy doing. You've got to come up with a mixture that you enjoy. . .and which at the same time does you good and doesn't leave you depressed with fatigue. So let's look first at the factors that make up fitness. These are the essential ingredients that should all be there, in some measure, in everyone's fitness mix.

STRENGTH Great strength and bulging muscles are often mistakenly believed to be sure signs of fitness, and from the days of Hercules the strong man has always been a figure of glamour. But in fact muscle bulk is one of the least important indicators of all-round fitness for modern living. The ability to push or pull heavy loads and to lift heavy weights is obviously useful when tackling tough physical work, or when competing in the power sports such as weightlifting, boxing or throwing, but big muscles–though impressive–are not essential to general fitness.

Almost any exercise programme will, and should, increase your strength–but often the effect will be to improve the trimness and tone of your muscles rather than to increase their size. No one wants flabby muscles, and women as well as men can benefit by taking exercise that will produce trim, rather than slack, muscle tone. But unless a statuesque beach-boy body is what you really want, you shouldn't bother with building great muscle bulk.

MUSCULAR ENDURANCE Muscular endurance is the ability of muscle groups to keep operating under the pressure of continuous use. This pressure can be anything from press-ups to painting the walls of the house. That ache that comes in the biceps or the shoulders, the dull pain in the thighs after prolonged physical work, mark the onset of localized muscle fatigue.

Endurance is one of the greatest human qualities, and is not something that disappears quickly with age. Many long-distance runners and walkers perform well into their forties, fifties and even later–and activities, sports and games that require endurance can be enjoyed long after your strength and speed seem to have deserted you.

The building of muscular endurance should be an essential part of your exercise programme, as it can ease the burdens of everyday life and take the stress out of heavy housework or the daily trek to the office. Muscular endurance is something that takes a long time to build up, but once you've got it you can generally keep it for life.

FLEXIBILITY One of the greatest differences between the young and the old is the way they move. Watch the young at work or at play and you'll see the beauty, the agility, the grace and the efficiency with which they move. But all too often growing old means growing stiff.

In our car-bound, desk-tied, armchair world people forget how to move. They lurch or they creak, until suddenly their joints tell them they're old. Yet there are plenty of gymnasts, acrobats, yoga-lovers and professional dancers who daily demonstrate that by regular stretching and mobility exercises the shuffle into premature old age with its loss of elasticity can be happily deferred. So include flexibility exercises in your fitness programme.

WEIGHT Fitness and fatness just don't go together, and one of the chief reasons why people take up exercise is because they are overweight. Certainly body-weight is an important aspect of physical fitness, and control of your weight is one of the most important ways in which exercise can benefit your health. The evidence of your own eyes will tell you that people who take regular exercise don't generally have great weight problems.

Paradoxically, exercise is not on the face of it an efficient way to lose weight. The statistical equations are discouraging. Eat a cheese sandwich and you've got to play almost an hour's squash, for instance, to burn off the effects! One pound of fat equals about 3,500 stored Calories, while jogging–which a lot of people take up to lose weight–burns up around 100 Calories per mile. So apparently you'll have to jog 30-plus miles to lose a pound of fat by exercise alone.

Of course, the simple equation tells only part of the story. The best way to keep your weight where you want it is to change permanently both your exercise *and* your eating habits. A regular fitness programme will help you do both. Also, a lot of people have found that regular exercise appears to have an effect on the metabolism beyond the simple burning of calories during the exercise programme. It's as if, having cranked up your body during a session of exercise, it goes on functioning as the body of an athlete for 24 hours or so after you've stopped exercising.

Certainly if you're trying to lose weight by dieting, regular exercise will help dramatically, and you can accelerate your weight loss by choosing a sport or activity, such as jogging, cycling, skiing or swimming, that really burns off the calories efficiently.

HEART-LUNG ENDURANCE Overall stamina should be at the centre of any exercise programme aiming at a high level of general health and wellbeing, for stamina involves the whole body through the heart, the blood vessels and the lungs.

It is generally reckoned by medical specialists and professional sports coaches to be the single most important of all the physical fitness factors—and it is today generally accepted that of all the muscles in the body, none is more vital than the heart. Heart disease has become the Western world's biggest killer, particularly among men, and one of the greatest miracles of sensible exercise is that it can condition the heart to cope with extra stress.

The best activities for strengthening the heart and lungs are those which make you work your whole body, rhythmically and continuously for a good stretch of time. Activities such as swimming, cycling, jogging, hill-climbing that keep the pulse rate some 75 per cent higher than its normal rate at rest are the ones that really produce this endurance—and everyone should include this sort of fitness training in their overall exercise programme.

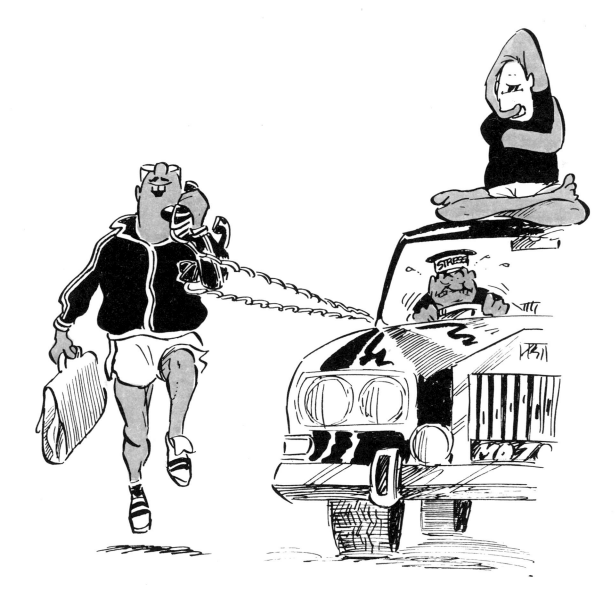

HOW FIT ARE YOU NOW?

The chances are that you'll have a pretty good idea of how you shape up at the present time. You'll know which of the fitness ingredients you're short on, and you'll have your own ideas about which areas you'll want to stress when it comes to putting together your own exercise programme.

But what about doing a test to establish firmly the shape you're in? Is it possible? Is it necessary?

There are certainly whole batteries of sophisticated and expensive tests that can be carried out to assess physical fitness – but mostly if you're unfit you know it anyway. Moreover, some tests can be dangerous (if not carefully supervised), and even the relatively mild ones can by their nature turn you off the whole idea of exercise.

For instance, one of the best-known measures of a beginner's physical fitness is the 12-minute test for joggers devised by an American, Dr Kenneth Cooper. It sounds simple enough. You just go to a running track and see how far you can jog, walk or crawl in 12 minutes. The result is matched up against charts devised by Dr Cooper to show how fit you are. There is an adjustment made for your age and sex, but generally if you cover less than a mile, you are in the 'poor' category; if you cover between 1 and 1½ miles you are 'fair', and so on. The trouble is that the very people who need it most are unlikely to want to be seen on a running track. And I know of very few people who have gone through this sort of initiation into jogging.

If you feel you need this sort of test it's probably better just to assume that you're *unfit* and start from there. But there are some very simple tests that will help you to assess your fitness – and point out where your weaknesses lie.

1 How long can you hold your breath?
Take a few deep breaths, then fill the lungs and try holding your breath. Fifty seconds is a good average. If you are really fit you should be able to manage about 70 seconds. Thirty seconds or below means you need some exercise.

2 How is your pulse rate?
You'll need a watch with a second hand for this. Sit or lie quietly for a few minutes, then take your pulse. It should be 80 beats per minute or less if you're in reasonable condition. Then stand up and take it again. It should rise, but not by more than 24 beats per minute. If you remain standing, the pulse should slow down to no more than 12 beats per minute over your resting rate.

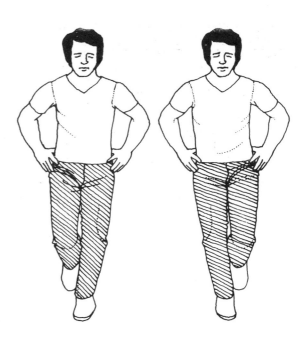

3 How is your balancing ability?
Stand with your feet together, hands on hips. Close your eyes and raise one knee. Hold the position for five seconds. Then, without opening your eyes, reverse the position of the feet – raising the other knee – and hold for five seconds. You should be able to do this without loss of balance.

TAKING A CHECK-UP

Exercise will help you slim if you're overweight, help you put on muscle if you're bothered by your scrawny image. It will keep you topped up with vitality, and, if you keep at it, it will give you a body that can look and perform as if it were a decade or more younger than your actual age.

But fitness is not the same as health. Fitness will almost always bring you better health, but before you embark upon your programme of exercise you should try to make sure that you are free from ill-health.

If you are over 40, if you haven't taken any regular exercise for a couple of years, or if you have any doubts about your health, then it is only good sense to see your doctor before starting on a programme of exercise. The chances are that whatever your condition, your doctor will be eager to encourage you to take some exercise. Show him this book, and listen to his advice.

Too many people get quite needlessly worried and put off by the thought of getting a medical check-up before they start on an exercise programme, but you'll feel much happier and safer if you replace fear with caution by going to your doctor and getting the all-clear before you start.

YOUR OWN FITNESS PROGRAMME

Almost all exercise, done in moderation, is beneficial. But most exercise programmes are too difficult, too discouraging and too boring for the average person. So the trouble with a lot of physical fitness programmes is that they are not likely to be followed by the very people who need them most.

Many of us eat too much, drink too much, and smoke. Exercise, when we try it, seems too hard and to take up too much time and energy. A lot of people plunge into exercise programmes just like they start diaries and journals at the start of a new year. They keep the programme going for a few days, perhaps a few weeks, and then suddenly it's over.

So when it comes to working out how you are going to keep fit there are some essential points to bear in mind. Whatever the form of exercise you choose, it must be:

1 Enjoyable If you don't have fun doing it at least some of the time, you'll soon find excuses enough to be doing something else.

2 Balanced It should cover the various ingredients of fitness examined in this chapter, giving you the mixture of strength, endurance and flexibility that you want.

3 Economical on time If you lead a busy life you aren't going to be able to devote hours every day to exercise, so you've got to get the most out of the minutes you do have available.

4 Practical Your exercise has got to be something you can do either at or near your home or place of work. If you have to travel for hours every time you want to exercise, you aren't going to exercise as often as you should.

5 Habit-forming A little exercise done regularly over a long period is a lot more beneficial than a huge dose of exercise taken over a short period and interrupted by long stretches of inactivity.

THE ROADS TO FITNESS To help you build up your own balanced fitness programme, we will be looking at three broad areas of exercise:

1 Exercises that can be done by all the family in and around the home.

2 Activities that will get you out into the open air, and which if followed regularly will build up a high level of fitness.

3 Games and sports. . .some of which will get you fit, and some of which you will need to get in shape for before you attempt to play them.

But whatever form of exercise you choose there are some basic points that you should remember.

START EASY There is no great mystery about how to begin. You simply start slowly, exercise gently and regularly, and gradually increase the amount you can comfortably handle.

If you think of training and conditioning as being like sunbathing you will soon get the idea. With sunbathing, you must start cautiously or you will burn. So, too, with exercise. Start slowly and build up. Too little is better, especially at the start, than too much.

MAKE IT REGULAR Try to exercise at least three times a week—every other day is a good target that some use. Many athletes exercise six or seven days a week, but research has shown that excellent results can be had from three exercise sessions per week each of around 20 minutes.

A lot of sports and games—cricket and tennis for instance—have the disadvantage that even those who play them seriously don't take part the whole year round. So if you're using a sport to keep fit, you'll have to work out how you can keep in shape during the off-season.

It's a matter of personal preference and lifestyle whether you choose morning, evening or the lunch-hour for your exercise. But, once again, habit can be a useful ally in your fitness programme, and it's best to establish as regular a fitness routine as you can.

DON'T EXERCISE AFTER EATING Don't try to exercise straight after a meal. It's not much fun and it can be dangerous. Your stomach is busy digesting the food, and a lot of your blood will be concentrated there.

Animals generally lie down after eating; they relax and often sleep a little. It's an example worth following. Generally, $1\frac{1}{2}$ to 2 hours should be allowed before you begin an exercise session, though this may vary according to your digestive system and on what and how much you've eaten.

EXERCISE IN THE HOME Ever since people realized the value of exercise, men and women have been exercising behind closed doors—in bedrooms, bathrooms and in basements—and often with startling results. The exercises have ranged from the daily dozen physical jerks to the dynamic tension and isometrics of the body-builders. They have included the exercises of the East, such as yoga and Tai Chi, and the fads of the West, such as carpet-jogging and skipping. You can easily turn your own home into a fitness centre, and the exercise programme you devise for yourself can be as simple or as sophisticated as you wish.

A BASIC HOME PROGRAMME

Stretching. . .strengthening. . .and endurance building—all three of the basic ingredients of fitness can easily be produced behind closed doors in the comfort and privacy of your own home. A simple seven-part programme, as outlined below, is suitable for men, women and children, and can produce good all-round fitness with two or three exercise sessions of 15 to 20 minutes each week. The exercises can be carried out every day if you wish, and should be run through not less than twice a week.

THE STRETCH

Standing straight, lift your arms over your head, with your palms facing outwards. Stretch your arms upwards and slightly to the back until your fingers and hands touch. You should feel the stretch in your arms and shoulders. Bring the arms slowly to the sides to complete the exercise. Do the stretch 10 times, inhaling deeply each time.

KNEE LIFTING

Standing upright, bring the right leg up towards the chest, bending it at the knee. Grasp the leg with both hands and pull the knee up towards the chest. Repeat the exercise with the left leg. Do the exercise 10 times with each leg.

REACH FOR YOUR ANKLES

Stand with your feet wide apart, and both palms on the front of your right thigh. Reach for your ankle with your hands as far down your leg as you can stretch without forcing. Straighten up, stretching to your full height with your hands reaching upwards. Repeat the exercise with your left leg. Do the exercise 10 times for each leg.

SIDE TWIST

Stand with feet slightly more than shoulder width apart. Put hands on hips and bend to the right. (Do not lean forward.) Straighten up and bend to the left. Do the complete movement to the right and left 10 times.

RUNNING ON THE SPOT

Running on the spot has a long and distinguished history. Back in the 1880s the then greatest mile runner in the world, Walter George, who set records that lasted for many years, devised his '100-up' exercise so that he could get fit to race even when stuck behind the counter of the chemist's shop where he worked. He chalked a line on the floor and ran vigorously on the spot, lifting his knees as high as possible, and pumping his arms energetically. He counted each completed step, and usually ran 100 steps at a session. It helped him run a world record mile in 4 minutes 12 seconds, which was years ahead of his contemporaries, so it must have been effective! The great Olympic multi-medallist Emil Zatopek is also reported to have run on the spot when doing army

sentry duty. And once, when unable to train outdoors, he's said to have filled the bath with dirty washing and to have run while treading the linen.

These days you can get a variety of sophisticated jogging machines that count the steps you take and convert them into 'distance' covered. Some of the machines also have a bleeping device that allows you to set a rhythm for your jogging. But jogging up and down on the carpet can also be quite effective. You can count the steps as you go, or simply jog for a predetermined time. You can watch TV or set your own jogging to music from the radio or record player. It's the simplest and most immediate of all exercises. You get out of the armchair and jog. You can start as easily as you like and for really good results you should work up to 10 to 15 minutes a session.

SIT-UPS

Lie on your back, then rise without using your arms, until you almost reach a sitting position. Your hands should reach down your thighs to touch your kneecaps. Return to the horizontal position to complete the exercise. Start with five sit-ups, and try to add five each week until you can manage 25.

PUSH-UPS

Place your hands firmly on the side of a bath, or the seat of a chair, with your arms straight directly under the shoulders. Slide your feet out full length so that your arms and toes support your weight. Lower your chest down towards your hands and then straighten the arms to complete one movement. Begin with five push-ups and add five each week until you can do 25 comfortably. At this point the exercise may be made more strenuous by performing the same movement but with the hands on the ground.

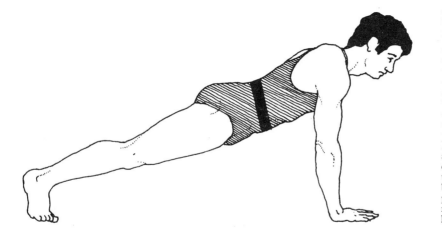

SOMETHING EXTRA ?

The basic exercise routine is a good package for all ages and both sexes. But once you are basically fit you may wish to try some of the more vigorous exercises that follow.

SQUATS

This is an exercise to strengthen the muscles and joints in the legs—and if done rapidly it will also give the heart a good workout. Stand about 45 cm behind a chair with your hands resting on the back, as shown. Bend the knees and lower the body into a squat. Return to the standing position to complete the exercise. Begin with five squats and work up to 20.

SQUAT THRUSTS

From a standing position bend to a crouch position with hands on the floor. Shoot the legs backwards until they are fully extended. Return to the crouch position and stand up to complete the exercise. Ten of these is a good workout, but as you get fitter you can build up to 25 or more.

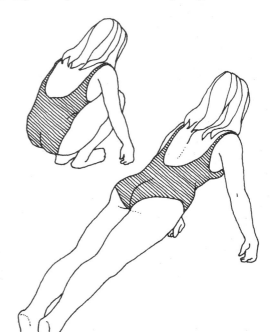

LEG-LIFTS

Lie on your back with your arms by your side. Raise both legs slowly off the ground until they are vertical. Lower them slowly to the floor. Begin with five and build up to 25.

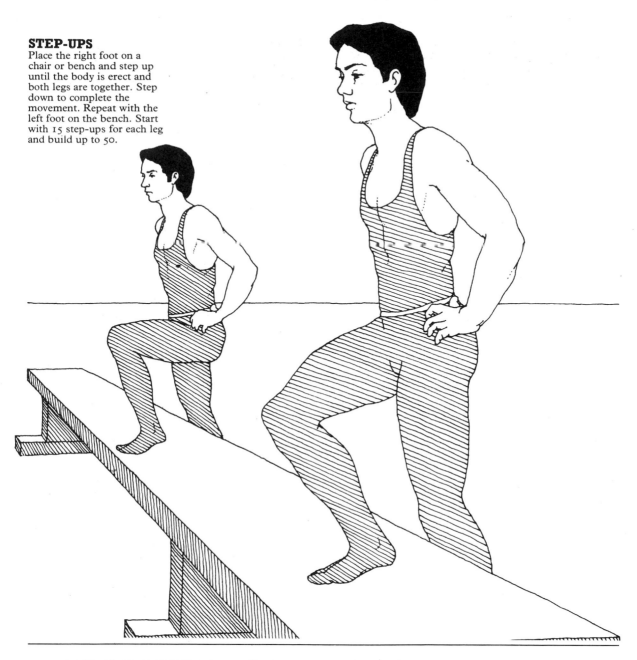

STEP-UPS
Place the right foot on a
chair or bench and step up
until the body is erect and
both legs are together. Step
down to complete the
movement. Repeat with the
left foot on the bench. Start
with 15 step-ups for each leg
and build up to 50.

ISOMETRICS

In the 1950s a group of West German
physiotherapists made one of the most exciting
discoveries for the struggler-after-fitness. They
pronounced that you can actually increase your
strength without moving a muscle.

In 'isometric' exercises the muscles
are contracted in a fixed and static position.
This happens naturally if, for instance, you try
to move an immovable object. Try pushing
against a wall or uprooting a tree, and you'll
realize that muscles can get worked quite hard.

Tests have shown that holding a

static muscle contraction for just six seconds
can produce measurable increases in strength.
You can work your muscles either by pushing or
pulling against something that won't move, or
by pitting one set of muscles against another.

For instance, link your fingers firmly
together in front of your chest and then try to
pull them apart as hard as you can for six
seconds. In another exercise, while sitting in a
chair press your hands down on your knees and
then try to raise your legs. Next, interlock your
hands behind your head, and then pull forward
while resisting with your neck and head; hold
each contraction for six seconds.

Of course, isometrics won't do

everything. While they can increase strength, they do nothing for stamina and flexibility. So if you include isometrics in your programme, you should balance your exercises with endurance training and mobility exercises.

Here are some simple isometric exercises that you can try.

FOR THE SHOULDERS

Stand in a doorway with your arms at your sides. Place the back of the hands against the door frame and press outwards as hard as possible for six to eight seconds.

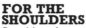

FOR THE NECK

Interlock your fingers and place your hands behind your head. Pull your hands and arms forwards while pressing back with your head. Hold the tension for six to eight seconds.

FOR THE ARMS

Sit at a heavy desk or table and place your hands under it. Using your biceps, press upwards trying to lift the table. Hold the contraction for six to eight seconds.

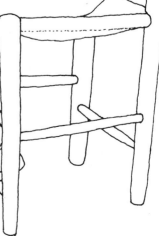

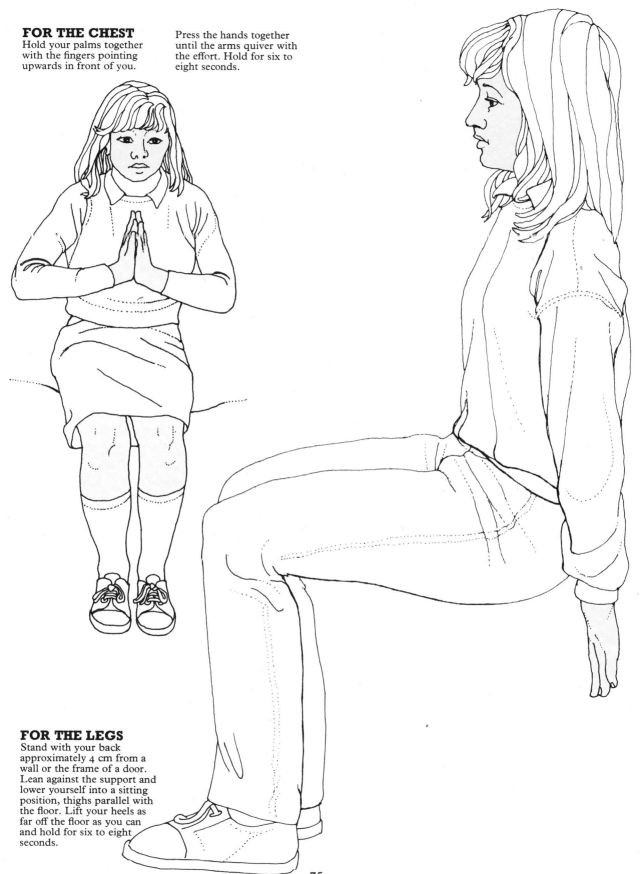

FOR THE CHEST
Hold your palms together with the fingers pointing upwards in front of you.

Press the hands together until the arms quiver with the effort. Hold for six to eight seconds.

FOR THE LEGS
Stand with your back approximately 4 cm from a wall or the frame of a door. Lean against the support and lower yourself into a sitting position, thighs parallel with the floor. Lift your heels as far off the floor as you can and hold for six to eight seconds.

HOW TO
EXERCISE
ALL DAY LONG

As well as the routines of free exercises and isometrics it is very easy to incorporate a minimum fitness programme into the odd pockets of your everyday life. You don't need any special equipment, you don't need to be a fitness freak, you don't even have to get out there and shock your neighbours by jogging—though once you are fit the chances are you'll be happy to be seen exercising anyway.

The secret is to weave exercise into the very fabric of your everyday life. If you choose to be fit, and if you choose to make exercise a habit, you'll soon come to realize that the whole world can be your gymnasium.

I know of one man, a librarian now in his 50s, who boasts that he never takes any exercise at all but is as fit and well as he was at 25. What he means, of course, is that he doesn't lift weights or play rugby. . .what he does do is to walk the half-mile to and from the railway station each day, to spend several hours each week on his allotment, and to walk his dog each night before he turns in for sleep.

So what must you do? And how can you be sure it's doing you any good?

The truth is that if you take no exercise at all at present, almost any exercise will do you good; and there are many simple ways in which you can make sure that you get the minimum exercise your body needs by making it a part of your everyday life.

If you're already doing exercises or taking part in sport, you can supplement and improve your fitness by incorporating these same ideas into your programme.

There are a number of opportunities to improve fitness that crop up in the daily lives of just about everyone, and the secret is to grasp these opportunities and to realize that they can add up to a considerable amount of exercise.

Here are some of the ways you can exercise all day long:

JOG ANYWHERE, ANYTIME You can get in a surprising amount of exercise simply by jogging whenever there's an opportunity. It's often the quickest way to cover a short distance in a town, for example, or to get yourself to the nearest railway station.

In his book *Jogging, The Anytime Exercise*, Harcourt Roy advocates 'functional jogging'. 'Basically,' he writes, 'jogging can be done wherever you please. After all, it is simply a matter of breaking into an easy trot, and no one's going to mind that. Plenty of people do it

to catch buses and to make appointments on time, while being conscious of the need to avoid perspiring noticeably, or getting into a flustered untidy state. It's a question of using your judgment and sense of pace. . . This is functional, opportunist jogging. Jogging to get somewhere faster than walking.'

Bruce Tulloh, in *The Complete Jogger*, has a section on how to keep fit when you really have no time to spare. 'Run everywhere,' he says, 'or walk fast. Even when crossing the yard, you can break into a couple of fast running strides. This has the effect of maintaining the muscles you use in running.'

TOWEL EXERCISES For many an old-time sportsman of the 19th century the 'rub down' after exercise was an essential part of the training. Certainly you can get useful exercise by vigorously towelling yourself after a bath or shower. Take the opportunity to twist and stretch, and to loosen up muscles in your legs, arms and back. By gripping one end of the towel in each hand, passing it behind your back, and employing an action rather like 'The Twist', you can get in some quite hard exercise.

STRETCH AWAKE LIKE A CAT Watch a cat or a child waking up and you'll get a good lesson in how to exercise your body without really trying. A cat in good condition will stretch its legs, arch its back and neck, yawn and ease its way into relaxed wakefulness.

It's a delightful way to greet the morning, and it will give your body a gentle overall workout. Make it a long and lazy stretch, reach out in slow-motion, work your jaw and neck muscles with a deep yawn.

Once out of bed, stretch your arms and fingers towards the ceiling and feel your shoulders and spine stretching. Reach out with each leg in turn and point and flex your toes. There's nothing formal about this kind of exercise. Just stretch and enjoy it.

A LITTLE HARD LABOUR Saw some wood, dig the garden, clean the car, polish the woodwork. . .and discover that there's not only dignity but good exercise to be had in manual labour. A lot of chores around the home and the garden can become more enjoyable once you're aware of the exercise potential of the activity. So don't be afraid to turn otherwise routine jobs into part of an exercise routine. The chances are you'll not only get a workout, but you'll get through the work quicker, too.

LIE BACK AND TURN OFF Relaxation is a much neglected, but essential element in any fitness programme. Much of the tiredness and tension of life can fall away if you can master relaxation. This theme is developed more fully in the next chapter, but in the meantime here is a suggestion for your all-day programme:

Lie on your back on a carpet or a

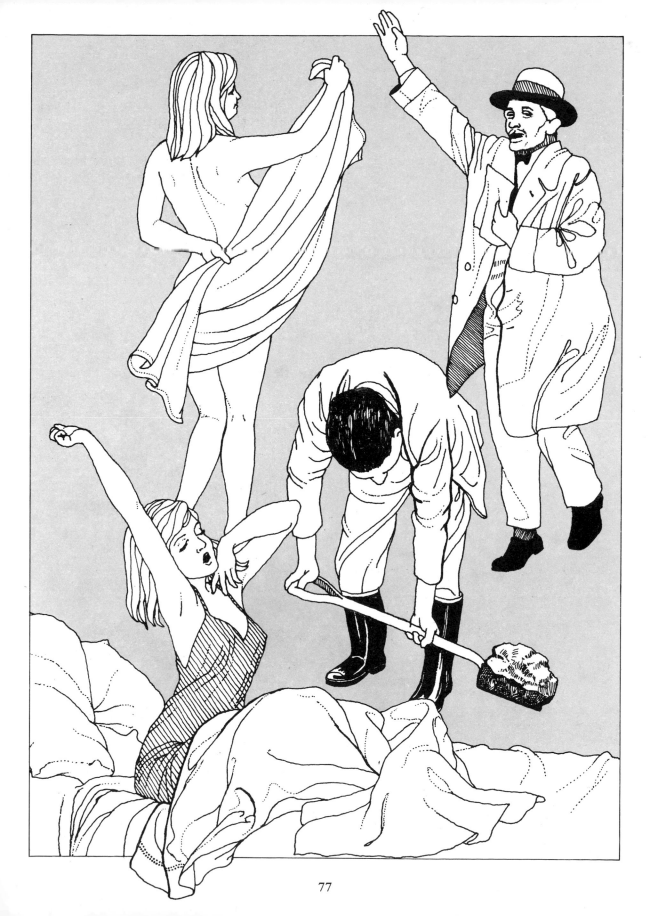

firm bed, with your arms at your sides. Make sure the room is comfortably warm, not too brightly lit, and quiet. Then, by first tensing your body and afterwards letting the tension go, you can start to learn how to relax. Tackle one area of your body at a time. Tense an arm, then let it go as limp as you can manage. Go on to your legs, feet, neck, face, eyes and so on.

Constantly monitor your body as you lie there for areas of tension, and then relax that tension away. Concentrate on your breathing, let it be slow, deep and relaxed. The more you unwind both body and mind, the better you'll become at the art of exercise.

LIFT A LOAD You don't have to be a weightlifter or take yourself off to a gymnasium to benefit from the exercise you can get daily by lifting something heavy. Lifting up a child, or carrying a large load of shopping or a suitcase can be useful everyday ways of maintaining minimum levels of strength, and should not be avoided—provided you've no trouble with your heart or your back.

When lifting almost anything remember *not* to bend over to pick it up. Squat down, keep your back straight and let your legs do the work. Your legs will enable you to lift and carry quite heavy loads, and the legs along with your heart and lungs will benefit from the work.

If you use your imagination you can make the most of any opportunity that comes along for keeping your body and your mind in shape. Making love, pushing a pram, playing football with the kids, dancing at the disco. . . they're all good opportunities for increasing your fitness and for supplementing your personal exercise programme.

EXERCISE AND THE GREAT OUTDOORS

Most people who get hooked on exercise, who really make keeping fit an integral part of their lives, are those who opt for exercise in the open air. . .and often as close to nature as they can get. The walkers, the joggers, the cyclists, the climbers and the swimmers are generally less likely to give up their exercise programme than someone bashing their way through a daily dozen.

Walking, running and swimming are the natural activities—the fitness routines that man took naturally for millions of years. These are the exercises that the animal bodies of men and women really crave. They are also the exercises that many experts believe will get you the best return for your investment of time.

They need a minimum of skill, and they can usually be done alone with very little in the way of facilities. Almost anyone can and will benefit from these activities, however young or old and whether man, woman or child. They can be carried out almost anywhere and kept up throughout your life. And, what is most important, these activities give you the sort of fitness that is of most value. The old concept of the muscleman as an ideal of physical fitness is now as outdated as those advertisements that promise: 'You, too, can have a body like mine.'

Nowadays most people have sensibly replaced concern with the bicep with concern about another muscle—the heart. The need to exercise the heart is behind the revolution that seems to have got half North America out on the pavements and into the parks. . .jogging.

Certainly, running is an excellent exercise for the heart. But it's not the only one. There are others. Swimming, cycling, skipping, energetic dancing, and vigorous walking are among the best. The idea behind all of them is to get your heart rate up, and keep it up during the period of exercise. It is this sort of exercise that makes the heart grow stronger.

As a rough guide most people will get the best results from endurance training if they can get their pulse to between 120 and 150 beats per minute. You will be able to note the effect of this sort of training upon your body if you regularly take your pulse when at rest. Most people have a rate of 60–80, but one of the effects of endurance training is to slow this down—and many top athletes have rates per minute of around 40 or even below.

YOU AND YOUR PULSE Your pulse is probably the most important rhythm in your life. You can learn a lot from your heartbeat and taking your pulse because it can tell you so much about your physical condition and the effect of exercise upon your body.

Taking your pulse with a wristwatch is easy. You can take it at the wrist or at your neck just below the jaw. Count for 15 seconds and multiply by four to give you the number of beats per minute. Most adults have a pulse rate at rest of between 60 and 80 beats per minute. Exercise will send the rate shooting up, but in the long run regular endurance activity will bring the pulse down to a less dramatic, steady throb.

But how high should you push your pulse rate when training for endurance? As an approximate guide you can work out your own maximum and minimum 'exercise heart rates'. This gives you two figures, and you should try to keep your pulse rate in this range to get the best results from, say, running or cycling. There is no need to take your pulse every time you train, but a check, perhaps once a week, can be useful. Calculate as follows:

Your minimum exercise heart rate =
170 minus your age.

Your maximum exercise heart rate =
200 minus your age.

A 45-year-old, for instance, should try to keep his exercise pulse rate between 125 and 155 beats per minute during active exercise.

Now we look at some of the activities that will get you fit by setting your pulse racing and by working wonders for that most important of muscles – your heart.

WALKING You must be able to walk before you run. . .or indeed before you cycle or swim. For anyone who has not been taking any regular exercise, walking is hard to beat. In the days before athletics training became a year-round activity, the out-of-condition athlete would always begin his training programme with walking – and sometimes in prodigious amounts.

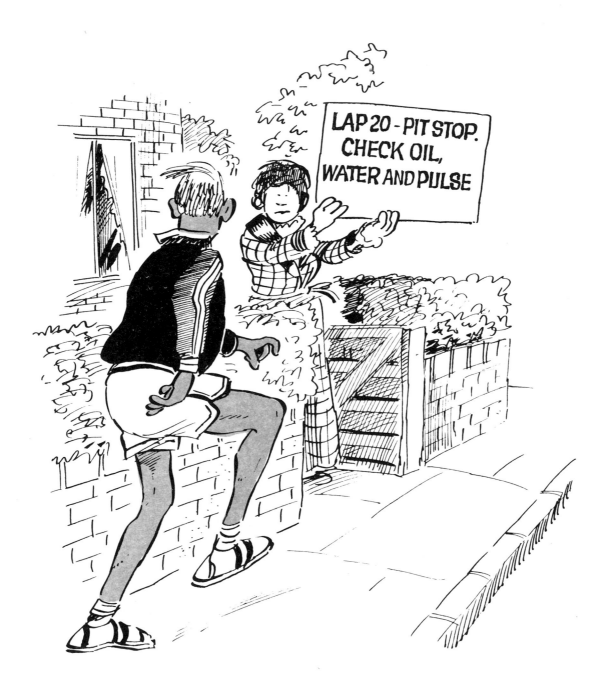

One of the great advantages of walking is that it can be woven into your day without even looking like training. You can use footpower to get you to the station, to the shops or to the pub. And you can soon build up the ability to handle quite long walks of 10 miles or more at weekends.

You can walk almost anywhere, anytime. And you don't need any special equipment beyond a comfortable pair of shoes. Paradoxically, more and more of those who are walking for health and fitness are wearing *running* shoes to walk in. But provided they are comfortable, you can walk in almost anything.

If you do enough of it, walking can be a helpful calorie burner—for instance, you'll burn approximately 300 Calories in 60 minutes by walking at 3½ miles per hour—and so it can help in any weight control programme you're following.

Perhaps the greatest thing about walking is that it's an exercise programme that people find they actually stick to. It's comparatively easy to make your walking into a habit—and if you choose your routes with care it can be one of the most stimulating ways to exercise.

You should start slowly, with walks that you can easily handle, and build up gradually. Your walks should leave you feeling exhilarated rather than shattered—that way you'll be building up your endurance to levels that you never dreamed were possible. As well as working a walking routine into odd corners of the day, those who wish to use walking as a serious exercise programme should plan to build up to 3 sessions a week of 45 to 60 minutes.

JOGGING Jogging and running, both for fitness and pleasure, are something of a boom activity at the moment, particularly in North America, as more and more people become aware of the dangers to health of sedentary living. It's certainly an excellent exercise for almost everyone, whatever their age and sporting ability, and it's perhaps the most efficient exercise of all for improving the fitness of your heart, lungs and circulation.

Running is one of the most natural of all forms of exercise, and its great advantage is that it can be done just about anywhere and at any time without any special equipment. It's a great way to burn off calories—you can get rid of around 800 to 900 an hour once you're fit—and for this reason it's an invaluable exercise for anyone trying to control his weight.

You can wear almost anything to go jogging in, though a tracksuit is the most practical all-weather clothing, but the one item you should be careful about choosing is your footwear. There are plenty of good running shoes to be found in any sports shop, and although they are comparatively expensive you should take the trouble to find some that are really comfortable with plenty of thick soft rubber on the sole. Nylon or suede leather uppers usually give the best comfort, and most runners wear socks to cushion the feet. If you're troubled by blisters, try smearing your feet with vaseline or covering the trouble spots with animal wool or plasters.

Many beginners are put off running because of the aches and pains that follow their workouts. These are usually caused by trying to do too much too soon, and can generally be cured by easing off, taking hot baths and stretching exercises, and jogging more gently next time.

Almost everyone who takes up jogging tends to try to run too fast at the start. Don't be in a hurry. Prepare yourself for a jogging programme by at least a week of regular and energetic walking. When you're ready to start jogging, run slowly and take frequent breaks for walking. It's best not to worry about how many miles you're covering. Instead just go out for a given number of minutes. Grass is probably the best surface for jogging, but in good shoes you can jog on just about anything.

The beginner-jogger who is looking for a simple schedule to follow should aim to get out for three 20-minute periods a week. For the first three weeks the greater part of the 20 minutes should be taken up by walking, with gentle runs of one, two and three minutes injected as you go. These initial periods should not leave you exhausted, just pleasantly tired.

After the first three weeks you can gradually decrease the amount of walking and increase the amount of time spent running. But, again, don't rush it. A 20-minute continuous run, however slowly you go, is good tough exercise. And the most pleasant and beneficial way to get to the point where you can handle such a run is to get there slowly, steadily and without strain.

SWIMMING Many fitness experts reckon that there is no other single activity to compare with swimming, both for the pleasure and the benefits it brings. You can do it alone, age and gender are no barriers, and it works a very wide range of muscles—including the most important of all—the heart muscle.

It is best to find a pool where you can swim regularly, and to set aside a period—at lunchtime, in the morning or evening—when you can take your workout. Overcrowded pools can be a problem, so try to pick a time and place when the pool is not being overused as a playground.

As with other endurance exercises it is advisable to plan on two or three periods a week. The stroke you use is really up to you since all the well-known techniques provide a good all-round workout.

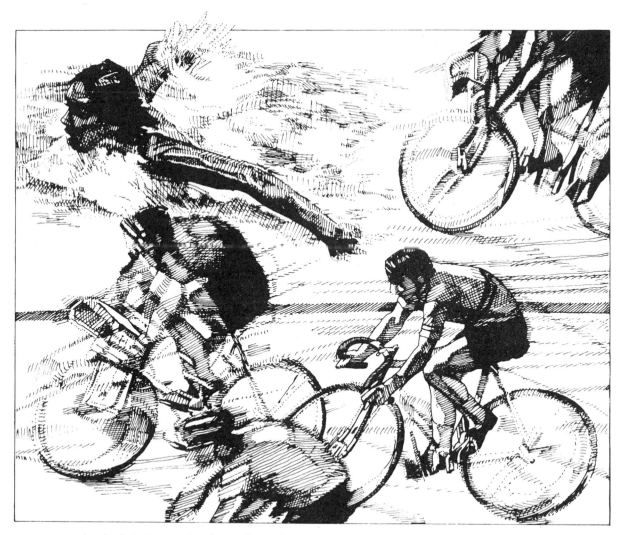

Again it is best to begin easily and increase your efforts gradually. One good and simple plan is to start with 30-minute swimming periods and initially to break the 30 minutes up with rests. For instance you might begin by swimming 25 yards, resting for approximately a minute, and repeating the effort until pleasantly tired or until the 30 minutes are up.

You can increase the severity of the exercise over a number of weeks by increasing the distance you swim—and cutting down on the rest periods. But don't overdo it. Swim for pleasure, rather than to exhaustion—and the fitness will inevitably follow.

CYCLING Like walking and swimming, cycling is one of the best keep-fit activities for the person who wants to take exercise without appearing to the neighbours to have become a fitness freak. Your bike can be used as a very efficient form of transport as well as a machine for exercise and pleasure. Either way it will work your heart, lungs and legs and burn off unwanted pounds. At around 9 miles per hour you can reckon to use some 400 Calories every

60 minutes, and at 13 mph you'll be burning 660.

Cycling is a wonderfully flexible exercise in that you can do it anytime and almost anywhere—and enjoy it to any age.

Bikes can be very expensive, but unless you're planning really quite ambitious tours or going in for cycle racing, you can get all the exercise you need from a comparatively inexpensive machine.

A tracksuit and windcheater or anorak are usually quite suitable clothing—though when you're using a bike as transport, for shopping or going to work, you'll find that you can cycle quite comfortably in your ordinary clothes as the movement of the bike can keep you comfortably cool if you don't go too hard!

For purposes of keeping fit your target should be to establish a routine of approximately 30 minutes of pleasantly vigorous cycling three times a week. Build up to it gradually by riding gently to begin with, and for a shorter time if you haven't touched a bike for years, or if your early rides leave you tired.

EXERCISE AND THE SPORTING LIFE

In looking at various sports it's impossible to say that any one sport demands more or less fitness than any other. Different sports require different kinds of fitness. Even when you're very fit for running, for instance, a hard swim or a game of soccer can leave you tired and sore.

In choosing and assessing the value of your sport it will help to group the most popular sports according to their demands and effects upon the body. Much research has been done into the relative values of different sports and although it is difficult to compare them, it is interesting to look, for instance, at the energy demands of various sports and activities.

HOW MUCH ENERGY DO YOU BURN UP?

When sitting down, a person weighing 70 kg uses approximately 100 Calories an hour. The more strenuous the exercise the more calories you use up, and the figures below provide an approximation of how many calories per hour will be burned up by various activities.

In terms of fitness benefits, rather than pure enjoyment, sports can be roughly classified according to how much of a workout they provide.

Any recreational activity is likely to be of benefit in keeping you fit—and if it gets you out into the open air it's likely to be doubly good.

Choosing your game or sport is an individual matter, and obviously age and gender must play a part. Rugby and boxing, for instance, are both sports for young men—so if these *are* your sports, you should think of developing alternative activities that you can take up later.

In choosing a sport there are a number of questions you must ask yourself. Do you want to be a serious competitor? Do you want to take part in a sport or game that you can share with your girlfriend, boyfriend, wife, husband or children? Is your sport to be your only way of taking exercise? Or will you take exercise to keep in shape for your sport?

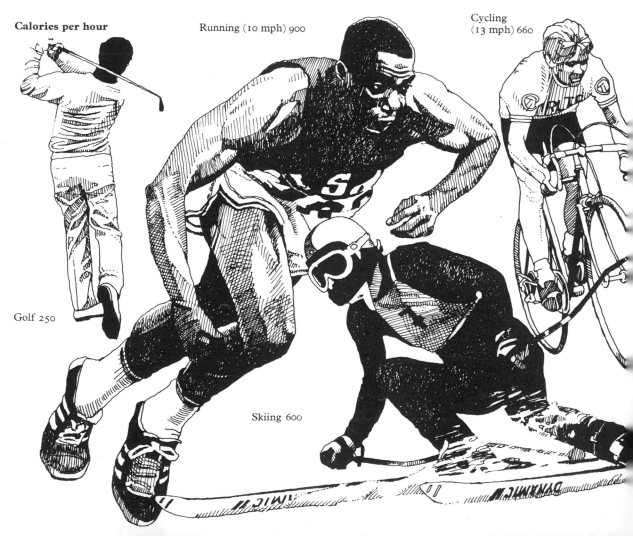

Calories per hour

Running (10 mph) 900

Cycling (13 mph) 660

Golf 250

Skiing 600

THE GOLD MEDAL SPORTS In this group are the sports that will be of most direct benefit to the body in terms of heart-lung training and calorie consumption. By their nature these sports can be tough (sometimes too tough) on the unconditioned body. They include: running, rowing, cross-country skiing, fast swimming, squash, energetic cycling and skipping.

THE SILVER MEDAL SPORTS These, while taxing, are not quite so demanding as the gold medal sports and include: badminton, tennis, skiing, basketball, hockey, horseriding, soccer, rugby, orienteering and jogging.

THE BRONZE MEDAL SPORTS These are essentially recreational—though if planned in conjunction with exercises such as those outlined earlier they can be a valuable part of a fitness programme, especially for the not-so-young and for those of us who are really out of shape. They include: bowls, cricket, sailing, recreational walking and golf.

Below, in random order, we look at some of the most popular sports and games that you may be considering as part of your exercise programme. Don't forget that in choosing a sport you must ask yourself:

Are you fit enough to play and enjoy playing it?

Is it a sport that you can keep up over a number of years?

Is it a sport you can afford?

Is it enough to keep you fit or will you need extra exercise?

Does it have an off-season?

TENNIS A good all-round exercise for all ages, provided that you have plenty of access to a court. It demands speed, stamina, mobility and concentration. It's a popular sport in which both men and women can play separately or together—which means that it's got a good social life attached to it. Most courts are outdoors, so it is primarily a summer sport—and you need, of course, to exercise in the winter too.

Taken with jogging in the winter and a set of the Basic Home Programme exercises, tennis is excellent for fitness.

GOLF Essentially, golf is a game of skill, not of strength or endurance, and if you want to get fit you are going to need more than a few rounds of golf to achieve it. It has the advantages of getting you into the open air for long periods

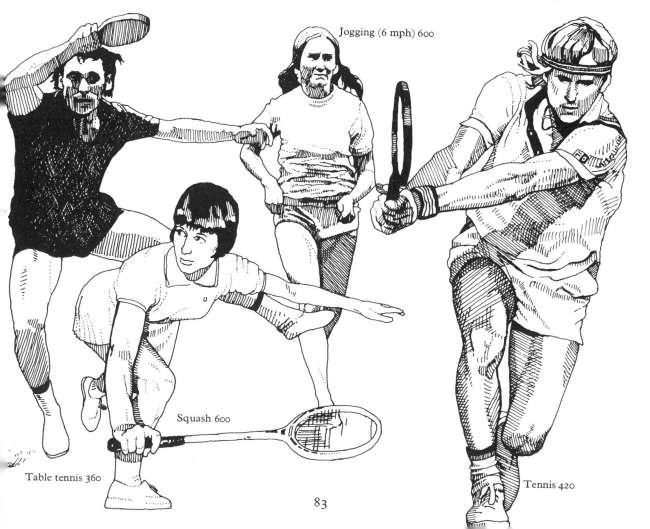

Jogging (6 mph) 600

Squash 600

Table tennis 360

Tennis 420

and of being a first-class relaxation, but puts too little stress on the heart-lung system to achieve a real training effect. It is also, unfortunately, a great consumer of time that might otherwise be spent on more demanding exercise.

If you're a golfer try to add some form of endurance exercise to your sporting life by jogging, cycling or swimming—and, if you hope to improve your game, use exercises to add strength and mobility to your shoulders.

SOCCER Soccer is probably the world's most popular team game, and is an excellent exercise requiring coordination, balance, speed and stamina. To play good soccer you must be in good shape, and professional players supplement their games with large doses of strength, mobility and endurance exercises.

The problem for the amateur player is that one game a week is not enough to improve physical conditioning, and that fitness can rapidly be lost during the off-season. You should supplement a weekly game with a couple of periods of jogging—and keep in shape during the summer either by exercising or taking up a second sport such as squash.

CRICKET Cricket is really a game rather than a sport that will provide you with demanding exercise. At a casual level it can be played by all the family and into middle age or beyond. The emphasis, whether played on a perfect grass wicket, on a beach or in a garden, is on skill, coordination of body and eye, and fast reactions. With the exception of bowling (which for a fast bowler can be a tough physical workout) cricket has little value in the maintenance of physical fitness.

But it does provide great pleasure and relaxation and can do much to extend your interest in active sport long after you've stepped out of more vigorous games. So play cricket for exercise by all means, but balance your programme with more concentrated exercise taken regularly throughout the year.

BASKETBALL This is a tough team game that can be played all the year round, both indoors and out. Essentially it's a sport for the tall, fit young man. It requires strength, endurance, agility and tough joints and ligaments. Nearly all successful competitive basketball players are very tall—generally well over six feet. Most serious players also

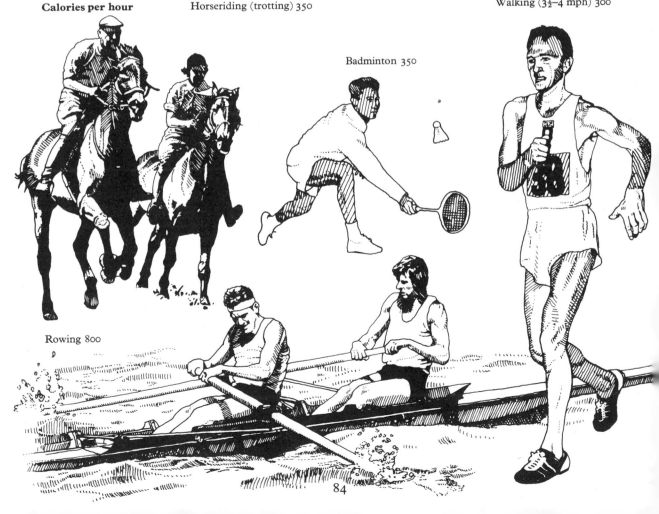

Calories per hour   Horseriding (trotting) 350   Walking (3½–4 mph) 300

Badminton 350

Rowing 800

condition themselves off-court by running, weight-training and gymnasium work.

Played hard and regularly (at least one hour three times a week) basketball is certainly an excellent fitness exercise in itself—and is often used by sportsmen to help them train for other games.

ROWING Rowing is a tough sport, requiring more fitness than skill—and the best rowers will inevitably be strong, tall and heavy. Both men and women row competitively, and boats range in size from single sculls to full eights.

As a fitness activity rowing is excellent, providing all-round strength and stamina. It can give you all the exercise you need, provided you have access to facilities that will allow you to row at least three times a week.

SKIING Although skiing itself is an excellent exercise, its greatest drawback, especially for those who live in Britain, is that it's difficult for most people to ski for more than short and intermittent periods. Skiing demands skill, balance, suppleness, strength in the legs and stamina. The skiing holiday, though relatively expensive, can provide an excellent incentive for people of all ages and both sexes to keep fit.

Regular all-round exercises (as outlined earlier in this chapter) together with running or a substitute endurance activity will enable you to get the best out of your skiing—and to return from it fitter and uninjured.

BADMINTON This is a game suitable for both men and women, and as such can be played at almost any age and at any level of skill. Good players need the stamina for sustained rallies and the agility for quick changes of direction. The singles game makes considerably more demands on your stamina. To improve your game you should exercise for flexibility and stamina as well as improving your badminton skills.

As a fitness activity the game is not enough in itself, and should be supplemented by exercises or one of the endurance activities.

ORIENTEERING This energetic sport involves running or walking from point to point, finding your way using a map and compass. At the highest level, orienteers are top-class long-distance runners who also display extraordinary skills at map reading. But because of the mixture of skill and fitness required by

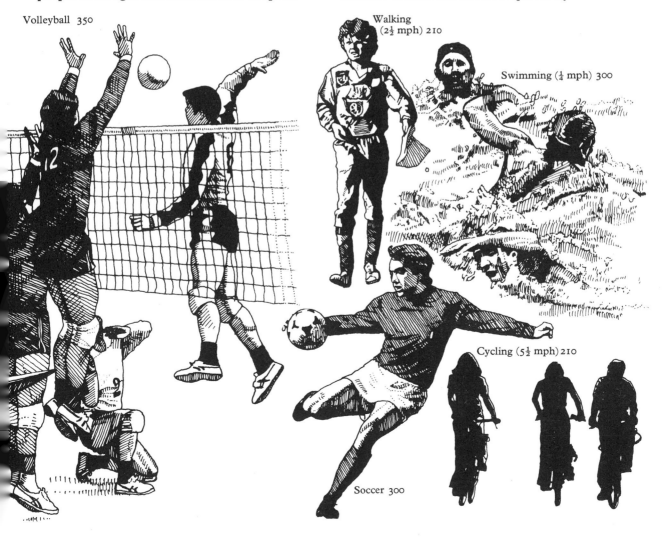

Volleyball 350

Walking (2½ mph) 210

Swimming (¼ mph) 300

Cycling (5½ mph) 210

Soccer 300

orienteering, the sport—which originated in Scandinavia—can appeal to all members of the family and is building up a very strong following.

The courses are generally laid out in beautiful natural surroundings, with the control points hidden in woods, hills and moors. A weekend orienteering event can provide the ideal family outing, with plenty of exercise for everyone.

Because the sport involves a lot of running, most orienteers are keen to improve their fitness by supplementary running between events, so building up to a good level of physical fitness. Orienteering events have classes for all ages and both sexes and the beginner, of whatever age, will find it relatively quick and easy to join in and compete.

HOCKEY Hockey is a good, tough running game that can provide first-class exercise for both men and women (who sometimes play together). If played hard and regularly throughout the year it would bring excellent all-round fitness. But the problem is that, all too frequently, players settle for one game a week over a limited season. Players should either aim to play more often, or top up their fitness with other exercises.

VOLLEYBALL Volleyball is an increasingly popular team game that demands coordination and speed and gives you a moderate exercise workout. It is often played by sportsmen as a relaxation from more vigorous training, and is an enjoyable game that all age groups can take part in.

Top-class volleyball is played by teams of six (men or women) but at a more casual level the numbers in the teams are often varied. It can be played on almost any flat surface, indoors or out. Its demands on your stamina are not heavy enough to make it a good all-round exercise, but volleyball is a useful supplement to any fitness and exercise programme.

GYMNASTICS The televising of Olympic gymnastic competitions has led to an enormous rise in the popularity of gymnastics, particularly among young girls. The many different movements, and the development of balance, mobility and strength make it an excellent form of all-round fitness training; the only aspect it does not cover is high-level heart-lung endurance. The gymnast who wishes to balance his or her fitness programme should therefore try to supplement gymnastic routines with an endurance activity.

It's a sport that really needs to be started very young—and although the adult will benefit greatly from taking up gymnastics as a fitness activity, the newcomer is unlikely to match the early starter in the demanding routines.

FENCING Fencing is a sport which requires great balance, speed, suppleness, skill and concentration rather than strength. It's a good sport if you have ready access to a club where you can meet and train regularly, and it's one in which men and women can compete on virtually equal terms. As a fitness activity it is short on stamina and strength training—so you should run, swim or cycle as well to add to your endurance, and exercise at home or in a gym to add to your strength.

Fencing is a sport you can continue with for many years if you keep in good shape. One of Britain's best-ever fencers, Bill Hoskyns, who competed in the 1956 Olympic Games, was still in excellent condition, and an international-level fencer, more than 20 years later in the late 1970s.

BOXING Boxing is an activity that is clearly limited to the young, fit and strong. It should never be practised without the supervision of an expert, as there is an obvious risk of serious injury. One of the greatest values of boxing as a sport is the amount of exercise that most boxers take before they ever clamber into the ring.

Boxing alone will not get you fit, but the road running and gymnasium work that boxers put in to condition their bodies is generally an excellent fitness programme.

YOU AND THE SPORT OF FEELING GOOD

If you exercise and play a sport or game regularly, the chances are that you will awake one day to the sudden but pleasant realization that *you* are a sportsman, and that keeping fit has become something very important in your life.

You're almost certain to find also that the benefits of exercise aren't just physical: psychologically you'll be more alert, aware, relaxed, cheerful and optimistic. In North America there has been much talk of the so-called 'runner's high'. This is the sensation—the release of mental energy and the sense of feeling good in both body and mind—that a lot of joggers get after their workouts. But the joy in movement, the relaxation of tension by physical effort, and the release of mental energy are really nothing very mysterious or new.

The athlete Roger Bannister, the first man ever to run a four-minute mile, writes graphically of what he calls the 'sense of exercise'. In his autobiography he says: 'I can still remember quite vividly a time when as a child I ran barefoot along damp, firm sand by the seashore. . . I was startled and almost frightened by the tremendous excitement a few steps could create. It was an intense moment of discovery of a source of power and beauty that one previously hardly dreamt existed. . . The sense of exercise is an extra sense, or perhaps a subtle combination of all the others.'

The good news for us is that we can all enjoy that 'sense of exercise'. It is not something that is the monopoly of the Olympic gold medallist or the world champion.

So don't be put off by your age, or what you believe to be your lack of physical ability. If you exercise regularly, there's no reason why you shouldn't enjoy all the benefits, physical and mental, of being a sportsman. You don't have to be going for Olympic gold to triumph in the sport of feeling good. . .you just have to know that fitness matters to you, that you are committed to it, and that you have joined the millions of men, women and children who have found that they can change their whole lives by exercise.

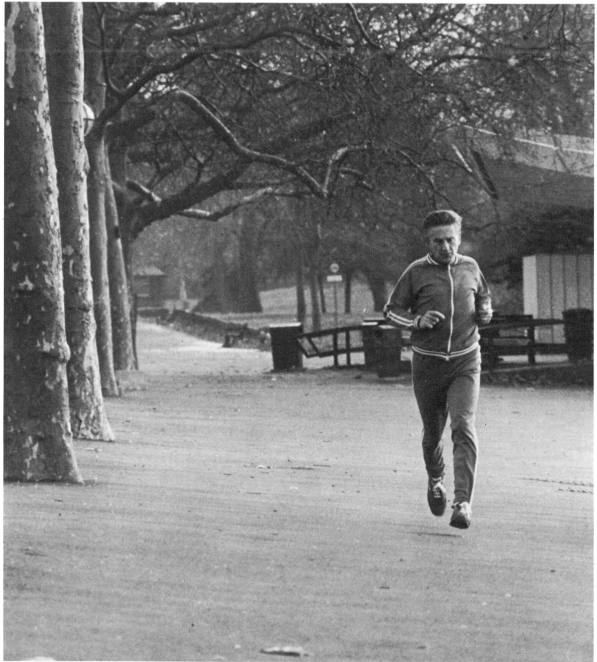

RELAX

All of us are exposed to stress in some form, physical, emotional or psychological. But what exactly is meant by stress? It is a difficult concept to describe in a scientific way but the best anyone has come up with is the 'rate of wear and tear on the body'. We all suffer this wear and tear but what matters is how we react to it and not all of us react in the same way. The difficulty is that little research has been done into our responses and all we have to go on is experiments with animals.

These experiments have shown that under prolonged and intense stress the animal has a common reaction–called the triad response. This is in addition to any reactions associated with any specific kind of stress. The triad response involves three changes. First there is an enlargement of the adrenal cortex. The hormones produced by this part of the adrenal gland help the normal body defences in times of stress. In order to produce more hormones to cope with the increased demand the gland enlarges. If the stress continues too long the gland cannot keep pace and eventually loses its ability to produce enough hormones. Secondly there is a shrinkage of the lymphatic tissue. The lymphatic system is intimately involved with the production of our immune cells which help us fight disease, and one type of immune cell may disappear completely from the body. Thirdly there may be ulcerations in the lining of the stomach and duodenum. These are, in themselves, only minor, but potentially dangerous and even life-threatening.

It is not yet clear if any or all of these symptoms occur in man under similar situations but it is reasonable to assume there will be some common features. For example, there is some evidence linking ulceration of stomach and duodenum in humans to excessive emotional or psychological stress. If similar changes do occur after prolonged stress you can see that the human body will soon lose its ability to adapt to the stress and may well break down either physically or mentally.

It obviously follows that it is very important to avoid too much stress and so not suffer the consequences. However, it is also important to remember that the body *has* these adaptations and therefore is designed to cope with them. A small amount of stress, particularly of the physical kind, is not only a good idea but of real benefit. The chief problems are how to reduce its harmful effects and how to cope with it.

At this point it is worth mentioning that the use of tranquillizers, alcohol and other drugs does not help to reduce stress in the long run. They will certainly reduce, or mask, the symptoms but they will not in any way *cure* the problem, and may well produce other damaging effects.

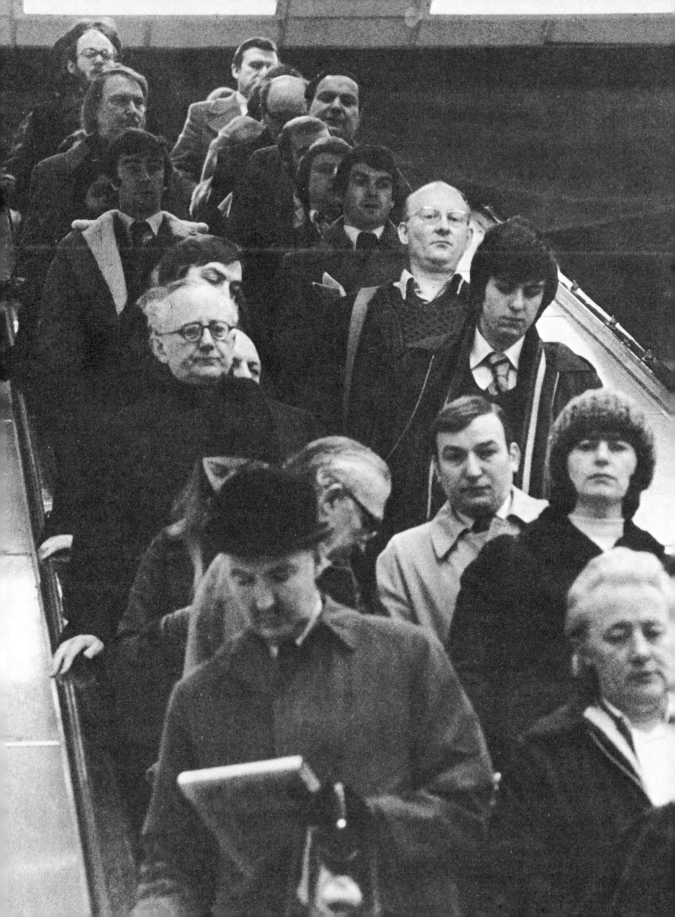

EFFECTS OF STRESS

How do we learn to recognize the effects of stress? This is not easy, largely because any visible signs take a while to appear and are individually difficult to spot. The most common features are a feeling of tenseness, difficulty in sleeping and being obsessive about problems. The heart rate returns to normal more slowly after any form of exertion and there is a continuous state of tiredness. Work becomes less interesting and may become a chore even for the 'workaholic'. What we have to do with stress is to learn to cope with it so that we don't have too much or too little.

The pressures of modern life are such that stress has become part of our daily bread. We need to learn to relax. There are many ways of doing this, some more efficient and some much easier than others, but they all have one thing in common—they aim at helping your body to relax and giving your body time to recover. The first and most important feature of any method is that it can be fitted in to the normal day without it itself becoming an additional burden.

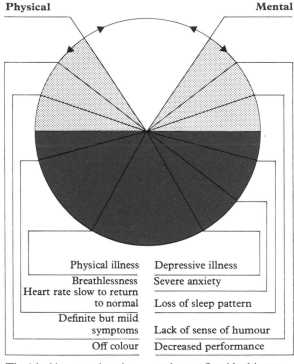

Physical   Mental

Physical illness	Depressive illness
Breathlessness	Severe anxiety
Heart rate slow to return to normal	Loss of sleep pattern
Definite but mild symptoms	Lack of sense of humour
Off colour	Decreased performance

The 'clock' summarizes the effects of stress on the body. The extent of the clear patch at the top (threshold) will depend on individual characteristics, i.e. the person's genetic and physical make-up. Outside this area the harmful stresses exceed the beneficial stresses. Below the horizontal line the physical and mental effects may grow to merit specialized treatment.

PHYSICAL EXERCISE

In many ways the simplest to start with is physical exercise. This can be done at some stage in the day and can range from simple jogging on your own to participation in a team game involving considerable activity (see previous chapter for ideas). The body is adapted for physical activity and both needs and thrives on it. Mild forms of physical stress will help because they will stimulate the heart and lungs and strengthen the muscles. This in turn will help to reduce tension in the body which is found in overstressed people. It will also help to encourage natural sleep as tired muscles will reach a point of exhaustion and so demand total relaxation.

SLEEP

The amount of sleep each person needs varies a great deal between individuals. To a certain extent the amount we sleep is determined by how much we think we need. As a very general average some six to nine hours a day would cover most of us. However, if we believe that we actually need more than eight hours, say 10, we will probably feel tired after sleeping for eight hours! Many people find they can reduce their time asleep with no ill effects and find the extra hours most useful.

About 75 per cent of the time we spend asleep is called Orthodox Sleep. A short time after we fall asleep (this varies between about 10 and 90 minutes), a different kind of sleep happens. This is called Paradoxical Sleep or Rapid Eye Movement Sleep—REM for short. During this time the eyes move rapidly behind the lids, hence the name. Throughout REM the muscles are very relaxed and we are dreaming. These periods of paradoxical sleep will be repeated perhaps four or five times a night, each one lasting for about 10 to 20 minutes at the beginning of the night but for 45 to 60 minutes at the end of the night. The use of many drugs such as barbiturates reduces the number of REM periods and so reduces the amount of dreaming that occurs.

Evidence on sleep studies has shown that we need to dream. Volunteers prevented from dreaming—this is done by waking them as soon as their eyes start to move rapidly—show on subsequent nights, when their sleep is not interrupted, a greater number and length of dreams. Although we sleep for nearly one-third of our life we still know relatively little about it. We are still not sure why we need to sleep and dream. However, it seems likely that two

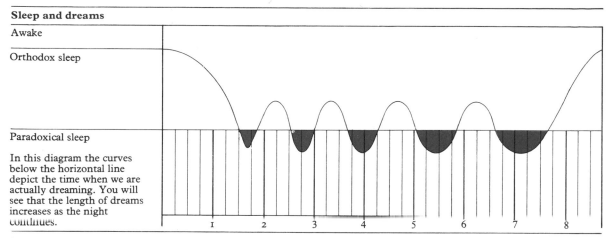

Sleep and dreams

Awake

Orthodox sleep

Paradoxical sleep

In this diagram the curves below the horizontal line depict the time when we are actually dreaming. You will see that the length of dreams increases as the night continues.

1 2 3 4 5 6 7 8

important things happen. During orthodox sleep hormones are produced which are involved with bodily growth so this may be a time when cells are repaired and reorganized. During REM or Paradoxical Sleep the brain itself is being repaired or growing. This goes some way to explaining why young babies sleep for so long and why sleep is vital throughout our lives.

Scientists found out about REM by placing electrodes on the head and eyes and recording the patterns of movement associated with sleep. Some further interesting discoveries were made about brain activity by this method. This brain activity was shown as a series of waves on a moving sheet of paper. One of the waves is called the alpha wave or the alpha rhythm. When we are awake with the eyes open but thinking deeply about a problem the alpha rhythm is very irregular. When resting with the eyes shut and with the mind wandering aimlessly these waves become regular at about 10 per second. When asleep they reduce much more in number and depth and eventually take on a flat or at most a sinuous record with the occasional burst of activity. In fact the first signs of drowsiness can be recorded electrically and are seen as a reduction in the

alpha rhythms. To achieve sleep, it is necessary to encourage the reduction of these alpha waves. This can best be done by shutting the eyes and attempting to empty the brain of all thought. As suggested earlier, extreme physical tiredness will make this easier.

There are probably more home-made remedies for sleeplessness than for any other condition. It is perhaps easier to give a few 'don'ts' rather than a long list of 'dos'. Don't attempt to complete solving the problems of the day. Don't drink a stimulant before going to bed; stimulants include coffee, tea and many soft fizzy drinks. And don't worry if you do not get to sleep immediately. This is important because worry will cause brain activity and make it even harder to doze off. However, you may like to try the following 'dos'. Take a warm drink of milk with you to bed; imagine a blank wall or a white sheet hanging on a line against a clear blue sky; slowly and carefully imagine that each part of your body is going to sleep. Start with the toes and slowly go up the whole body leaving the head, eyes and brain till last. And remember that the expression 'I was just too tired to sleep last night' is not true. Take comfort from the fact that if you can't go to sleep it may be that you don't really need it.

MEDITATION

It is possible to promote those alpha wave rhythms by meditation. It has been reported from studies on monks who practised a form of Zen meditation that their alpha waves appeared as little as 50 seconds after the start of their meditation—and despite the fact that they were meditating with their eyes open and so could easily be disturbed by external influences. This would suggest a possible link with sleep or relaxation and meditation.

When a person is resting quietly and doing little physical or mental activity the rate of oxygen consumption drops; this is measured

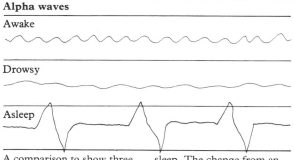

Alpha waves

Awake

Drowsy

Asleep

A comparison to show three alpha wave patterns recorded from electrodes placed on the brain during wakefulness, drowsiness and sleep. The change from an irregular pattern during wakefulness to a regular pattern during drowsiness is clearly shown.

in part by a slowing down in the rate of breathing. In fact during the sleep period oxygen consumption reaches its lowest level in the full 24-hour cycle. During the first few minutes of meditation oxygen consumption has been found to decrease by as much as 18 per cent. Further experimentation has shown that this is not in any way harmful and in fact gives

The graph compares how the rates of oxygen consumption drop during sleep and Transcendental Meditation.	Notice the different amounts of time taken to achieve the lowest consumption rate and the lower rate during TM.

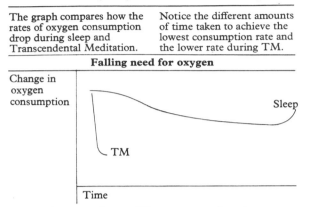

Falling need for oxygen

the body a good rest. The output of carbon dioxide which is usually roughly equal in quantity to the input of oxygen stays the same so the body apparently must slow down its rate of activity. There is also a similar drop in the workrate of the heart during meditation and the rate of the beat drops by about five per minute. These phenomena are characteristic of sleep but whereas it will take some hours to achieve this state in sleep, a similar state can be reached by meditation within a few minutes—or less for the experienced practitioner.

The graph shows the sudden and dramatic drop in breathing rate shown by	expert practitioners of Transcendental Meditation (TM).

Fall in breathing rate

Another proof of the benefits of meditation has come from a series of experiments of which the Galvanic Skin Response (GSR) is probably the best. In this test the resistance to a mild electric current is measured by placing electrodes on the surface of the skin. The GSR decreases with states of anxiety or stress and increases during relaxation, and this has been generally accepted as an accurate measure of the degree of relaxation present in a subject undergoing the test. It was found that over a period of 10 minutes non-meditators produced galvanic skin responses that were irregular and unsteady, whereas those of meditators were higher and steadier. It was also shown that people untrained in meditation techniques were able, after only two weeks' training, to increase their GSR by nearly 50 per cent.

All the research done so far shows that meditation gives many of the same benefits as sleep and is one of the best ways of relaxing. What, then, is meditation and how can we learn to do it? First of all you must appreciate that there are a number of different types of meditation all involving their own different techniques. Essentially, though, they all involve similar approaches although inevitably their end-points are different. The two most commonly used are Transcendental Meditation and Contemplative Meditation. It is not the purpose of this article to give a comprehensive account of the methods, techniques or customs involved but a brief summary will give some idea of what each is trying to achieve.

Transcendental Meditation or TM is neither a religion nor a philosophy—but it is considered to be a simple way of improving one's life in all ways. It is a very ancient practice originating in the Far East. It has become well known in the West recently, largely due to the influence of one teacher, the Maharishi Mahesh Yogi, and a number of his followers and disciples. It is not tied to any one particular culture or dependent on any one philosophy. Why is it called 'transcendental'? The idea is that if you can achieve the state of pure consciousness, then by this stage you will have gone beyond or transcended every thought or image. Maharishi chose this term to indicate that the practitioners are taken beyond the familiar level of their wakeful experience to a state of profound rest coupled with heightened awareness of their surroundings and thoughts.

Transcendental Meditation requires an initial training in its techniques before full benefit can be obtained. This involves two introductory lectures, in the first of which the nature of TM is described and a second which outlines the techniques needed to apply it. This, of course, means that in the beginning if you wish to participate in TM you must find the time to do so. For many people suffering from overwork, and living under stress because of it, time is a real problem. However, once the decision to join in has been taken—usually the hardest part—the time can and will be found. After the initial introductory lectures instruction carries on for about three days until the individual is able to leave the teacher and meditate alone. To achieve the full and proper benefits of this technique proper teaching is required. However, in very simple terms, this is what happens.

An appropriate 'mantra' is chosen. This is a Sanskrit word which means a 'thought the effects of which are known', not on a level of meaning but on a level of sound quality—what is called the vibratory effect. (The actual mantra or word usually has no meaning in a traditional sense.) By sitting comfortably and quietly and concentrating on your mantra your thoughts turn more and more inwards. The mind remains active but in a totally random way. Eventually the awareness achieved settles down, becoming less random and eventually transcends thinking altogether, thus reaching the state of pure awareness or consciousness. In the early stages TM involves time to acquire the technique and understand what is involved. As practice becomes perfect so TM can become the answer for the person suffering from too much stress. The act of TM can then be pursued for as little as five minutes a day.

Contemplative Meditation, although similar in basic techniques, has a different end point. TM is aiming for total awareness while contemplative meditation has a sacred as opposed to a secular aim. Contemplative Meditation is a method practised by certain members of the Roman Catholic Church to achieve an awareness and greater communion with God. It also uses a mantra but this may be a biblical phrase or word. Again its actual meaning is unimportant; the purpose is to retain it and so quieten the imagination, allowing inner awareness to develop. Although prayer might be considered a similar process, the mind is far more active than in meditation and so its value as a pure relaxant is far smaller.

In both types of meditation the aim is to achieve harmony within oneself. Moments of peace and serenity can be obtained and there are distinct physiological and psychological gains to be made. Neither is a game, to be played frivolously, but is an approach to a different way of seeing things and as such needs to be correctly taught, and learned, to derive full and lasting advantage.

MASSAGE AND SAUNA

Other forms of achieving complete relaxation also need expertise, either your own or someone else's. Consider the state of the muscles. Most of us have seen domestic animals such as cats and dogs stretching themselves when they wake. We also do this and its biological purpose is to increase the blood flow to the muscles and loosen up the joints. There

are times when the body is under such a strong degree of stress that the muscles become tense and tight and almost seize up. They need help to relax them again, and turkish baths or saunas can help enormously. The heat applied to the body during the treatment increases the flow of blood to the skin in an automatic effort to reduce body heat. This diverts blood away from the muscles and the gut, and in turn makes it harder for the muscles to function so well, and they get temporarily sluggish and/or lazy. This creates a period of relaxation during which time the muscles can reorganize their structure and rest and so work better and more efficiently in future.

There are times when the muscles need some form of massage to loosen them up. Imagine a piece of elastic that has been stretched in the same position for some time. It will slowly lose its elasticity and eventually become useless. Fortunately the muscles are made out of living tissue and will repair themselves so they will not become totally useless. But, like the elastic, they need to be loosened occasionally and sometimes massage will do this. By massaging the muscles, particularly the ones in the small of the back, the fibres making up these muscles will be loosened and exercised. Movement becomes freer, and the muscles more flexible. Massage also helps to remove or redistribute any toxic waste products which may have built up over the years when the muscles were under continual tension.

There is another valuable side effect to both massage and the hot atmospheric conditions of the steam bath. It is much harder to concentrate on your troubles and problems when somebody is pummelling your back or you are sweating profusely.

YOGA

Like TM there is another Eastern way of obtaining complete relaxation. This is yoga. Unlike TM, yoga can be described as a philosophy because its adherents believe that mind, body and spirit are not separable but can be one. However, like TM and Contemplative Meditation, very little is required of the practitioner. For a few minutes a day you have to hold various body positions, breathe correctly and meditate quietly. In order to benefit fully from yoga it is necessary to study the practices and techniques of experienced teachers, or gurus. They will also teach you about the rules of conduct called yamas and niyamas. While these are of fundamental importance to a full study of yoga, for our purposes they can be set aside. Complete and absolute awareness and fulfillment will only come from a total comprehension of all aspects of yoga but this is outside our brief. As with TM, we must be content with making a few general points about yoga breathing and exercises.

The relaxation position for yoga starts with what is called the Corpse Position. In this you lie flat on the floor on your back with your feet slightly apart and the hands and fingers held limply. The head should be resting gently on the floor so there is no tension in the neck muscles. If you find this uncomfortable then place a towel or jumper under the neck and/or small of the back to make it easier. Make sure that any support you use is as small as possible to maintain as horizontal a position as you can.

From here on you concentrate on relaxing all the parts of the body, starting with the feet, one at a time, and working slowly up the body. (You will notice the similarity with one of the methods to fight sleeplessness.) Despite the apparent paradox of having to concentrate in order to relax it will come more and more easily with practice until you will be able to do this anywhere and, importantly, without having to lie down. In the early stages sensory perception of your surroundings may prove to be too much of a distraction for you to succeed in relaxing yourself. If this happens

then turn down the light and try to find as quiet a place as possible. This may actually send you to sleep—which is not to be encouraged as a yoga technique but is valuable to you in its own right.

Even in the early stages your body temperature may drop slightly and you may feel cold. This does not matter, but if it worries you then make sure that the room temperature is slightly above normal.

Once you have mastered or at least organized this relaxation technique you can move on to breathing properly. Ideally the two should not be separated and each helps the other, but the Corpse Position is probably easier to achieve in the beginning.

Normally you will be unaware of your breathing rate, except after some form of exertion. However, as soon as you begin to think about it you will find the rate becomes uneven and goes up and down. Since natural breathing is controlled unconsciously, it should be possible for you to monitor your own rate without too much difficulty, and without causing changes in the rate. As you are relaxed, or trying to relax, the rate will tend to be slower than usual as your oxygen demands are less than usual. At this point you should try to slow down the rate of breathing by using the diaphragm as

Corpse Position

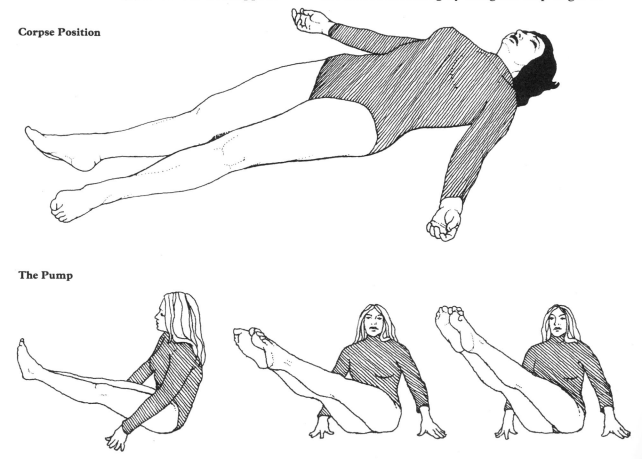

The Pump

94

much as possible. This will pull the air deep down and really fill the lungs. In a fairly short time it should be possible to achieve this combination of physical relaxation and reduced breathing rate and so introduce you to the simplest elements of yoga. It is impossible to say how long it will take because it depends largely on your initial state of tension and on how often you practise.

The postures adopted in yoga are designed to increase suppleness of the joints and to increase the blood supply to all the body organs. In this way stiffness and tension will be considerably reduced or even eliminated, and the whole system will work with much greater efficiency. Provided the following simple exercises are done carefully, there is no danger of tearing or straining muscles. They should not, however, be done after a meal, and clothing should be as loose as possible.

The Rock and Roll posture involves you sitting on your back with your arms crossed and gripping the toes of the opposite feet. Now gently rock backwards and forwards without letting the neck touch the floor.

The Pump (sometimes informally known as the Gut Buster) will help to increase hip strength and reduce excess fat from the buttocks. Again sit on the floor but this time

place your hands on either side of the hips. Raise the legs a few centimetres off the ground and swing them from side to side as high as possible, three to one side and three to the other. At the apex of each swing hold them for a few seconds while you exhale slowly. The length of these 'few seconds' will increase the more you practise these exercises and your breathing.

Finally, in this brief introduction to yoga positions, there is the Head Roll. This is simple and relies on the ability of the head to swivel on the neck. Allow the head to fall forward. Breathe in deeply and raise the head. Now turn the head as far as possible to the right and breathe out slowly as you hold that position. Repeat the whole exercise turning to the left. Finally return the head to its position on the chest. Now rotate the head and the neck in this position stretching as far back as possible, breathing out when the head has returned to its original position.

Meditation and yoga both require expert teaching and guidance if their full value is to be realized. So is there any simple way of relaxing which does not involve great commitment to teachers, gurus or experts? Fortunately the answer is yes, although they will not all be as tried and tested as other methods so far mentioned.

Rock and Roll

The Head Roll

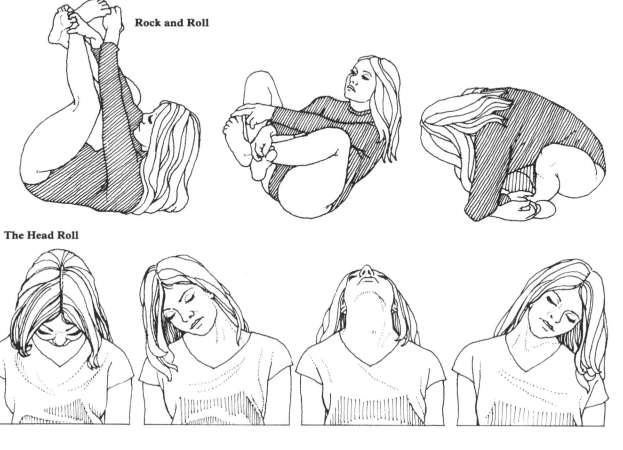

TAKE
A BREAK

One obvious way to relax is to go on a holiday. A change is as good as a rest, it is said. Is it? Holidays usually involve considerable organization by someone and are normally for a short time only, say two or three weeks. The first week is almost certainly spent still thinking about the problems which have been left behind and in generally unwinding. The second week is fine until the time to return to work approaches, when all the tension and worry are likely to start again. A longer holiday would probably give a space in the middle when full relaxation could occur, but longer holidays are not that commonplace – not yet, anyway.

The timing of the holiday is also important. The body has not evolved over the last two billion years to work at an unfair pace for 50 weeks of the year and then recover totally in two. A reduced pace throughout the year would seem to be a better and more sensible approach. But what about those people who never seem to take holidays or, alternatively, those who do so regularly? Kings, Presidents and Prime Ministers seem to live for a long time. This is not scientifically proven but think about such people as Mao Tse Tung, Churchill and Adenauer. How did they survive the strains and stresses of their jobs? Possibly because they had the kind of body metabolism which enabled them to cope with the pressures of their life, or possibly because they too had discovered their own means of relaxation. Churchill, for instance, was able to 'take forty winks' during the daytime. They were also continuously under the watchful eye of their own personal physician. For those of us who have neither that built-in resistance to stress nor personal medical supervision, relaxation in some form becomes an essential part of our life.

What about those who have regular holidays? Schoolteachers are the obvious example of people who work hard during termtime but who also have long holidays in which to relax and 'get away from it all'. They too seem to live longer than the person we may call the executive. One simple conclusion which may be drawn from the above examples is that relaxation is a thing to be taken seriously and not just for a couple of weeks each year. Of course, in theory weekends are also holidays or breaks from work. But for those people under extreme pressure weekends are similar to other days and complete or even partial relaxation is seldom achieved.

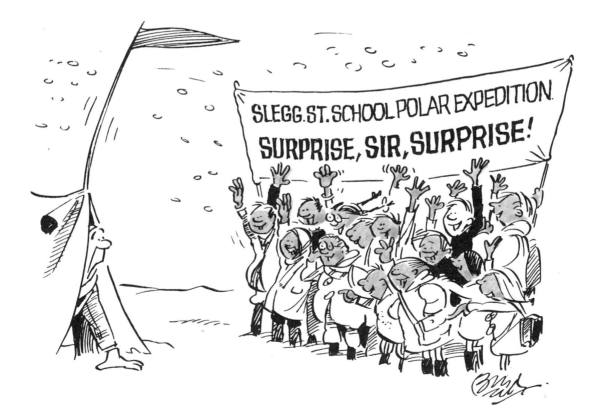

SLEGG. ST. SCHOOL POLAR EXPEDITION.
SURPRISE, SIR, SURPRISE!

HOBBIES

For many people one way of relaxing is merely to have an alternative way of spending time. One of the great modern methods of relaxing is to sit in front of some undemanding television programme and allow one's thoughts to be taken over by the picture and dialogue. The flickering lights also help to encourage relaxation, and provided the brain is allowed to 'drift' both enjoyment and relaxation can be had without effort.

Other hobbies, if we can call watching television a hobby, can also be used as means of relaxing. Reading a book, which takes the mind off other matters, is useful and usually involves sitting down comfortably which in turn helps to relax the body muscles. Gardening has the added advantage of involving physical exercise as well as providing an escape from other pressures. Going out to the cinema and theatre have relaxant value provided the cost doesn't cause too much anguish!

All such pastimes can help, but, as always, prevention is better than cure. The first important step should be to get a job which you enjoy and at which you are prepared to work hard. An enjoyable occupation should also be one which you can leave at the end of the day, putting its problems behind you for the time being. Second, make sure you are healthy in body. This will be helped, as stated earlier, by gentle to hard exercise taken regularly and not just on an occasional basis. The 'overworked businessman' derives much more benefit from playing golf than may at first appear. He can expel some of his physical energy on the walk around the course and some of his fury can be vented on the little white ball. Even though the amount of energy he burns up may be relatively low – 250 Calories per hour – compared with more energetic sports, he is nevertheless getting into the Great Outdoors and giving himself a chance to relax and divert his mind from the disagreeable strains of office or factory.

Third, it is essential that diet should not be overlooked. The link between diet and certain diseases such as coronary thrombosis is fairly well established. You will find on page 42 of this book an account of foods, nutrition and general dietary habits, and observation of these will have a beneficial effect on your health and well-being. Remember, though, that however well-ordered your life may be, there will be times when you need to switch off. This is when knowing how to relax can help – but you will have to make a conscious effort to join in.

PERSONAL HYGIENE

'Cleanliness is next to godliness' is a well worn expression. Whether it is mostly used as a kind of bribe to make children wash themselves or merely as an exhortation to us all is here irrelevant. Our main concern is to emphasize the importance of keeping our clothes and bodies clean. We are all exposed to dirt and dust from the atmosphere and the bacteria, fungal spores, and other disease-causing organisms or pathogens that they contain. The human animal no longer indulges in the kind of communal grooming seen among our relatives the apes and monkeys, so we have to do this cleaning ourselves.

This might all seem fairly obvious but the very considerable increase in dermatological complaints suggests it is not. None of the suggestions for improvement made here costs very much provided simple instructions are followed. Some of the problems do need specialized medical treatment, but as a general rule it is not necessary to go to the doctor for every minor complaint. In any event, prevention is better than cure and a basic understanding of the care that our bodies need is a necessary first step in the right direction.

Included here is a separate subsection on the health and hygiene of the sexual organs. Despite plenty of freely available information, much is still inaccurately known or understood. There is a steady increase throughout the world in Sexually Transmitted Diseases, and only with better knowledge and more sensible attitudes can we hope to reduce this trend.

CLOTHES

Our outward appearance is important. Dirty, unkempt clothing, smelly bodies or hair can be very off-putting when we meet strangers. Why man alone needs clothes or, to put it another way, why we are virtually the only mammalian species which has a lack of adequate personal body covering is not at issue here. Suffice to say that while we are not totally hairless we have evolved from hairy ancestors whose need for clothing was nil. We, on the other hand, need it for three biological reasons—warmth, protection and recognition. Only birds and mammals are able to maintain their body temperature at a constant level, and a change in this temperature, in man about 37°C, will lead to a less efficient system. So far as is known, clothing in man for what we may call purposes of modesty is, in the long history of mankind, a very recent innovation. The use of fashion as a recognizable sign, however, is neither new nor unique to man. Many animals, the birds being probably the best example, use colours and patterns to identify themselves, as did early man. There are important connections between fashion and health and hygiene, as we shall see.

In primitive man clothes were simple and made of readily available materials—initially of animal skins and later from plant extracts, e.g. cotton and linen. Their function was essentially twofold—protection for the skin and warmth for the body. Today the situation has radically changed. Apart from the natural fibres and materials we now have available to us a wide range of artificial or synthetic fibres such as rayon, nylon, polyesters and acrylics. Each type has its own merits and disadvantages. Synthetics, for example, are still relatively cheap and can be mass-produced. They wash easily and can be dyed all kinds of colours. They tend not to shrink or change their shape when washed, but some of them build up an electrostatic charge and to some people their texture has an unnatural feel. Natural fibres and materials, for example leather, are generally more expensive and limited in availability (with the exception of cotton), but they do absorb sweat and allow the skin to breathe. They too can be dyed with a wide range of colours but unlike synthetic fibres are vulnerable to attack from organisms such as the clothes moth. As fibre technology improves so, no doubt, some of the associated problems will be overcome, but

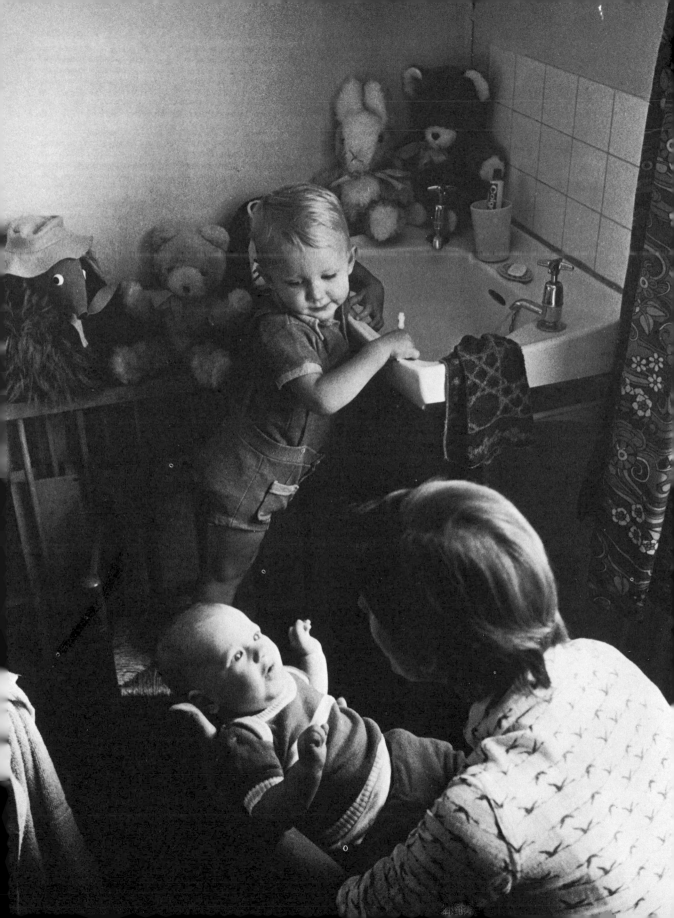

at present the choice is a mixture of cost and personal preference.

Once you have sorted out what kind of clothing suits you there are a few basic rules to follow. As with all things careful treatment will prolong their life and keep them looking good. Washing or cleaning regularly to remove accumulated sweat and dirt, and putting them away carefully so that they are not squashed or crumpled will help to retain their shape and texture.

Remember that one function of your clothes is to help maintain body warmth, and keep your body at a comfortable temperature. Loose-fitting, lightweight materials and pale colours are cool to wear whereas heavy and well-fitted clothes are warmer. The apparent paradox of a 'string vest' or stockings or tights being warm is due to a layer of warm air being retained at the skin surface. This will insulate the body against the colder air outside and thus retain body heat.

Clothing must obviously fit well, and children's clothes need especially careful watching because of their rapid growth rates.

Over-tight clothes can cause pressure in the groin and armpits and such clothes should then be discarded for that child.

Shoes are a still greater source of danger. They are relatively inflexible and stretch little to allow for growth, so care must be taken to allow for this. Pressure on the feet can cause ingrowing toe-nails and corns – conditions which may well persist into later life. Very high heels or 'platform shoes' may induce back pain, because of the unnatural posture adopted by the body, and weak ankles from high heels which have pushed them into an unnatural position.

You can also suffer from general instability if you wear platform shoes, since the thickness of the sole makes it harder to feel where your foot is on the ground. Worn for short periods the risks are minimal, but shoes or any form of clothing which cause any restriction in movement or bodily distress are best avoided.

Fashion, in other words, should be modified to suit your body, not the other way round.

THE BODY

If the clothes are clean what about the next part of the frame? As with your clothes your hair, mouth and skin should be kept clean to stay healthy.

HAIR

Man is not only not a 'naked ape', he has as much hair as a chimpanzee. The difference is that human hair is much finer and shorter so you don't notice it. Growth rate of hair varies according to where it is on the body and also according to your state of health, but on average head hair grows about 12 cm in one year. At the base of each hair is a small muscle capable of causing slight movement – goose pimples – and an oil or sebaceous gland.

HEAD HAIR People know a great deal about hair care today, probably because of the concentrated advertising of hair products over the last 20 years. You probably know that hair should be washed at least once a week, more frequently if it is greasy or you are working in a dusty environment. What is not publicized so well is that over-washing can damage the hair as well. It is better to wash your hair in running water than in a bath so all the dirt can be removed completely. Dry it thoroughly with a soft towel or hair dryer and brush it occasionally while doing so. Shampoos are most efficient for cleaning your hair, but remember that most contain detergent and will remove along with the dirt the natural oils produced by the sebaceous glands. Hair conditioners, which many people use after washing to give their hair a sheen, will not replace the oil although they may make your hair shine.

In the same way, hair creams and lacquers are of little benefit to the hair other than acting as a kind of glue and holding it in place.

One of the most common hair problems is dandruff or scurf, caused by small flakes of dead skin produced in excess. Medicated shampoos, which are made up of proprietary preparations, can help to contain the condition. Another problem and one that is commoner than many people realize is that of head lice. These are small wingless insects about 1–3 mm long whose eggs are called nits. In themselves both are harmless but they irritate the scalp, cause scratching and so may lead to secondary infection. They can usually be removed by washing in proprietary lotions and/or using a specially fine-toothed comb (see also page 168 for treatments).

SHAVING Research in the USA showed that when shaving off facial hair all that was needed (apart from the razor) was hot water and time. The hotter the water the softer the bristle became, and the longer the time available for shaving the wetter the bristle. The use of soaps and creams merely speeds up the process and makes it easier to see.

BALDNESS Although not exclusive to males, baldness is probably genetically determined and to date the only sure preventive measure is castration. Removal of the testes before puberty prevents the production of the male hormones and baldness does not occur. A sudden and fairly considerable loss of hair is due to other factors than age and should be treated by a doctor.

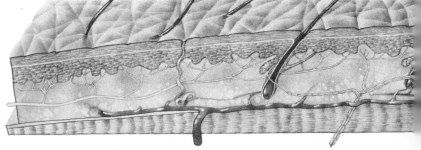

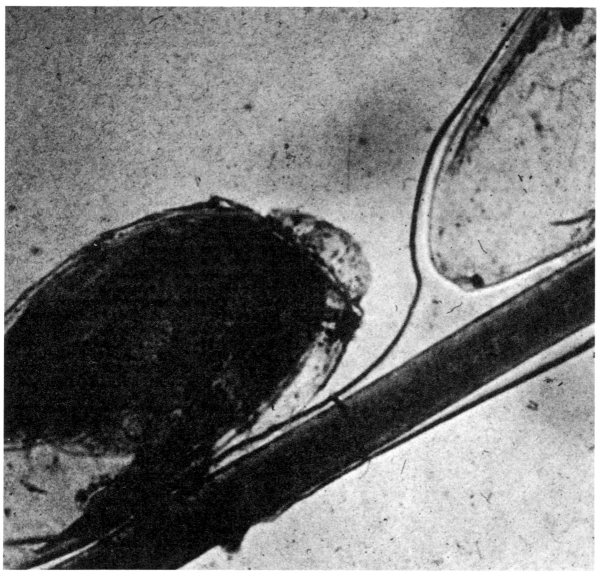

Photograph showing the nit
of a head louse.

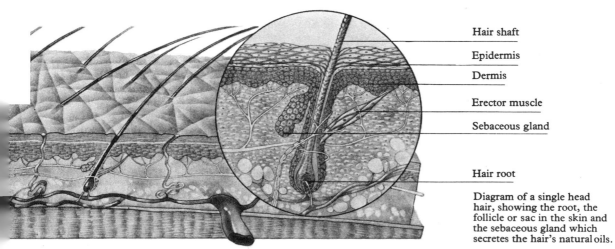

Hair shaft

Epidermis

Dermis

Erector muscle

Sebaceous gland

Hair root

Diagram of a single head
hair, showing the root, the
follicle or sac in the skin and
the sebaceous gland which
secretes the hair's natural oils.

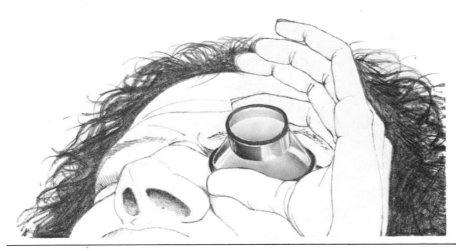

EYES

The eyes are unusual in that they largely provide for themselves. They are protected by the eyelashes and the blinking reflex, and particles of dirt are usually only temporarily present and will normally be washed away by tears. Particles which do enter the eye are best removed by bathing the eye in warm water cupped in the hand or a small glass. See also page 183 for first-aid routines for larger objects in the eye.

The eyes are so delicate that it can be dangerous to use other methods—any infection of the eye should be examined by a doctor.

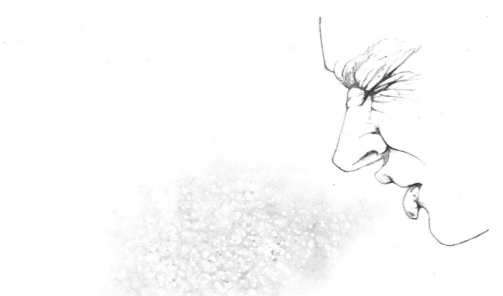

NOSE

Like the eyes the nose is well protected. The entrance is guarded by small hairs and if something does cause irritation there is a reflex action, sneezing, which helps to keep the nasal passage clear. Internal secretions of mucus which build up during infections such as colds can be blown out. Always use a handkerchief or tissue to collect the mucus as it may contain pathogens which may infect other people. Similarly, both nose and mouth should be covered while coughing to prevent the thousands of minute droplets being spread around.

Each of the tiny droplets expelled when you sneeze may contain infectious pathogens. It is important that you should try to trap them in a handkerchief or, preferably, a disposable tissue.

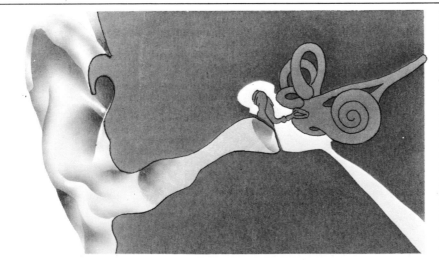

EARS

Sound waves travel along the ear passage and hit the ear drum or tympanum before they are transmitted across and into the inner part of the ear and heard as sounds. The ear is protected from infection by a waxy secretion which lines the tube. A build-up of this wax (see left) will inevitably cause a reduction in the flow of sound waves and thus poorer hearing sensitivity. Normal washing with warm water is usually sufficient to keep the passage clear. Excess wax should never be removed by any hard or stiff object; consult your doctor, who will probably remove the wax by syringing.

TEETH

Mammals have two sets of teeth, a primary or deciduous dentition and a secondary or permanent set. In humans the first permanent teeth normally start to appear at about 5–6 years of age and the last teeth, the so-called wisdom teeth, usually arrive during the late teens or early twenties, and bring the total number of teeth to 32. Structurally, each is surrounded by non-living enamel, the hardest organically produced substance, a living layer of dentine related to bone, and then inside this a pulp cavity containing nerves and blood vessels. Despite the enamel, teeth are very prone to infection. In a survey the average adult in England and Wales had 20 teeth which were either decayed, missing or filled, and in the last category two needed either further work or extraction. Each year in Britain children lose a total of 4 million teeth. You can do a lot to keep your teeth in reasonable condition. Foods containing sugar should only be eaten after a meal or before brushing. Brushing after every meal or, at the very least, last thing at night should be encouraged from an early age. The action should always be from the gums onto the teeth, and do not forget to clean the inside of the teeth in the same way. Small wooden sticks or dental floss should also be used to clean the areas between the teeth and gums; no tooth brush or paste can reach all the areas where bacteria thrive. Gum disease –pyorrhoca–causes more teeth to be lost than decay. It is commonest among the over-30s, and almost always develops in a dirty mouth where gums are neglected. The presence of the chemical fluoride at concentrations of one part per million in drinking water has been shown to reduce dental decay in children considerably and the use of a fluoridated toothpaste, while not as efficient, is still better than nothing. Other toothpastes are essentially a flavoured soap containing a mild abrasive.

Regular visits to the dentist will help to maintain the teeth in a healthy state and may well prevent many of the problems associated with bad teeth.

The photographs show two kinds of tooth decay: the kind resulting from negligence–and eating too much acid fruit, in this case oranges–and decay through exposure to industrial acids, such as might be found among workers at a battery factory.

The arrangement of the teeth in an adult upper jaw. The teeth on the lower jaw have the same pattern and fit into the gaps and depressions in the upper jaw. The amount of space between the teeth varies greatly among individuals, but these are the places where bacteria thrive.

Incisor

Canine

Premolar

Molar

Palate

Vertical section through a front tooth showing the arrangement and relative positions of the parts mentioned in the text.

Enamel

Dentine

Pulp cavity

Gum

Cement

Bone

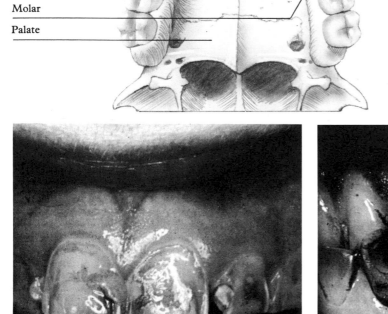

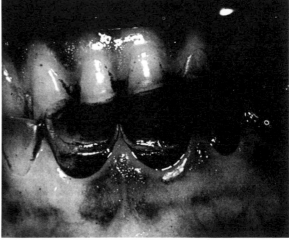

SKIN

The skin is the largest organ in the body with a surface area of between 1.5 and 2 square metres. It consists essentially of two layers—an outer epidermis and an inner dermis. The outer epidermis contains dead cells which through permanent pressure from the atmosphere and clothes are continuously being sloughed off. In fact a lot of domestic 'dust' is little more than a very fine layer of dead skin cells—hence the impossibility of keeping a house spotlessly clean! The inner dermis, varying in thickness from less than 0.1 mm to 3 mm, is a living tissue and it is in this layer that the major functions of the skin are carried out. These include temperature regulation, secretion of sweat, protection against invasion by pathogenic organisms, sensitivity to various stimuli such as pain, touch and temperature, and, of course, holding in the internal organs.

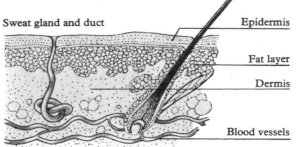

Sweat gland and duct — Epidermis — Fat layer — Dermis — Blood vessels

Skin colour is due to at least five different pigments of which the most important is melanin. The amount and distribution of these pigments causes some areas of the skin to darken more than others and the difference in skin colours in different peoples is due to the depth and variation in melanin concentration. A tanned skin is no healthier than a pale skin. The ultra-violet light in the sun's rays causes both a darkening and production of melanin. The only biological benefit to be derived from sunbathing is in an increase in the production of vitamin D. Since this vitamin is normally amply supplied in a good diet the advantages of a tanned skin belong more in the realm of the sociologist than to the biologist.

Such is the regenerative power of the skin that a healthy young adult can lose up to about 70 per cent of his skin by burning and survive. As you get older so the amount which you can afford to be damaged gets smaller. In people over 80 years old the figures are virtually reversed, and burning in excess of about 25 per cent is usually fatal.

The extremely rich blood supply to the skin, so important to its regenerative powers, can be seen when we get hot. At this time the blood vessels near the skin dilate so blood can flow more easily through them. This means we can lose heat to the atmosphere and of course our skin goes redder.

Healthy skin should be supple and kept clean by daily washing. Soap is not essential although it makes the job slightly easier. The dead cells and bacteria need to be removed from the surface. The oily secretions from the sebaceous glands have a slight bactericidal (germ-killing) action but the oil will also tend to retain the organisms and the dead cells on the surface. If you don't remove the oil properly it can cause a blockage of the pores and lead to unsightly blackheads. If these get infected with bacteria, a septic spot or whitehead may appear.

ACNE This is a condition commonest in adolescents and is certainly not due solely to a failure to keep the skin clean. While it cannot be cured, it almost always disappears in time, and some steps can be taken to minimize its effects, which tend to make the sufferer increasingly depressed if the spots persist for several weeks or months, as they often do. Woollen clothing should not be worn next to the skin, and girls should try and avoid make-up. The spots should not be picked as this may cause scarring. Washing frequently in mild non-perfumed or medicated soaps also helps. The commonest places for acne are the face, chest and upper back. Acne is unpleasant while it lasts, but the long-term effects are almost always slight. The photograph, right, shows a severe case.

BODY LICE Although these are less common than the head lice (see page 100), they are more dangerous in that they carry the organisms which cause typhus and relapsing fever. Other parasites living on the skin, known as ectoparasites, are human fleas. They suck blood and need food frequently. The bed bug is another blood sucker, but does not actually live on the body; even so it can cause irritation and thus lead to secondary infection. All lice and fleas can be prevented by careful and elementary hygiene and severe cases can be treated with insecticides. In the latter case it is safer to seek medical treatment since many insecticides are harmful to humans (see also page 168).

The finger and toe nails are, like hair, dead tissue continuously produced by living cells at their base. The rate of growth is about four times faster in the fingers than in the toes and even here depends on the particular finger and general nutrition. Growth rate for fingers is about 1mm every 10 days, a bit more in summer and a bit less in winter. Nails need little attention other than cleaning and cutting—toe nails are better cut straight across to prevent ingrowing nails. Nail biting looks bad but does no harm although it does, surprisingly, increase the rate of growth, by some 20 per cent. Split nails can be helped by keeping them very short; the little white spots sometimes visible are due to uneven growth and will eventually grow out with the nail.

ATHLETE'S FOOT The feet are an ideal breeding ground for fungal growth. They should be washed daily, taking special care to dry between the toes. Socks should also be changed daily. Athlete's foot (foot rot, also known as ringworm of the feet) can infect the areas between the toes and is easily and rapidly spread in places such as swimming pools. The use of sweat-absorbing socks will help to reduce the moisture which the organisms need and a mild fungicidal cream or powder will usually treat the condition. Verrucae, a form of wart, are also sometimes transmitted at swimming pools (see also page 156).

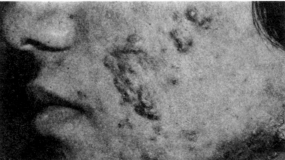

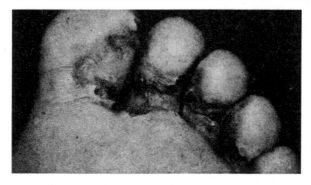

HEALTH AND SEX

There is one part of the body that deserves special treatment. This is the area around and including the genital organs. This part is prone to disease, has a unique physical development and is probably the area of the body about which the least is known by the average person.

PHASES OF CHANGE: PUBERTY AND MENOPAUSE

The genital organs are extraordinary in that unlike all other organs or tissues in the body they are not functional until a few years after birth. Other organs, such as the liver and brain, need time, in some cases many years, before they work at peak efficiency, but are still capable of doing their jobs at birth. The genital organs are physiologically useless until puberty.

This major and dramatic change occurs usually at about the age of 11 or 12 for girls and 12 or 13 for boys although, as with all body development there is considerable variation and the onset of puberty may be delayed until well into the teens. At this time, and it takes some months for the whole process of change to be completed, anatomical, physiological and psychological changes take place. Essentially they are all designed to convert a young sexually immature child into a sexually mature adult fully capable of reproduction and thus perpetuating the species. In man these changes are permanent, and provided he is in good health he retains his fertility until death. Women on the other hand undergo a second change called the menopause.

Naturally there is some variation in the age at which this occurs but it is usually around 45 to 50. After this change, which may take from a few months to a few years, the woman becomes infertile and can no longer bear children. Menstruation ceases and during this period, as the body hormones are disturbed, there may well be associated side-effects. The commonest are hot flushes. The normal sex drive is not impaired either during the menopause or afterwards, and for most

women the discomforts of menopause last for a short period of time only. The more unpleasant side-effects, such as insomnia, dizziness and depression, warrant seeing a doctor if they are prolonged.

There is one other major difference between the genital or sexual organs and the other body structures. For the sexual organs to do their job two individuals are necessary, not just one. In many low forms of life there is a kind of asexual reproduction in which one individual can produce offspring, but in all higher forms two are necessary. The only type of asexual reproduction which occurs in man is the formation of an identical twin from one fertilized egg. No other system in the body is dependent on a second organism and one of the reasons why the sexual organs take so long to develop is that you need both emotional and physical maturity to cope with the involvement of another person and possibly others too.

From birth until puberty the bodies of both boys and girls are fundamentally similar, the external genitals being the exception. Basic hygiene is therefore essentially the same—careful washing and drying of the skin around the organs and daily changes of underwear. Where male circumcision has been performed for medical or religious reasons, cleaning the tip of the penis is easy; where there is still a foreskin the process is a little more complicated. The foreskin and the tip of the penis are tightly joined together and it may take three or four years before the parts are freely moveable. Once this happens the foreskin should be carefully pushed back and the waxy-

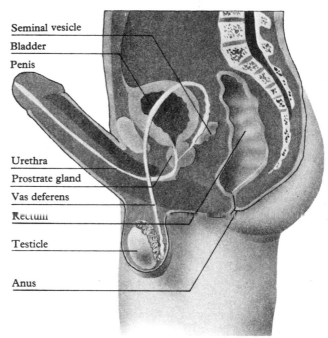

Side view of the male reproductive organs with an erect penis. Note the common opening for the excretory and reproductive systems via the urethra. Also the position of the prostate gland and seminal vesicles.

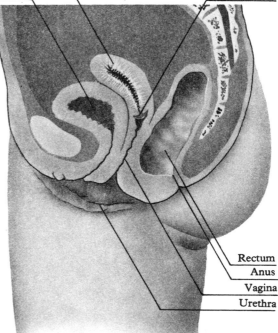

Side view of the female reproductive organs. Note the separate openings for excretory and reproductive systems. The oviducts and ovaries are not shown in this picture. The right-angled bend between the cervix and the uterus is one reason why amateur abortionists tend to damage their patients by perforating the cervical wall.

looking secretion called smegma removed by gentle washing. As this is an obvious area where germs may thrive, careful cleaning should be done regularly. For girls in the year or two preceding menstruation there may be an increase in vaginal discharge. This is quite normal and is only a sign that the body is preparing for full female maturity. During menstruation, and it is essential to forewarn girls of what is involved so it does not come as a complete surprise and thus frighten them, sanitary towels or tampons should be worn. These are to absorb the blood and tissue lost from the wall of the uterus. Tampons or internal towels should only be used where no suffering is caused. In some young girls the membranous hymen is still present and the use of a tampon may cause considerable pain and discomfort.

For boys there is also the possibility of a discharge. This happens at night during sleep and is called a wet dream or nocturnal emission.

Sperms are produced all the time by the two testes and are then stored in the seminal vesicles. Like all cells the sperms need to be alive to function properly. After about a month they build up in such a large quantity that unless they are released during normal sexual intercourse or by masturbation the body will release them automatically. This gets rid of 'old' sperms. Although in wet dreams there may be as many as 400 million sperms the wastage of cells is an efficient method of eliminating old and possibly diseased sperms and indirectly reducing the possibility of a deformed baby. There is some evidence which suggests that sperms maintained at a slightly higher temperature than that found in the scrotum, normally about 35°C, suffer from a greater number of abnormalities than do those maintained in the scrotum. This applies to sperms stored for some time inside the body in the seminal vesicles, where the temperature is around 37°C.

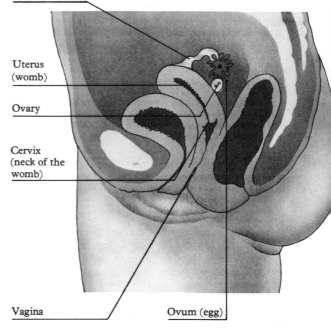

The diagram shows the elements of the female reproductive system and their relative positions in the body.

Fallopian tube

Uterus (womb)

Ovary

Cervix (neck of the womb)

Vagina

Ovum (egg)

SEXUAL DISEASES

The fact that it needs two people to perform the sex act brings special pleasures and problems, particularly the transmission of venereal or sexually transmitted diseases (STD). The first name is derived from Venus, the Goddess of Love, and although they are treatable the diseases are on the increase. People are often ashamed to admit they suffer from VD, which can become very serious if not treated properly and early. In this section we confine our remarks to social aspects of the VD problem; for advice about symptoms and treatment, turn to page 172. It should be stressed that none of the sexually transmitted diseases–chiefly syphilis, gonorrhoea and non-specific urethritis (NSU) can be caught other than by direct physical contact, and all have a clearly identified causative organism or organisms. Most can be treated with antibiotic or fungicidal drugs although resistant strains exist and are becoming more widespread. Physical contact with a carrier of one of these diseases is likely to result in

infection. Sitting on a lavatory seat or drinking from a dirty mug is not. In every case specialized medical treatment should be sought either via a general practitioner or at a local VD clinic where the patient's identity will be kept secret. Simple measures such as washing may reduce the chances of infection but will not kill the organisms responsible. Once VD is diagnosed, health authorities attempt to prevent further spread by contact-tracing. This involves tracking down anyone thought to have been infected, and checking and treating them if necessary. However, the much greater and freer movement of peoples around the world today makes it hard to carry out thorough contact-tracing. Sexual contact with one partner only cannot spread these diseases further than that person, and when treated the disease can be got rid of altogether. It is not easy, though, to ask a prospective partner if he or she is infected with a venereal disease, and a knowledge of his or her lifestyle and habits may help to prevent infection. The

organisms are no respecters of persons and anybody can become infected. Any group of people living close together in a free sexual atmosphere and lacking basic cleanliness is more likely to contain carriers than two people living in a clean environment who are sexually faithful to each other.

CONTRACEPTIVE METHODS

In the past certain contraceptive devices have been used as a prophylactic measure against VD. No doubt they have had some use in that the condom or french letter prevents physical contact between the two sets of organs. But the only true and certain safeguard against these diseases is not to have direct contact with someone suffering from them. Using contraceptives as a means of preventing infection is nonsense. Contraception fundamentally means 'against conception', not 'against disease'.

How, then, do contraceptives work? Basically they prevent the male gamete, or reproductive agent, the sperm, from entering the

oviduct and thus fertilizing the female gamete, the egg, or by preventing the release of the egg.

A primitive measure is coitus interruptus which involves withdrawing the penis from the vagina before ejaculation occurs. This is psychologically difficult and usually some sperms are released before ejaculation takes place. The second method, the rhythm method, involves exact knowledge of the date of ovulation. Using the 'safe period', as it is also called, makes certain that neither sperm nor egg is viable at the same time. The problem is that it is very difficult to determine the exact date of ovulation since each menstrual cycle is different, not just from woman to woman but also in the same individual woman. So, apart from the time when menstruation is actually occurring, the 'safe' period is too difficult to estimate with 100 per cent accuracy.

It is possible to make an informed guess at the date of ovulation by taking a daily body temperature. In the first half of the menstrual cycle, that is up to the time of ovulation, the body temperature follows a low level. At ovulation it falls by a small amount, then immediately rises a little above the pre-ovulation level and usually stays at this higher level until the next menstruation. The daily temperature must be taken first thing in the morning before any activity of any sort has occurred and before any food has been taken. Once the higher level has been recorded for at least four consecutive days it is fairly safe to assume that the egg is no longer viable. It is perhaps worth stressing that the rise in temperature is less than 1°C, and very careful measurements are essential. More modern methods are of two types—mechanical and chemical. The mechanical involves a condom or french letter being worn by the man over his penis. This collects the sperms as they are released, and so none can enter the female. Each condom has to be extremely thin to allow for the fullest possible physical satisfaction, and this carries a risk of permeability. Also, when they are improperly fitted or removed too early, sperm can enter the vagina.

The woman can also wear a barrier—a diaphragm or dutch cap. This, provided it is fitted correctly, will also prevent sperm from entering the genital tract. However, a sperm is only about one-hundredth of a millimetre long and about three-thousandths wide so a hole of microscopic size is all that is needed for entry into the female system. In both cases—condom or diaphragm—the use of a spermicide gel, cream or foam will give added protection by destroying living sperms released in the area.

All the methods described so far are either free or relatively cheap, but they share one major disadvantage. Most doctors and sex experts agree that sexual intercourse should be spontaneous, and the organization and planning involved when using these mechanical methods make spontaneity difficult if not impossible. There is, however, one mechanical method which allows for spontaneity. This is the coil or loop. Known by various

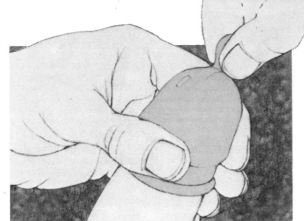

The condom should be positioned over the end of the erect penis. Pinch the teat-end to drive out air and unroll the condom down the length of the penis.

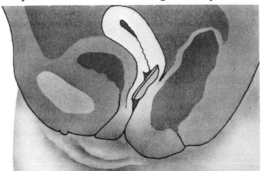

The diaphragm is shown in position. The fit, which should be as exact as possible, will always allow a small gap through which the microscopic sperm can swim and so fertilize an egg. This is why a spermicidal gel, cream or foam is recommended for use in conjunction with the diaphragm.

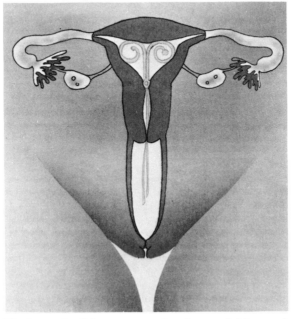

The loop and coil Intra Uterine Contraceptive Devices (IUCDs) are shown in position. The thin piece of cord suspended from each allows the wearer to check that the device is present and in the correct place.

names—the Intra Uterine Contraceptive Device, or IUCD, the Intra Uterine Device, or IUD, the loop or coil depending on its shape, the method probably acts by preventing implantation of the egg. Fitted by a qualified person it can be retained in the uterus for some months without needing to be checked and is an effective device. Unfortunately some women suffer excessive bleeding after insertion and some find it impossible to retain it, so it can not always be used.

The second general method is the chemical one. Using synthetic hormones, the 'Pill' can be taken daily or for a period of 21 days after the end of the last period. To summarize what happens, the introduction of hormones into the body upsets the normal balance; no ovulation occurs, and no fertilization is possible. The Pill is so far the most efficient contraceptive yet found. However, as with all drugs, there are drawbacks. First, it is quite easy to forget to take the Pill. Since the balance of hormones is so delicate, even one day of failure to take it may allow ovulation to occur so intercourse is best avoided in such situations. The Pill has also been linked with nausea, increase in weight and, most notoriously, a greater proneness to thrombosis. However, all drugs have side-effects and these must be weighed against what it would be like without them. Pregnancy itself causes nausea and weight increase, and more people die each year from being pregnant than from using contraceptives.

It is worth stressing that as yet no method of contraception has been devised which is totally effective. Each method has its own advantages and disadvantages and some methods are better suited to an individual than others. Failure rates are normally expressed as failure rates per year. The term used is 'pregnancies per 100 woman years'. This means the number of pregnancies which would be expected from 100 women using that contraceptive method for one year. The Pill achieves a failure rate of about 1–2, the coil about 2–3 and the others are rated worse. While these figures seem very good—a failure rate of 1 means only 1 pregnancy per 100 women using the system for a year, or 99 women still not pregnant at the end of the year—the fact remains that if it is you who is taking the precautions and you end up pregnant then the method is a total failure. The only true contraceptive device is abstention. Of course, sterilization can be used to prevent conception, but this is permanent and usually only used once a family has been produced and no further children are wanted. For the man it is a simple operation, done under local anaesthetic and called a vasectomy. It involves cutting the two vas deferens which are the tubes carrying sperms from the testes to the seminal vesicles where they are stored. Seminal fluid will still be produced, as will other secretions by glands such as the prostate, so that an ejaculation is still possible but this will not contain any sperm and so fertilization cannot occur.

In women the equivalent tube—the oviduct or Fallopian tube—is cut or tied. This prevents the egg from travelling down the oviduct and so again no fertilization is possible. In this case, however, the operation is not simple as the oviducts are deeply situated inside the abdomen. Both methods guarantee sterility, although for men there will probably be a short period of about two to three months before the surgeon is satisfied that no sperms are passing into the penis. Verification is a simple procedure and merely involves microscopic examination of the semen. The subsequent sex life of either partner is completely normal after such an operation and, particularly for women, may become even more satisfying with the risk of an unwanted pregnancy removed. Reversal of either or both of these operations is theoretically possible but the success rate is very low. Since the purpose is to cause sterility, the techniques involved are such as to make it very difficult for either tube to regrow naturally or after surgery.

Removal of either testis or ovary is not used as a means of producing sterility, nor is removal of the uterus. In the former case both glands have other functions and their removal would cause serious hormonal imbalances, the harmful effects of which totally outweigh any advantages gained by sterilization. Removal of the uterus (hysterectomy) will of course make it impossible for the woman to conceive but this is a major operation involving a major organ and would not be removed for such a reason.

Finally, once a woman has reached the menopause she will be unable to bear any more children. However, it is wiser to continue to use precautions for about two years after the last menstrual period in order to be sure that the risk of fertilization has passed.

The drawing shows the position of the cuts made in the vas deferens during a vasectomy. Both the seminal vesicles and the prostate gland are still present and so both can produce their own secretions and give an ejaculation.

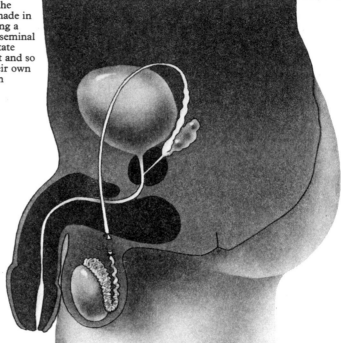

Here are shown the cuts made in the oviduct during an ovidectomy. As with men after a vasectomy, the gametes are still produced by the sex organs but—since their passage is blocked—they will be reabsorbed by the surrounding tissue.

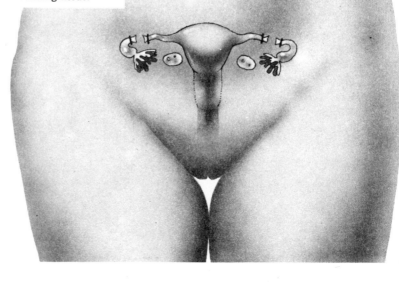

CHILDREN AND SEX

What should children be told about sex? The simple answer is: whatever they want to know. From about the age of four, children start to ask questions such as 'Where did I come from?' Simple and honest answers are best, keeping away from anatomical terms and long complicated explanations. Whether you choose to use family nicknames and abbreviations for the various parts of the body is a matter of personal preference. Later questions such as 'How did I get into mummy's tummy?' or 'How did I get out?' can again be answered directly. Any child old enough to ask this type of question is old enough to be given an answer in terms which can be understood. A long complicated explanation will probably bore the child and not answer his question. The child will not be embarrassed when he asks and nor should you be. There is no difference to an inquiring child between a question about sex and a question about the workings of the heart. Both systems are normal and probably interesting.

It is better to introduce the subject at some opportune moment if questions are not forthcoming. This will forestall inaccurate information heard at school. Some children are naturally more inquisitive than others and if there is a pregnancy in the family this affords a good opportunity to explain what is happening.

One of the hardest questions to answer relates to what can generally be termed 'abnormal sex'. The term is necessarily ambiguous but refers to those practices which are considered either criminal, such as paedophilia and child molesting, or are such as to offend our own decency. There are two main difficulties. One, the child comes from a loving family where such habits do not exist and most of us are unable to explain to ourselves the true meanings of the terms let alone inform a child about them. It is probably better, though, to attempt some kind of explanation along the lines that a very small number of people find normal pleasures difficult and therefore resort to other methods which may hurt or harm other people. Tolerance of *their* problems is unlikely to promote imitation whereas total condemnation and horror without explanation can produce an unwanted result. What about our own 'abnormal practices'? Masturbation used to come under this heading but is now accepted as an almost universal act indulged in by both sexes. It is not harmful nor does it lead to or signify anything 'wrong'. Babies touch or play with their genitals and the best way to deal with this is to ignore it. Babies and young children will probably play 'doctors and nurses' or 'mummies and daddies' among themselves but, like masturbation, it is best left alone. No harm will come of it unless *you* make a fuss. Finally, should you let your child see you naked? Remember, if you do, that your body is fully developed and different, and may well cause him or her to ask questions, especially about your genitals and breasts. As before, simple direct answers will not only satisfy the child's curiosity, they will also help him to gain an awareness of the human body and a respect for its functions.

SOCIAL STIMULANTS: THE DANGERS

Life in Western society today is difficult. To live successfully with others, whether in your own family or at work, or with people at large, can make heavy demands on people and institutions, especially in crowded towns and cities.

Since World War II our society has changed remarkably. There is greater affluence, but the fruits of affluence tend to subject the individual to more and greater stresses. The era of rapid transport, mass advertising and television—coupled with a pharmacological 'explosion' that has made the widespread use of drugs far more acceptable than formerly—has transformed the social lives of vast numbers of people. Increasingly, society pressures people into resorting to artificial means to help them to socialize with their fellows.

The use of tobacco, alcohol and other psychoactive drugs is not new. They are considered to be part of normal life. What is new is the ever-growing number of people who use these substances— the social stimulants—in order to *have* a social life, and who use them to excess. Pressure to compete with others, and to excel and be seen to excel, notably in the fields of sport, academic achievement and social expertise, contributes to a widening dependence on these stimulants. This pressure is most strikingly apparent in the wealthier countries, which is really another way of saying that natural selection is still operative. The fit survive, and the unfit struggle and may sadly fail to avoid unsupportable loneliness, depression and despair—conditions which may occur from time to time in all our lives. In this chapter we discuss the use of tobacco, alcohol, and drugs—those prescribed by your doctor and those which can be obtained from other sources.

TOBACCO

Smoking is reported to have been brought to England by Sir Walter Raleigh from the American colony of Virginia. King James I condemned and outlawed the habit. He called it 'a custom loathsome to the eye, harmful to the brain, dangerous to the lungs, and in the black stinking fume thereof, nearest resembling the horrible Stygian smoke of the pit that is bottomless'. How right he was! He would be still more horrified to know the complications that smoking has produced since 1600—the disease and the mortality, and the vast amount of money spent on it by an ever-demanding public.

The first smokers were usually men, and in polite society they smoked away from women. There were smoking rooms in hotels and clubs—there still are—and later came smoking compartments on public transport. The poorer smokers used clay pipes, and the richer smoked cigars from Havana, and it was not until the first cigarettes became available in the late 18th century that the smoking habit grew widespread. Two world wars increased its popularity, though it is still illegal to sell tobacco to children under the age of 16 and for them to smoke. However, some children now start at the age of five, and 80 per cent of those who smoke regularly when young continue to do so as adults.

Consumption in the United Kingdom at present is at the average rate of 56 cigarettes per week for men and 37 cigarettes per week for women. Eighty million pounds is spent annually on sales promotion and only £1 million is spent by the government on anti-smoking propaganda. At the same time, the death rate attributable directly to this habit is 25,000 per annum, with a further indirect mortality rate of 25,000. It has

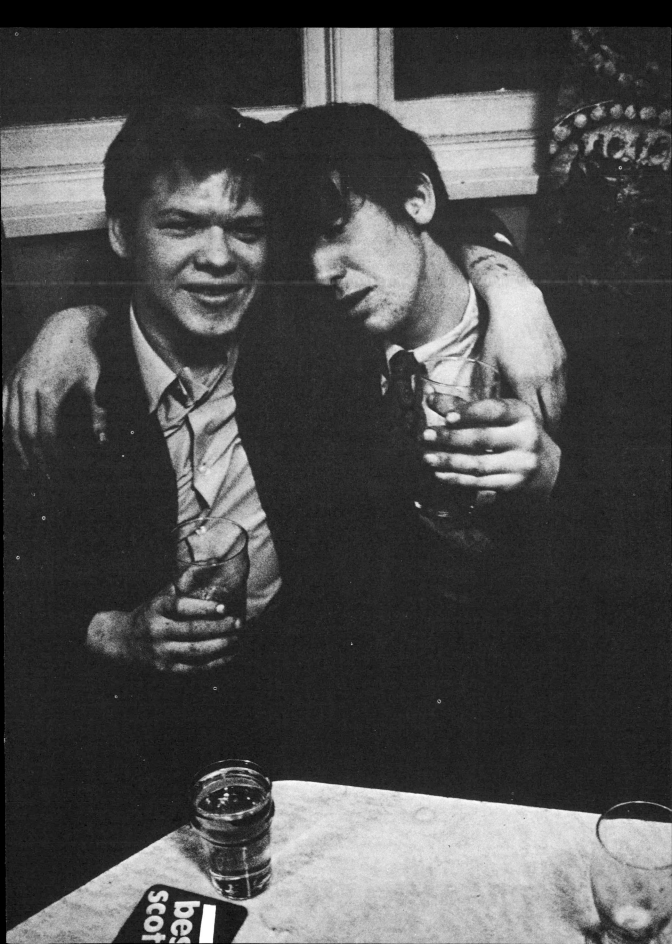

been calculated that each cigarette smoked shortens a human life by five and a half minutes. Smoking also loses the nation some 50 million working days a year.

These very serious figures have been investigated by the Royal College of Physicians of London and the Surgeon General of the United States of America, whose research and reports over ten years fully substantiate the connection between cigarette smoking and disease. It is the view of the Conference of Medical Royal Colleges and other Faculties in the United Kingdom that cigarette smoking today is the most important cause of preventable death and disease in the United Kingdom. The government has been urged to take vigorous measures, including legislation to prevent the tobacco manufacturers from promoting their wares in ways that undermine the impact of health education on both children and adults. At present rates, it is estimated that at least 1 million more people in the UK will die from cigarette smoking before the end of the century unless sales are somehow controlled, especially among children.

The governments of Norway and Finland have adopted comprehensive policies to reduce cigarette smoking, including phasing out advertising and promotion, and these are already beginning to show valuable effects, especially amongst the young. Yet successive governments in the UK have failed to take any such action, even though the death rate from smoking-related diseases is one of the highest in the world.

WHAT SMOKING DOES TO YOU The physical effects of cigarette smoking are:
1 Bronchitis, and the gradual deterioration of the lung tissue. This causes increased breathlessness which is later fatal.
2 Increased risk of heart disease, when the vessels of the heart cannot obtain enough blood and so the heart fails to work properly. This condition later produces heart attacks commonly called 'coronaries'.
3 Cancer of the lung. Virtually all cancer of the lung is caused by smoking.
4 Higher incidence of babies born abnormally or stillborn; the latter risk is increased by 30 per cent if the mother smokes after the fourth month of pregnancy.

The 1977 Report of the Royal College of Physicians named chronic bronchitis and emphysema—then claiming more than 27,000 victims a year—as one of the major killers in present-day society and representing 'one of the most cogent reasons for not smoking cigarettes'. The Report also showed that smokers under the age of 65 were about twice as likely to die of coronary heart disease as non-smokers—and for heavy smokers the risk was three and a half times as great.

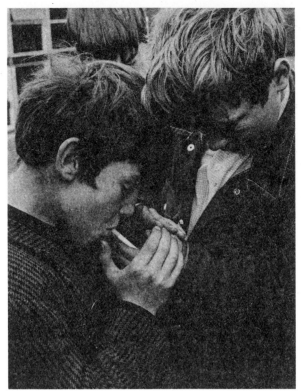

While the incidence of other forms of cancer seems to have decreased over the last fifty years, that of lung cancer is increasing and seems to run parallel with increases in cigarette sales.

As for the mother-to-be, if she smokes during her pregnancy she is at greater risk all round—of having a miscarriage or bearing an abnormal baby or one with retarded growth at birth.

THE YOUNG SMOKER The young smoker is the target at which most attention should be directed. The aims are to get those who smoke to stop, and to prevent others from starting. A report carried out recently in England and Wales on 5,600 young persons aged between 11 and 16 shows four major influences that lead them to smoke. These are:
1 Their circle of friends.
2 Their own desire to join in the social life of older teenagers.
3 Their parents' attitude to smoking.
4 Their own attitude to the health risk.

Smoking appears to be associated with 'toughness' and precocious maturity, and is often done to attract the opposite sex. Smoking can also begin for negative reasons, when it appears to take on a consoling role. The habit may be prompted, for example, by failure at schoolwork and sport. Parents may encourage smoking unwittingly. They may do this by leaving cigarettes around at home, and by not making it clear whether they actually

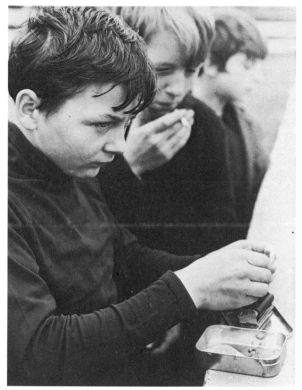

disapprove of their children smoking or not. Even though most parents express the hope that their children will not smoke (including 80 per cent of those who are regular smokers), as children become older restrictions against smoking tend to be withdrawn (31 per cent of 14-year-olds said their parents occasionally gave them a cigarette). What parents do not appear to realize is that in a large family the attitudes they adopt towards the older children are likely to affect the younger ones as well.

The majority of boys, i.e. 80 per cent, have tried their first cigarette by the time they are aged 15. In the first year 4 per cent smoke at least one cigarette per week, and in the fourth year 36 per cent smoke this same quantity but 14 per cent by then are smoking 20 or more per week. Most of them smoke filter cigarettes which they obtain from friends or slot machines.

Most, or at least 95 per cent, of schoolchildren have heard about lung cancer, and 78 per cent have certainly heard about the association between smoking and other kinds of damage to health. The main reason, however, that young smokers were not put off smoking, according to this survey, was because they enjoyed it so much. This enjoyment is closely linked to the gradual dependence of the smoker on his tobacco. It is a psychological dependence and it often makes the effort of giving up smoking very difficult. Some people are so seriously affected that they become addicted, and then special methods have to be used to help them over this dependence. No one knows why some people can smoke for many years and give it up without trouble, whereas others can become dependent very quickly.

WHY SMOKE AT ALL? Can smoking contribute usefully to a person's social life? It is certainly not *necessary*. It is pleasurable to some but not all, and indeed is an acquired pleasure–though it is easy to see why it is habit-forming. Many advertisements show people smoking–although there is a ban on TV cigarette advertisements–and they give the impression that these people are mature, have sex appeal and a better way of life. The truth is far from this: apart from expense, the habit destroys first smell, then taste, and after a while a smoker's cough begins that leads to chronic bronchitis. Studies show that children's growth, especially in height, is potentially decreased if smoking starts at an early age.

Therefore, in no sense can one maintain that smoking is part of a healthy social life. It is the opposite, it detracts from it by stunting growth, diminishing taste and smell and later causing irreversibly damaged airways and heart disease, and often cancer.

Another aspect of smoking is the effect the smoke has on those who do not smoke, or who are trying to give it up. Exhaled smoke has been shown to be three times as toxic as the inhaled variety, and may even cause bronchitis in the young children of smokers. It is also generally anti-social: it clings to clothes and furniture, it stings the eyes of non-smokers, gives the smoker bad breath, and its stale smell lingers unpleasantly in the air.

Is there any advantage in smoking? The actual drug in tobacco, nicotine, does stimulate the brain at first and smokers claim to feel a little more alert while smoking. Appetite is certainly reduced, hence the wails of those who have stopped smoking that they are gaining weight! In extreme cases later, and with novice smokers, the stimulation changes to paralysis, there is sweating, dilation of the pupils, difficulty in vision, nausea and vomiting. This is often, thank goodness, when the newcomer ceases his smoking experiments!

What about pipes and cigars? The facts are the same in general, with the one exception that fewer smokers inhale. This is to their advantage since the depth of inhalation is directly related to the bad health and diseases already described.

The smoker who can ration himself to one or two cigars or up to four pipes per day can be reassured that he is not increasing his risk of developing lung cancer. But beyond this ration the hazard increases and can eventually reach four and a half times that of the non-smoker. (The heavy cigarette smoker increases his chances by up to 14 times.)

STOP SMOKING How does one stop smoking? Society in general can help by taking a disapproving attitude, and parents and teachers should be restrictive rather than permissive. At the heart of the problem is education, and the first step in persuading a smoker not to smoke is to make sure that the seriousness of the short and long term effects is clearly understood. At the same time, encourage the smoker to see the gains that he or she may expect by not smoking.

When giving up is a problem—which it usually is—work with the smoker to assess his or her degree of dependence. For example, pipe-smokers do not generally inhale, and a pipe-smoker consuming only one ounce of tobacco per week is likely to have less trouble giving up than someone who is chain-smoking 60 to 70 cigarettes a day and inhaling.

Encourage the smoker to attend a Smoking Clinic. These are available on the NHS and privately. There the smoker will meet a group of like-minded people, similarly motivated, who together will assess the needs of individuals, with full discussion and reinforcement. This reinforcement is a key point, for it seeks to encourage by praising success in reducing or stopping, rather than censoring failure to do so.

Should smokers aim to stop suddenly —and for ever—or cut down gradually? It is best to look first at the nature of the individual's problem rather than try to follow one standard method. Ideally, however, the smoker should stop abruptly, and not smoke again.

Drugs, in the form of tranquillizers or anti-depressants, have little part to play in the smoker's problem since they tend only to smother his need and not remove it. It is easy to say that willpower is the absolute requirement: this is true, but the desire to stop smoking is also important, and although willpower may not be a particular person's strong point, a continuing desire to stop, with reinforcement from others, especially from the family, can make all the difference. As time passes, moreover, the victim begins to appreciate the bonuses of giving up. He has more money in his pocket, he feels healthier and more energetic, coughs less, can smell flowers, sees more clearly, and is generally an improved version of the person he was when he smoked.

Although mortality rates remain far too high, there has been some success for the anti-smoking movement in that the number of smokers in the professional classes has continued steadily to decrease since 1958. Such campaigns have not changed the habits of the working man, however, and the rate is still rising in working women. But perhaps the message is coming home to some of us.

ALCOHOL

Alcohol has been used in various forms, e.g. beer, ale, spirits and wine, for thousands of years, but it is only in the last 100 years or less that it has been produced and consumed in such large and increasing quantities that it has become a threat. Its apparently alleviating effect on anxiety, and promotion of relaxed relationships, is directly related in Western society to the stresses of everyday living. In the United Kingdom, it is only in the last ten years that alcohol has been recognized as the major hazard to health in the home countries, contributing to such diseases as liver failure (cirrhosis), malnutrition, impairment of intellectual function (dementia) and fatty degeneration of the heart.

Alcohol is a great socializing agent. Taken to excess, it reduces most drinkers to a common level of disinhibited behaviour. What is excess? This is an individual equation for each person and depends on many factors such as the mood of the individual, bodyweight, and whether the stomach is empty or not.

Anyone who drinks should understand the strengths of what he or she consumes, and the effects that alcohol exerts on the body. The accompanying diagrams, based on material devised by the Health Education Council, offer a basic guide.

How much is enough? 'Moderate' drinking should be the ideal, but this again is hard to define because alcohol affects each individual differently each time a drink is taken. On the one hand many people, by using alcohol in moderation, can experience feelings of pleasure and relaxation with no ill-effects, but in others the consequent loss of inhibitions may be potentially harmful and later dangerous. Therefore, it is more constructive and safer to stick to a specific limit which we set at two large whiskies or four pints of beer per day. Anything over that should be considered excessive. And indeed, even a *regular* intake of two large whiskies or four pints of beer per day is shouting a warning. It means that the drinker is developing a dependence on alcohol— and, more likely, has already become dependent.

ADDICTION TO ALCOHOL Nobody is satisfied with the definition of alcoholism, but it may be useful to consider it in the following contexts:

1 When you drink to feel better rather than to enjoy a drink.
2 When you feel the need to 'top up' every lunch time, and in some cases before breakfast.
3 When alcohol has caused trouble—road traffic offences, violence towards others and physical illness, e.g. liver disease.
4 When others feel that *you* have a problem with alcohol.

How strong are alcoholic drinks?

Note If the drink was bottled on the Continent, the degree figure on the label refers to the percentage of pure alcohol present, e.g. 10° for table wine.

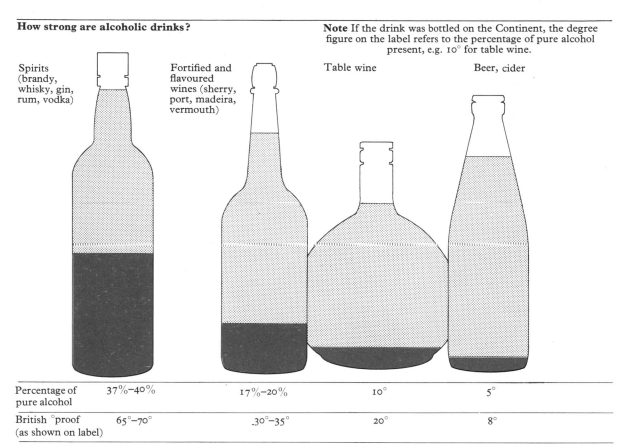

Spirits (brandy, whisky, gin, rum, vodka)

Fortified and flavoured wines (sherry, port, madeira, vermouth)

Table wine

Beer, cider

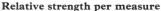

	Spirits	Fortified wines	Table wine	Beer, cider
Percentage of pure alcohol	37%–40%	17%–20%	10°	5°
British °proof (as shown on label)	65°–70°	30°–35°	20°	8°

Relative strength per measure

Each of these contains approximately ½ oz of pure alcohol, and this is roughly the amount that your liver needs 1 hour to digest (oxidize). The more you drink, the more you ask the liver to do.

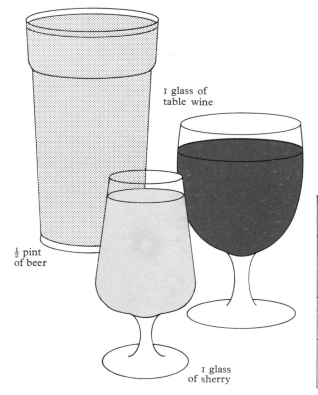

½ pint of beer

1 glass of table wine

1 glass of sherry

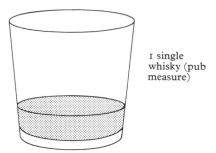

1 single whisky (pub measure)

Consumption of Alcohol in the United Kingdom in 1975 for a Population of 55.962 Millions (latest figures available)				
	Gallons per head	Alcohol content %	Alcohol in mls per pt (beer) or bottle (others) %	Increase in consumption in the last 10 years %
Beer	33.66	5	28.5	28.1
Wines	1.81	10	73	76
Spirits	0.74	40	302	114.4

A daily average consumption of 150 ml of alcohol is associated with high risk of cirrhosis of the liver, i.e. 5.35 pints of beer, two bottles of wine or half a bottle of spirits. In the last 10 years cirrhosis has increased by 27.3%.

Although much is known about alcohol, almost nothing is known of the mechanism of addiction and the cause of alcoholism. Thus it is that one man may be a heavy drinker all his life without incident, while another man may start drinking heavily in his twenties and in five years or less develop the signs and symptoms of the alcohol-dependent person.

Today in the United Kingdom alcoholism is running at the rate of about 700,000 (mostly undiagnosed persons), i.e. more than one in every 100 of the population, and rising. The number of driving offences committed under the influence of alcohol is now back to what it was before the introduction of the breathalizer (7,000 per year). It contributes to a massive loss in working hours; it is

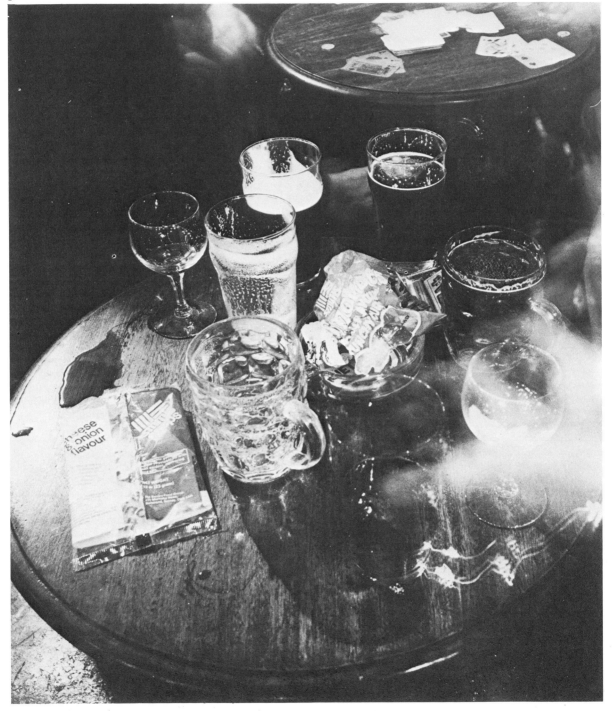

responsible for more broken marriages and disturbed families, and it is responsible for more violence than any other factor. It is also often involved either directly or indirectly in suicide attempts.

At the onset the victim does not realize, and indeed is not capable of realizing, what is happening to him. Loss of memory and concentration, with blackouts from what has happened the previous night, is so usual that the patient (and he must be considered that) vehemently denies what has happened, while at the same time he is drinking secretly and hiding bottles. The tragedy for so many alcoholics is that they are found too late, e.g. in a car crash, or in a hospital bed having been admitted for something else.

As with tobacco, dependence comes soon for those that are vulnerable, but affects almost every heavy drinker sooner or later. In extreme cases this means that if alcohol intake is reduced withdrawal symptoms are experienced: sudden fears, sleeplessness, shaking, sweating, panic, and in bad cases delirium tremens (referred to as the 'shakes' or 'DTs'), episodes of waking nightmares that consist of frightening visions together with fits. Without medical help the outcome is often fatal.

There is no really satisfactory method of ending alcohol addiction. Medicine does not have the answer, except to dry the victim out, which does not end the addiction. It is often a lifelong struggle to stop drinking, for alcohol to an alcholic *is* a poison. He must rearrange his lifestyle in such a way that stress is kept under control, or reduced, and those around him are not alienated but supportive.

So serious is the problem today that this grim picture would not be complete without a short account of the complications of excess alcohol. The most common alcohol-related disease is cirrhosis of the liver, which can be arrested, but not cured. In fact the rate of cirrhosis in a country is an indication of its alcoholism. France has the highest rate in Western Europe with 40,000 deaths per year. This condition, together with loss of weight, gastritis, sometimes haemorrhages and ulcers, is common in the excessive drinker; so too are deterioration of the nerves to the foot and hand causing weakness, and to the heart causing breathlessness. Mental complications can include impaired reflexes, loss of memory and premature senility.

You may wonder if this is all exaggerated. It is not. It is the biggest problem in the National Health Service, and it is made more difficult to treat because alcohol is almost universally regarded as an acceptable social drug. People drink and enjoy it because it is fun, or is thought to be sophisticated. Nor would governments wish to see consumption of alcohol reduced by any great amount, since without the heavy tax on alcohol the country would become bankrupt.

GUIDELINES FOR DRINKERS Alcohol in moderation can be a pleasure and help people to lead a pleasant social life, but the borderline between moderation and excess is narrow and the slope slippery. Alcohol is a *depressant*, not the stimulant that it first appears to be. In certain cultures, particularly in America and Scandinavia, it is a sad fact that people drink in order to get drunk, i.e. they deliberately consume enough to obliterate unpleasant memories and grant them a period of forgetfulness. They choose to disregard the complications that will inevitably follow the next day, or even during the time in which they are intoxicated. Among such drinkers the taste of the drink is unimportant; only the force of the alcohol matters.

Much more needs to be done to educate the public about the dangers of alcohol. This process should begin in schools, where much problem-drinking develops. Parents, too, should be wary of the examples they set. Studies of young problem-drinkers, i.e. below the age of 16, show that the families roughly conform to one of two types. One disapproves of alcohol so strongly that it prohibits drinking in the family while the children are still at home. This leads to the danger that the children will overreact when they leave home and become excessive drinkers. In the other type of family the parents drink freely at home and, tacitly or otherwise, encourage their children to do so.

Once drinking has been isolated as a problem either by the drinker or his family, it must be treated, not ignored. Professional advice must be sought. This can be obtained through the local GP or social worker. Some people are too self-conscious to seek help so near home. They can best be helped by one of two main bodies, Alcoholics Anonymous and the National Council on Alcoholism. Both have branches all over the UK, and one will very likely be listed in the local telephone directory.

Alcoholics Anonymous is an international self-help group which preserves members' anonymity while helping them to discuss their drinking problem and giving them the strength to abandon drink altogether. The UK headquarters are at 11 Redcliffe Gardens, London, SW10 9BG, telephone (01) 352 9779.

The National Council on Alcoholism offers a free advisory service to anyone needing confidential information about a drink problem. They will help the relations and friends of problem-drinkers as well as the sufferer. Their headquarters are at 45 Great Peter Street, London SW1P 3LT, telephone (01) 222 1056/7.

OTHER DRUGS

The main subject in this section is the range of preparations, other than tobacco and alcohol, to which people become addicted. Before we consider the specific natures of the 'hard', 'soft' and 'psychedelic' drugs, it is relevant to see their increased use against a background of mounting national dependence on drugs, pills and painkillers of all kinds.

People today are becoming more health-conscious than ever. Or, rather, they are becoming more disease-conscious than ever, and are in danger of reaching the point where they believe that every ache, pain, worry or queer feeling must be soothed away by taking some kind of preparation. This encourages the mistaken idea that every form of stress is harmful, and in years to come the tendency will become even more marked unless people become more independent of medicine, and learn again to put up with some discomfort, some strain, and occasional sleeplessness.

The general public has not formed this attitude unaided. It is backed up by a gigantic pharmaceutical industry with highly productive research laboratories and other facilities geared to easing numerous minor aches and disorders. This is not to belittle the many life-supporting and essential preparations, for example, diuretics for heart disease and antibiotics for infection, that have also emerged from the laboratories in recent years. These have revolutionized the expectation of life and have made it possible for many to live who otherwise would have died. It is also true that many people, including the young, are able to experiment with drugs without becoming addicted to them.

There is, nonetheless, a strong link between an overtly pill-conscious society and one that includes a growing population of drug addicts. Some varieties of sleeping tablets and tranquillizers, e.g. those in the benzodiazepine group such as Valium and Librium, demonstrate the connection by the pleasurable effects they can produce in vulnerable persons. Experience of these effects leads to dependence, and can bring with it all the complications of dependence on stronger drugs, including withdrawal symptoms if they are stopped and a desperate need to get more or lay-in a supply in case of need.

Let's now analyse the truly addictive drugs that are our main concern here. There are four principal types, as follows:

1 Narcotics These are the 'hard' drugs, e.g. heroin, morphine and opium.

2 Hallucinatory Drugs in this group produce 'unreal' sensations that are sometimes called 'psychedelic'. Examples are lysergic acid (LSD

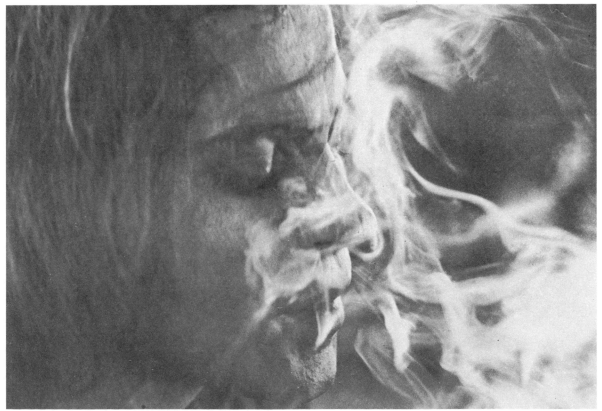

or just 'acid'), cannabis (marijuana, 'hash' or 'smoke'), and psylocin or psylocibin (the mushroom drugs).

3 Stimulants These are the amphetamines and appetite-suppressant tablets known as 'speed', 'sulphate' or 'dex', also cocaine.

4 Hypnotics In this group are the drugs that put you to sleep, e.g. Mandrax and the barbiturates.

The latter two groups are sometimes called 'soft' drugs, but if this is seen to imply harmlessness it is a serious misnomer. Barbiturates, for example, as the commonest kind of drug prescribed for sleep, are the commonest kind involved in overdoses and suicidal behaviour.

The effects of the various groups are as follows:

1 Narcotics produce sleep or doziness, sometimes a feeling of omnipotence or well-being.

2 Hallucinatory drugs give odd sensations, visions, distorted sight, voices in the head, and sometimes a 'vast understanding', really a bogus insight into life's problems.

3 Stimulants reduce sleep to zero, increase activity to such a point that the victim never sits down, never goes to bed and ends up doing everything at once in a welter of uninhibited chaos.

4 Hypnotics put the person to sleep, as already mentioned – sometimes into a very deep sleep, which, in the case of barbiturates combined with alcohol, may result in death.

HOW HABITS BEGIN Like most difficult problems, the mechanism whereby a person, often quite young, comes to use these drugs, is complicated. Studies of addicts suggest that the following factors can play important parts in starting a drug habit:

1 Curiosity, and the desire to imitate. These are especially strong pulls on children, as is the desire among adolescents to keep up with their friends, some of whom may be older.

2 Prohibition Because drugs are banned, they become desirable in circles where boredom, money and the wish for glamour and excitement are commonly felt. Such feelings are encouraged by suppliers.

3 Illegal contacts These are commonly made with suppliers of drugs in places like all-night discos and pop parties.

4 Depression Drugs may be taken as a means of getting over depression. Doubts about the ability to pass an examination may also start a drug habit.

5 Health problems People seek cures for states such as obesity, sleeplessness and pain. Drugs are often prescribed, in the first instance, by the medical profession.

6 Other factors These may be cultural, or merely a matter of changing fashions, a passing

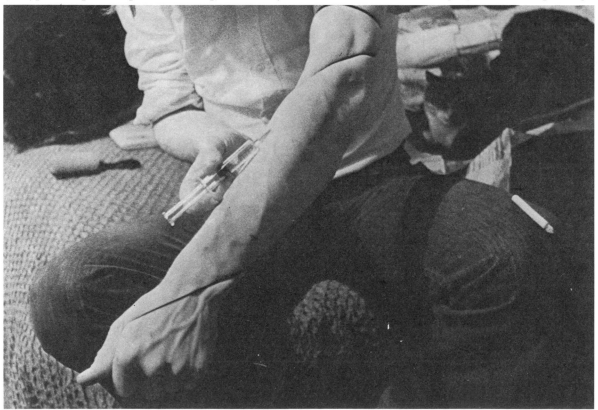

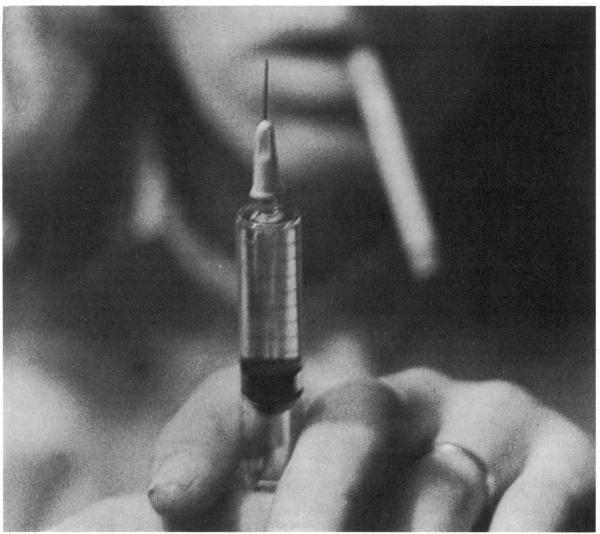

craze. While it has been established that drug-taking can be indulged in with no ill-effects, an implicit risk of dependence remains.

AVOIDING DRUGS The 'Golden Rule' for avoiding offers of drugs is simply not to accept any substance that may seem suspicious. This is best done by avoiding places where drugs are commonly in circulation. You should be aware of the dangers surrounding all drugs in the groups listed above. Take only the minimum of medication prescribed by your doctor, and make sure you understand what he is prescribing them for. Do not succumb to the persuasive efforts of others to 'con' you into taking drugs—even to 'get by' on a very temporary basis, say to pass a test or an exam.

RECOGNIZING A DRUG-TAKER IN TROUBLE This advice about avoiding drugs is all very well, you may say, but it does not help people to detect the ill-effects of drug-taking in others, nor tell them what to do. This probably applies most of all to parents, made

anxious by the behaviour of a child whom they suspect of experimenting with drugs.

First of all, it is important to recognize that after the age of 14 or so the young cannot be protected for 24 hours a day. It is therefore impossible to prevent experimentation. What is important is to detect any harmful effects quickly. There is no single pattern of behaviour that will give away the drug-taker, but one or more of several changes usually occur. Late hours are kept; general behaviour deteriorates; friends are not so much in evidence, or are unsuitable or different in some way; performance at school falls off. Parents, teachers and friends can detect such signs—if only they have eyes to see. The next step is harder.

Behind every so-called victim of a drug problem there lies an emotional problem that has not been resolved, or a need that has not been met. Possibly advice has not been taken, or not been given when it should have been. When a parent or friend detects that something is wrong, the drug itself may seem to have become the greater problem—or the problem itself. But do not be deceived. The emotional problem is the underlying cause and must be dealt with. The difference between a young and an older victim is that the young one may be facing a particular problem for the first time and cannot cope. The older victim is often only too aware of the trouble that is developing and is ready to accept help if it is offered in an understanding way.

TAKING ACTION If you witness an emergency, medical help must be sought. Where the victim is unconscious, treat as described on page ooo. If there is no emergency, but the problem has somehow been exposed, try to get the person talking. Emphasize that your discussion is confidential. This is important, because drug-takers are secretive for various reasons. They are afraid of the police being told, or of word reaching their parents. Neither of these steps may be necessary unless further serious risks are apparent. If in doubt, consult the family doctor, if you know or can identify him. He will be able to advise you how and when to take matters further should the need arise.

How can the misfortunes of drug abuse be prevented? Once again, it is to the young that the message must be relayed. Health education classes in schools must be beneficial. There is currently a great need for well-informed people who can give factual information in a non-sensational manner and who are willing to answer questions.

Parents meanwhile can contribute by accepting that experimentation is a feature of youth, but that some experiments are more dangerous than others. They should be prepared to give their adolescent children positive guidance: allowing a glass of wine at home, for example, but making it clear that pill-taking is not permissible. Many drug-takers are using drugs to attempt to solve personal problems rather than as ends in themselves. The great task for friends and parents is to remove their need for more drugs.

AGEING

AGEING It is impossible to define old age, though most of us think we know what it means. In fact there are no constant body or mind changes, and certainly no definite number of years which characterize what we call the elderly. The simplest thing to say is that with advancing years, and apart from any specific illness or disability, we find a restriction of physical or mental power. When the restriction is great enough to interfere with normal work or social activity, then we are old.

The best attitude to old age is a double one. We should accept it as inevitable and not resent or fight the natural limitations it brings. However, we must not equate an impressive number of birthdays with relegation to a background state of inactivity. This applies not only to our advancing years, but importantly to the many aged people who surround us.

And indeed they are many. Not because science has increased the natural span of life. This averages around the psalm's 'threescore years and ten'. What medicine and social welfare have done is to better a person's chance of reaching that age. The journey's length has not really changed; it is simply that travel has been made easier and the hazards on the way have been reduced. Four centuries ago the average age of death was about 30. Today it is 70 for men and 77 for women, and the numbers exceeding these ages are increasing.

Thus the proportion of the elderly in the population has become higher. At the beginning of this century every seventeenth person was of pensionable age. Today the figure is approaching that of every fifth person.

THE PHYSICAL CHANGES

We can think of ageing as a process which begins when growth ceases. The process is by no means a steady one. Changes, limitations or deteriorations often happen in stages, with quite quick transitions. Other health factors seem to play a fairly large part here. The elderly person hitherto unusually vigorous and young in mind or body may suddenly and permanently bear the physical attributes of his age after a severe illness or emotional upset.

Yet it is not all that easy to list what these attributes are. There is no 'normal' for any decade in old age, unlike the case of children where paediatricians have more or less absolute medical measures of normality. Medically old age is a mixed-up condition with no clear-cut standards.

The physical alterations to body physiology as age advances can be listed, but we must remember that not all of them happen to everyone, and that the changes vary in degree, occurring in different people to a lesser or greater extent.

Arteries harden and also tend to thicken up inside. This means a less free circulation of blood, some diminution in its capacity to supply oxygen to all parts and a poor response to any sudden bodily demands for an increased expenditure of energy. Reserves are great and in many cases this is of small moment, except for the brain whose cells are extremely sensitive to its oxygen receipts. The heart has to work harder pumping blood through the narrowed arterial spaces, and blood pressure may rise. Another factor which can reduce the intake of oxygen is the fact that the elasticity of the tissues about the microscopic air sacs of the lungs decreases; respiration is marginally less efficient.

The endocrine glands, those organs which secrete the hormones (chemical messengers acting through the blood stream on varying parts of the body) reduce their secretions. To make matters more difficult the tissues in these parts respond less sensitively to

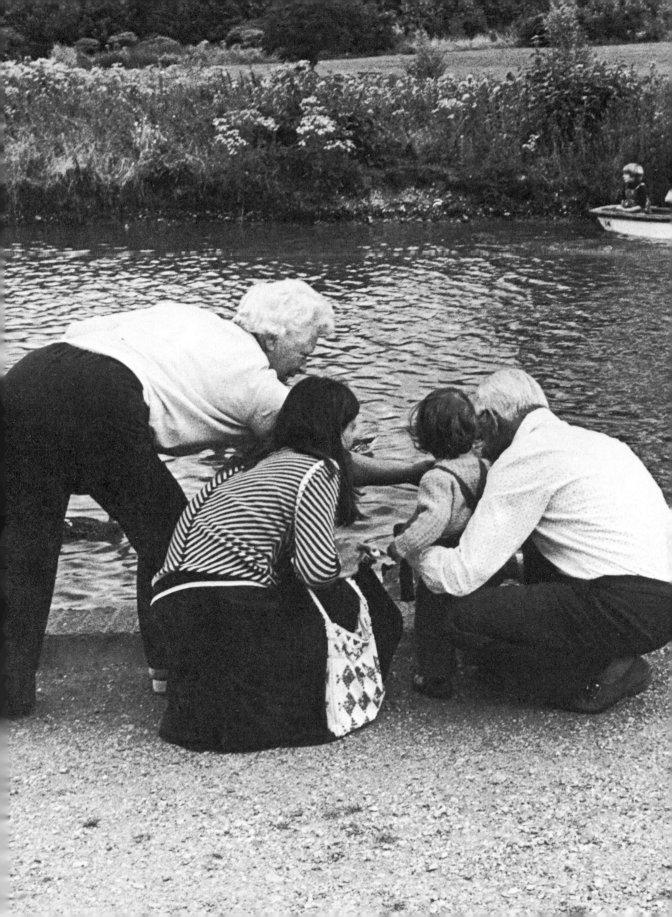

the hormones which reach them. A common example is the thyroid gland in the neck whose secretions govern the rate of metabolism (the sum of the energy and chemical changes in the body) and play a part in the transport of calcium to the bones.

Fat immediately beneath the skin decreases. Not only is it a helpful insulator, but also its presence helps to give the rounder contour of youth. The skin itself becomes drier and loses some of its elasticity and wrinkles mark our seniority.

Many of the above factors explain the frequent complaint voiced by the elderly of feeling the cold intensely. With a reduced intake of calcium the bones become relatively brittle and thin. They have a greater liability to fracture, and if fractured they take longer to heal.

As they grow old muscle fibres become thinner. Muscles lose their tone and the limbs become weaker. Collagen, that part of our body's connective tissue which fills some spaces and binds together many parts of our frame, loses its flexibility so that movements may be not only weaker but also stiffer. The body becomes less limber.

Loss of height is common in the elderly. Some stoop because of muscle weakness. In many cases the backbone shortens from shrinking of the discs between each vertebra.

Many other functions, such as the excretory efficiency of the kidneys, are reduced. Other alterations are more obvious: the hair changes colour, the lenses of the eyes lose some of their suppleness and ability to focus, and there is a decrease of hearing power, especially to higher pitches. Receding gums may loosen and teeth fall out.

More recondite is the steady degeneration of brain tissue and of some of the important chemicals it produces. In all other parts of the body there is a constant loss of tissue cells with regeneration of new cells to take their place. The brain is an exception; gradually through life the brain cells die off but are never replaced. The brain, in fact, decreases in size as we grow old. Just what significance this has is not yet clear, and research on the problem continues.

The elderly may take some comfort in the theory that many of the changes may be due not just to increasing years but to a poor habit of diet and to lack of exercise in younger years. Better attention to the latter may be very important in minimizing this sad catalogue of changes. The foundations of a strong senescence may be laid in the teens. The task of the adult is then to maintain the body in the best possible order, in preparation for an eventual decline in its powers.

FACULTIES

One of the commonest age disabilities is difficulty in remembering recent events. Often this is only a minor handicap. In an extreme case the old person will be able to recall accurately many trivialities from youth and childhood, but be powerless to recall that he has just been given (and eaten) his meal, or has received an important visit. In conversation he may continually repeat himself. If he is very confused this differential memory will make him believe he is living in a place and circumstances of many years past, and the failure of current happenings to fit in will confuse him further.

In less severe examples the elderly person tends simply to dwell on past aspects of his life. It is a way out of facing the fact that he cannot keep up his memory for events around him.

However, many aged people do have good memory recall for the immediate past. We must beware of the generalization that the elderly are poor learners. There are splendid examples ranging from the Open University to Adult Evening Centres to testify that they can be excellent students. They tend to apply themselves more methodically to their work than when they were younger; intuition and sudden perception now play a far lesser part than do system and pertinacity.

They are slower. They take longer to react to outer events, and they are less able to face suddenly the challenge of a new set of ideas. But they are amply able to use skills and experiences developed during their life. In general they can offer their own special expertise with great success.

As a rule they are less successful in work where time is important and likely to cause stress. They like to plan, even if this is a matter of seconds only. They take longer than the young to do a job, not because they move more slowly, but because they spend longer thinking. Age tends to give priority to assessment and to accuracy.

Many of the elderly also become more introverted, withdrawing into themselves and being less aroused by the outside world. This seems to be not merely a consequence of reduced physical and social circumstances, but a normal psychological evolution. We should, of course, offer them as much stimulation and chance to be interested in events as possible, but this must not be forced. If and when it appears we should respect the natural change.
SEXUAL ACTIVITY Sexual interest never switches off. It may with advancing years reduce its urges; it may command less forcefully and less frequently. But in the elderly it does not necessarily disappear entirely.

This is not sufficiently recognized. The sexual feelings of young people are regarded as natural to youth, but the older man may be distressed to find himself categorized as an example of the 'dirty old man'. On the other hand, he may accept society's verdict and anxiously wonder why he should be so abnormal as still to feel sexual forces which so many people wrongly regard as normal only for his earlier years.

The sexual peak in males is reckoned by doctors to be in the late teens, and in women to be at the age of about 40. The decline thereafter is generally so slow and gradual that reports of activity and interest into the seventies and beyond should cause no surprise.

The major problem for elderly women is a relative dryness of the vaginal lining. This can be coped with by the use of simple lubricants obtainable at chemists. In some cases doctors may find it appropriate to prescribe hormone preparations.

Men may face more obvious problems concerning erection and ejaculation. Frequency and force certainly do tend to be lessened and the elderly male may be discomfited by the way his performance does not measure up to his feelings. A few failures then might convince him that he is past sexual congress. He approaches each new attempt with anxiety and is likely to fail again mainly from psychological reasons.

Let him relax but certainly not give up. Sex does not always or necessarily mean firm erection. The partners can enjoy each other's persons and bodies without his having to achieve full penetration and ejaculation. Once he can take his mind off what he had regarded as a humbling problem, he may find that the problem corrects itself spontaneously.

When health allows the elderly should, in sex as in other matters, continue with what they feel they wish to do and not give up for false reasons.

MEDICAL PROBLEMS

Never discuss an abnormal condition of body or mind with that unfortunate phrase: 'What can you expect at his (or "her"–or even "my") age?' Every symptom demands a medical check and very often responds splendidly to treatment. It is true that the elderly tend to accumulate disorders, but even if they cannot all be put right the majority of them can be alleviated. Swollen legs, breathlessness, poor sight, failing appetite, unsteadiness, bad gait are just a few of the handicaps which old people disregard because they consider them their lot.

The medical miseries listed in this section are not specific to old age; they occur in the young as well. Nor are they an inevitable part of being old. But we know that, statistically, they occur more among the elderly.

FLUID INTAKE Perhaps because they are worried about bladder weakness, and they wish to reduce the number of journeys to the lavatory (especially at night), many old people cut down the amount they drink. Unless they are otherwise advised by their doctors they should be encouraged to take daily at least 3.5 litres of fluid either as part of their meals (e.g. soup or stewed fruit) or separately. This total should include half a litre of milk, either drunk with or without flavourings such as cocoa or incorporated in a recipe for a cooked dish.

NUTRITION Diet should be watched with great care (see page 42 for detailed information). Undernutrition is a word suggesting a desert land of drought. Yet it is all too possible to achieve in a community of many shops and full supplies. The elderly person living alone, who cannot be troubled to cook for one, buys easy 'convenience foods' and gradually, from apathy, increased by inadequate feeding, slips into the habit of an enfeebling diet. Progressive weakening is blamed on 'old age'. Relatives, friends, doctors and social workers, after inspecting the tell-tale barren larder, must act firmly and tactfully to correct the situation. A helpful and inexpensive book is Louise Davies's *Easy Cooking for One or Two* (Penguin).

OBESITY Excess food on the other hand is all too common. A drop in working activity after retirement, a sedentary life, some handicap to mobility (including obesity itself, acting in a vicious circle) is very often not matched by a corresponding reduction in food consumed.

Too much food, which does not match the body's expenditure of energy, has no alternative to being stored as fat. This applies even to proteins, though the more usual fault is the eating of high amounts of carbohydrate. Bread, biscuits, cakes, pastry, flour (in soups and sauces, for instance), jams, sweets, chocolate, sugar are so easy to house in the kitchen; they need no larder or refrigerator; they keep a relatively long time; they are quick and easy to turn to for the occasional nibble which soon turns to a frequent habit. And by their bulk they displace the really valuable items which should be forming part of the daily menu.

Narrowed arteries, a raised blood pressure, a weakened heart, breathlessness, arthritis of weight-bearing joints like the knees, diabetes and gall bladder stones are all conditions in which obesity can play a causative role. No specific diet instructions can be given in these pages. The general practitioner's advice should be sought for each individual case. The overweight person, and especially the overweight old person, must accept the challenge of obesity and valiantly battle against it, under the command of his doctor.

TEETH It is common when a patient is admitted to a geriatric hospital to find, on routine medical examination, that he is in need of dental attention. All too often old people lose interest in the condition of their teeth and allow an unhealthy and inefficient method of chewing to develop and persist. Some who have lost all, or almost all, their teeth do not seek dentures. Others who have had dentures do not wear them. With increasing age the shape of the jaws may change so that dentures which were correct in the past become uncomfortable or insecure.

The elderly should get regular dental checks and treatment. There are rewards to be had: their appearance may improve, and they may once more enjoy food in ways they had forgotten.

EYESIGHT In the same way many old people neglect their teeth, they allow their eyesight to weaken without seeking help. Very often reduction of vision develops insidiously and is barely noticed. A yearly test in old age is perhaps a counsel of perfection, but a check every three years at least is sensible.

The two major abnormalities are cataract and glaucoma. Both words need explaining. Cataract is derived from an ancient name for portcullis, the barrier at the gate of a castle. In the eye the penetration of light becomes barred by densities forming in the lens; vision gradually becomes less and less distinct.

Glaucoma is quite a different matter. The term comes from the word glaucous, meaning grey or blue which is said to be the appearance of the pupil of the affected eye (but which, in fact, is a quite unreliable sign). The eyeball becomes tense from excess accumulation of the fluid which it normally contains, bringing damage to its internal structures. Reduced definition of vision may be a feature, but even more important is loss of part of the area visualized. This should be tested with one eye at a time, the other being covered up. A 'shadow in the eye' is a very suspicious symptom.

Sometimes glaucoma gives sudden severe but transient troubles which include one or more of the following: blurred vision, the impression of coloured rainbow or halo effects around lights, headache and vomiting. Any suggestion of glaucoma needs medical advice. If left untreated this condition can cause irreversible damage.

At the other end of the scale is the instant improvement to vision obtained simply by cleaning the spectacle lenses. Old people are not the only ones who let their glasses get grubby, but it seems to happen to them more often.

If new frames are ordered, avoid the heavier types which are more likely to bother an elderly skin.

Make certain that electric lighting in the home is really good, and that if possible favourite chairs are placed so that the light comes at an angle from behind. Finally, there is a wide range of literature available in large-print books for those who cannot cope with ordinary type-sizes.

THE FEET Decades of wearing tight shoes (and socks) and of bad attention to nails may produce cramped and buckled toes, bunions, corns, thickened or ingrowing toe nails. With advancing years the feet tend to splay if their owner is overweight, and correspondingly wider shoes are needed. Many an old person will benefit from chiropody.

The foot is an outpost of the circulation and prone to difficulties if the blood supply is poor. Small injuries or infections here take longer to heal. The diabetic is particularly at risk and he needs to be very careful about foot hygiene, and to seek immediate medical attention for any foot trouble.

In general shoes need to allow good room for the toes, especially if they are deformed. They should fit snugly round the heel, and they should not be so long as to let the foot slide within them at each step. Shoes ought to give a firm comfortable all-round support, and the habit of slopping around in slippers must be avoided. If the wearer has difficulties in tying shoelaces, he can use an elastic lace, which is permanently tied and will stretch as the shoe is put on.

HEARING With old age some loss of hearing is natural. It is then thoughtful to speak to the sufferer clearly and directly while facing him, and without drawing attention to the fact that a special effort is being made. We can help also by beginning any conversation with the less important, more 'expendable' statement, to give our listener the chance to concentrate on and gather what follows. And we must bear in mind that background noises, which younger people can dismiss, may create a total obstruction to understanding in the hard of hearing. When the television is shared we must accept that the sound volume be raised above our normal. In extreme cases, and in certain types of deafness, special earpieces can be worn by the deaf which have leads to the set.

Not all forms of deafness will benefit from a hearing aid, and medical advice must be sought before any trial or purchase. Aids are available in Britain through the National Health Service or through commercial firms. Most makers allow a trial of one or two weeks, and the wearer should test the aid at different points outdoors and indoors. He may be disappointed at first to find that the sounds seem bizarre. The aid is designed mainly for receiving the speaking voice; music will not come through faithfully. Background noises, which normally we can exclude by act of mind, may be magnified to be a nuisance at first. To a great extent, awareness of which direction a sound is coming from depends on the configuration of the external ear and its canal, and this can be obliterated by the aid. Most aids have control buttons for volume and sound pitch: their use has to be learnt.

The part of the aid which fits into the ear itself should be specifically shaped for each wearer, and the canal which receives it must be clean and dry. The outside section may be worn on clothing or, if miniature, behind the ear: the rub of material or of long hair can cause unwanted noise. If the aid is allowed to grow too warm through contact with clothes, its efficiency may be reduced.

Other mechanical forms of help for the deaf include door or telephone bells which are specially loud, or which are coupled to room lamps which light up when they ring.

THE DANGEROUS BED For anyone whose movements are handicapped the bed should be easy to get into, that is 45 cm high, the same height as a chair seat. If necessary use blocks (or a saw!) to adjust the height. Or an extra mattress may solve the problem. In any event seek firm unsagging mattresses.

The bed-fast or those who remain an abnormally long time in bed run very real risks. The body's chemical and mechanical processes are such that prolonged immobility can lead to the following unpleasantnesses: congestion and inflammation of the lungs, muscle weakness, stiff joints, loss of calcium from the bones which become fragile, clot formation in the blood

vessels, kidney stones and bedsores. Every effort, compatible with comfort and safety, must be made to keep an old person out of bed and active.

PRESSURE SORES The bedsore is a breach of the skin, often an infected ulcer, developing where bodyweight has produced sustained pressure against the bed, or where one hard part of the body lies against the other, as with the insides of the knees when lying on one side.

The bedsore is worse in the immobile, especially those under strong sedatives, in very thin or fat people or those with puffy skin, in the undernourished and in the incontinent, and heals with difficulty.

Not only beds can give pressure sores. Chairs are just as bad for people who sit for long without changing their position.

How can we avoid pressure sores for those who are chair- or bed-fast? Advice from a doctor or nurse is essential. Some basic principles include: good nutrition; keeping the handicapped person as active as possible within his limits; frequent changes of position, or two-hourly turning from side to side; meticulously keeping the skin and the bed, or chair cushion, clean and dry; keeping pressure off the heels by using a bed cradle that will relieve the weight of covers, and placing rubber foam at strategic points to ease pressure or to keep threatened areas raised. Heel rings or rubber ring cushions are of limited help for they may create their own pressures. In some cases a ripple bed or chair cushion can be provided. This mechanical aid has separate air-filled compartments which gently alternate in their degree of filling, constantly varying the pressure. Sheepskin makes a comfortable cover to lie on, is simpler to use and often very successful.

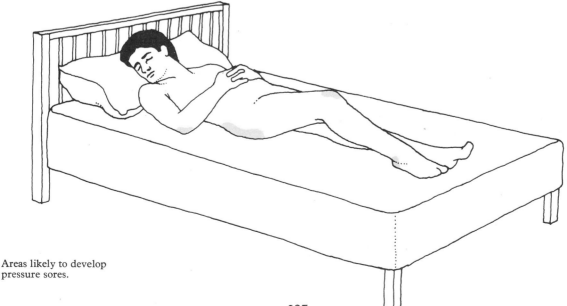

Areas likely to develop pressure sores.

HYPOTHERMIA All too often the body reactions of the elderly are reduced in very cold atmospheres. In cold weather they may be found white, inert and even unconscious with a temperature far below that which the ordinary clinical thermometer will register. The condition can be fatal and is discussed in the First Aid section (see page 186).

INFLUENZA Winter attacks of influenza are harsh and dangerous for old people, especially for any who have chest troubles. Immunization against influenza at the beginning of the cold season is often, though not invariably, a successful protection. It is worthwhile getting the doctor's advice about this.

INCONTINENCE Lack of bowel or bladder control is intensely distressing to an old person who sees it as another ignominious sign of slipping dignity and independence. It must be taken seriously with full medical consultation.

Broadly speaking, incontinence has two principal causes, an abnormality in the bowel or bladder itself or a disturbance of brain and nerve control to the organ.

The **abnormality** could be infection, weakened organ muscles, the presence of a bladder stone or of hardened stools wedged in the bowel ('impacted'), an enlarged prostate or a tumour.

The **nerve disturbance** might be the result of a stroke or of some trouble in the spinal cord.

For the first group treatment may be successful but the outlook is harder for those in the second group.

There are two other much simpler causes of incontinence. Slow in action and perhaps stiff of joints, the old person just may not be quick enough to reach the lavatory in time. Planning access to this or to a commode and the wearing of easily adjustable clothes is the answer. Then many of the elderly are necessarily on diuretics, medicines or tablets which stimulate the kidney to form urine and also are often prescribed for their effect in controlling blood pressure. Some of these are very rapid in action. If this seems to be what is happening, it is worth asking the doctor whether slower-acting, but no less effective, preparations could be substituted.

How to cope with intractable cases? The psychological attitude of the sufferer is important. Discuss the problem in a simple factual way with him; with sympathy, but without hint of worry, work out routine measures to deal with the situation.

Usually restriction of fluid drunk is of little help. It is wise to drink plentifully until two hours before bedtime.

A catheter, a tube inserted into the bladder, can drain away the urine into a collecting bag worn under the clothes. But only the doctor can decide whether this would suit the patient.

Wearing plastic pants with padding (e.g. Kanga or Maxi-Stretch) is a common solution. There are small urinals available in many forms. That for men is well known. For women some ingenious designs are now available (e.g. Suba-Seal, St Peter's Boat or Feminal); these are small and easy to handle by a patient who cannot reach the lavatory or get out of bed in time. The bed itself can be covered by protective underpads (e.g. Kylie or Polyweb).

Much equipment of this type is available through the medical and social services. It is important to get a doctor's or nurse's opinion before selecting any. They will also advise about care of the skin. A final simple point: do not overlook keeping windows open for good ventilation.

A helpful book is *Incontinence* by Dorothy Mandelstam, published by Heinemann Health Books and available from the Disabled Living Foundation (see page 132).

BODY REACTIONS TO DRUGS AND ILLNESS What would be normal doses of some drugs for the average adult may produce unpredictably heavy and untoward responses in the elderly. Ordinary amounts of tranquillizers, for instance, could cause considerable mental confusion and even hallucinations. Tablets for heart conditions often have to be prescribed in forms appropriate for children. Geriatricians take great care in assessing these factors. The layman looking after an old person should not offer him a trial of, say, his own sleeping tablets without first consulting the doctor.

Another problem is that the elderly body often demonstrates fewer features of acute illnesses. An abdominal emergency such as appendicitis or obstruction of the bowel has its very marked characteristics in the young. The same severe afflictions in an old person may show misleadingly mild signs and symptoms. All concerned should be on their guard not to overlook this danger.

FALLS AND ACCIDENTS Here are three simple statistics. 70 per cent of falls in the home and nearly 90 per cent of deaths from such falls affect the age group of 65 or over. Falls occur twice as often with women as with men.

Falls carry with them a big risk of fractures. Quite often light bruising and relatively slight pain may cover damage of a severity of which even the victim is unaware.

Defective vision and hearing play their part in many falls, and people taking tranquillizers or hypnotics are more at risk than those not taking such drugs. Other factors are weakness and stiff joints, preventing the quick correction which could come easily to younger people in a slip or loss of balance. There are also what are known as **drop attacks**; quite suddenly the legs weaken and give way and the victim falls to the ground without losing consciousness. The legs may remain weak for some minutes afterwards.

The cause of drop attacks is still uncertain. General reduction of brain cells with age may be a factor. Another may be the way arteries to the brain pass by the bony structures of the vertebral column in the neck. If these vessels are sufficiently narrowed or the bone deformed, sudden or sustained movement of the head sideways or upwards can obstruct the circulation to the brain. Also some falls have been attributed to miniature strokes.

Lifting someone from a fall This demands a little planning rather than an immediate rush to action. First check as best you can that there is no likelihood of a fracture (see First Aid section, page 184). If you suspect a fracture leave the victim on the floor in the most comfortable position, cover him with a blanket

and call a doctor without further delay.

If there seems to be no severe injury clear the area around and proceed as in the diagrams. If the victim has strength in his arms and legs turn him gently on to his face and stand across his feet. By holding and pulling him at the hips get him on all-fours. Bring a firm stool or chair in front of him and help him to bend over it kneeling on one knee, with the foot near the chair and his hands on the seat. Now get to one side of him: one of your hands supports his elbow and the other is tucked under his armpit on the same side. He pushes himself into a standing position as you help him.

If the victim's legs are not strong enough to accomplish this, get him sitting on the floor with his legs straight out. Immediately behind him put a very low stool on to which he puts his hands. He pushes with his arms to get himself sitting on the stool. Now put a low chair behind him; he then repeats the manoeuvre to get himself sitting on the chair.

Helping the victim to his feet

1 Pull at the hips to raise him on all-fours.

2 Help him to bend over a firm stool or chair.

3 Support and help him to push upwards into a standing position.

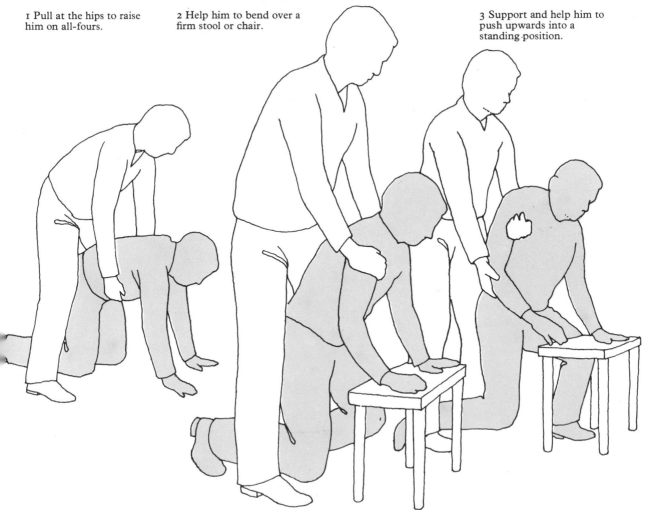

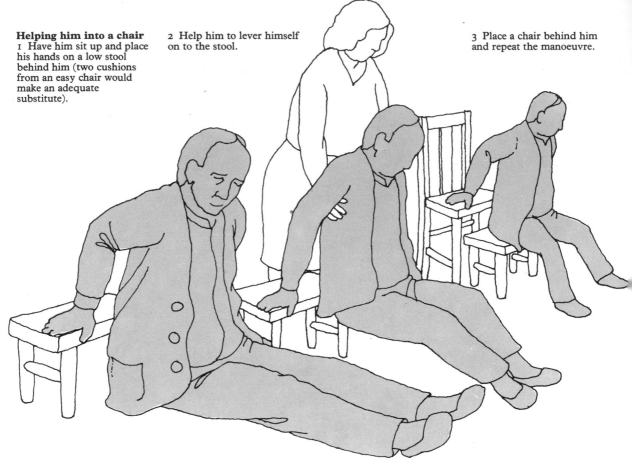

Helping him into a chair
1 Have him sit up and place his hands on a low stool behind him (two cushions from an easy chair would make an adequate substitute).

2 Help him to lever himself on to the stool.

3 Place a chair behind him and repeat the manoeuvre.

Accidents are rarely the result of pure mischance. They are caused. They generally arise from human mistakes or lack of care and foresight. And the elderly are much more prone to this. They share this failing with the very young. But the elderly are far more fragile than the young and are more likely to be killed or injured.

As the middle column shows, the elderly and the very young share a high tendency to suffer accidents in the home. But (right-hand column) it is the elderly who are considerably more likely to die from these accidents.

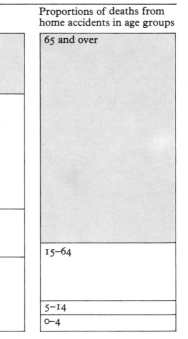

Proportions of population in age groups	Proportions of home accidents in age groups	Proportions of deaths from home accidents in age groups
65 and over	65 and over	65 and over
15–64	15–64	
	5–14	15–64
5–14	0–4	5–14
0–4		0–4

What can we do to mitigate the likelihood of accidents? The picture here summarizes the conditions leading to accidents.

It is up to all who look after old people to study it carefully and meticulously and to take the necessary precautions.

Hazards in the home
Use this picture to make your home accident-proof— or the home of an elderly relative or friend. Remember that any one of the 20 hazards shown here could cause a death.

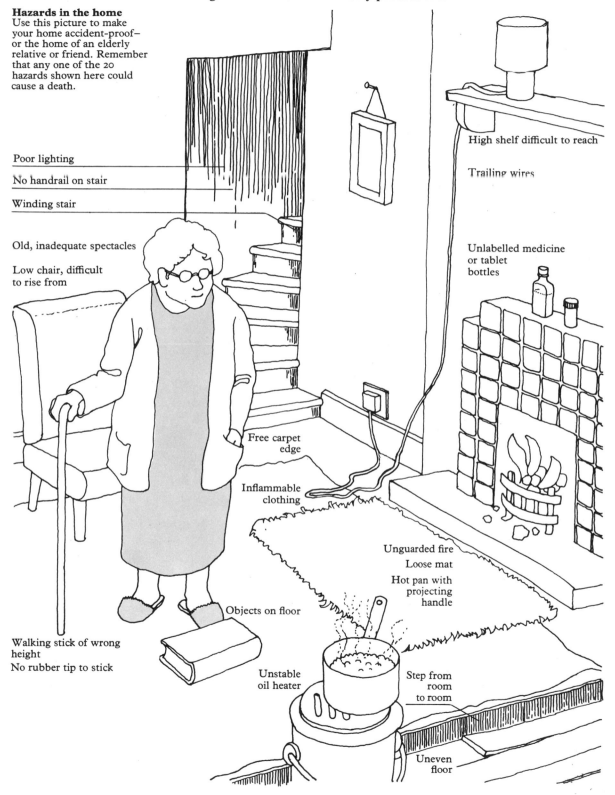

Poor lighting

No handrail on stair

Winding stair

Old, inadequate spectacles

Low chair, difficult to rise from

High shelf difficult to reach

Trailing wires

Unlabelled medicine or tablet bottles

Free carpet edge

Inflammable clothing

Unguarded fire

Loose mat

Hot pan with projecting handle

Objects on floor

Walking stick of wrong height

No rubber tip to stick

Unstable oil heater

Step from room to room

Uneven floor

OVERCOMING HANDICAPS

Rheumatic stiffness, loss of function from strokes or just generally weakened powers affect many of the elderly and limit their activities. A rich assortment of aids has been devised to help them. Many are not sufficiently known, and a few are illustrated in this section as typical examples. There are many others not shown.

You can get more information from your doctor, from the social services, and in the UK from the British Red Cross and from such excellent institutions as the Disabled Living Foundation, 346 Kensington High Street, London W14 8NS. But if you contemplate getting any aid always make sure you consult the doctor first.

MOBILITY

All too often one finds a small-statured widow inefficiently relying on the tall and quite unsuitable stick of her late husband. A walking stick should be of correct height, with its handle at hip-joint level. It should also be comfortably shaped to accommodate an ailing hand.

Some handles have a leather covering over sponge rubber cushioning.

Greater stability is obtained from the tripod stick or the walking frame; both of these should have adjustable heights so that the user does not crouch over them. A small basket fixed to the frame for carrying objects is a good idea. One form of frame incorporates a folding seat.

As for wheelchairs, do not try to obtain one without expert advice. In the UK they can be obtained free under the National Health Service. Remember that inside the home they may have to negotiate small halls and corridors, pass through narrow door frames and turn in small spaces. Outdoors, if motor powered, they may be subject to Ministry of Transport regulations.

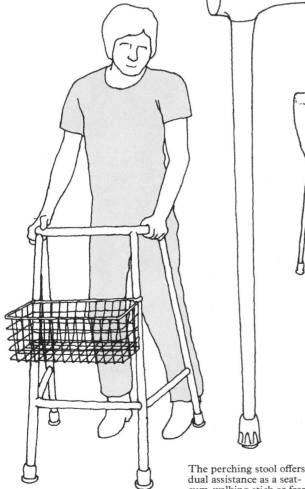

Walking frame for someone needing a lot of stability; a small carrying basket can be fitted to the front.

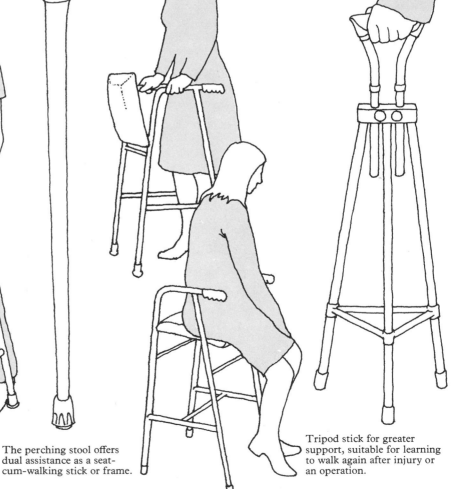

Walking stick with shaped handle. The handle should be at the level of the user's hip joint.

The perching stool offers dual assistance as a seat-cum-walking stick or frame.

Tripod stick for greater support, suitable for learning to walk again after injury or an operation.

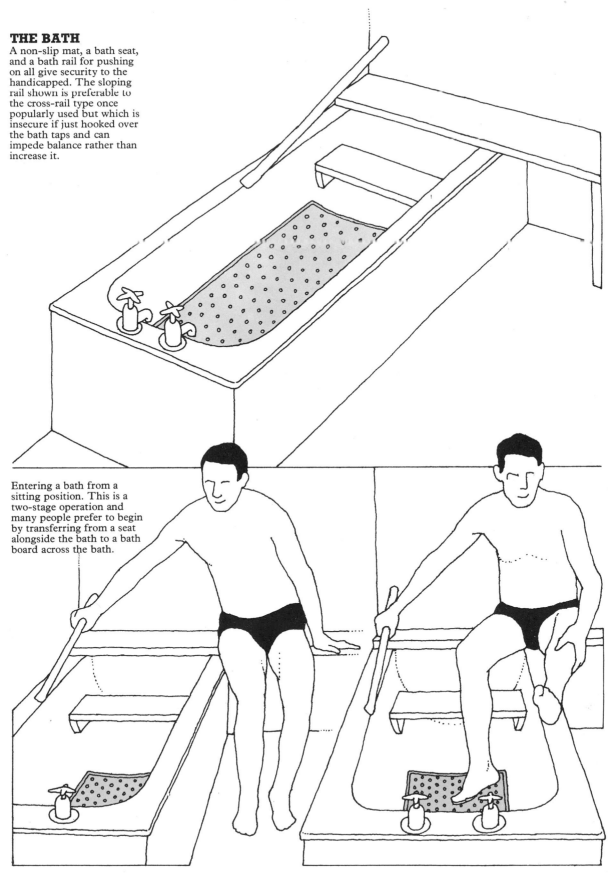

THE BATH

A non-slip mat, a bath seat, and a bath rail for pushing on all give security to the handicapped. The sloping rail shown is preferable to the cross-rail type once popularly used but which is insecure if just hooked over the bath taps and can impede balance rather than increase it.

Entering a bath from a sitting position. This is a two-stage operation and many people prefer to begin by transferring from a seat alongside the bath to a bath board across the bath.

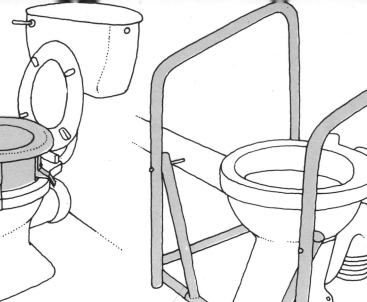

THE LAVATORY

Handgrips and a raised toilet seat for help in rising are frequently used. The handgrips can be fixed on the wall or be in the form of a stand around the lavatory pedestal.

GROOMING AND DRESSING

Difficult taps can be turned by 'keys' designed to fit them. Long-handled hairbrushes, combs, sponges and even lipstick holders help those with stiff shoulders who cannot fully raise their arms. Where only one hand can be used, objects like nailbrushes may be fixed by suction cups. Those who are unable to bend to their feet need stocking-pulling gadgets, long-handled shoe horns, and for their shoes elastic laces which do not need tying.

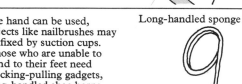

Long-handled sponge   Tap turner

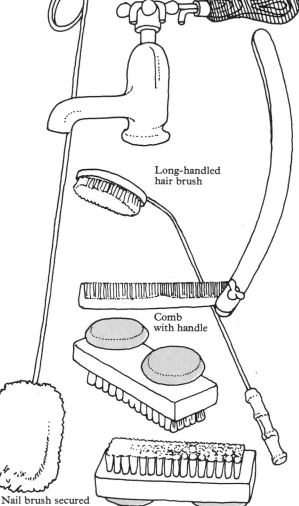

Device for pulling on stockings

Long-handled hair brush

Comb with handle

Nail brush secured by suction pads

COOKING AND EATING

Hands with poor grip need cutlery with thickened handles; bent handles help those who have limited arm and shoulder movements. When only one hand is in action a vertical shield on the edge of the plate helps the food to be scooped up. Other aids are an egg cup anchored by a suction pad and a spiked board to hold a slice of bread for buttering. Some independence in the kitchen can be obtained by such items as easy-to-turn cooker switches, mixing bowls set on non-slip mats, a non-slip tray fitted with a single-handed carrying handle, a board for holding down a loaf to be cut, and a grater to peel potatoes.

THE INTERESTED LIFE

Let us encourage mental and physical activity among the elderly—within their abilities. All too often, though, they and their relatives do not realize the extent of these abilities. Below are a few useful liberating devices. Chairs should be high (about 50 cm), with tall protective backs and with good arm rests. Some chairs have spring lifting seats which help a weak user to get up. Small keys can be gripped easily if fitted with wide holders, and lever door handles are much easier for weak hands than round knobs. In some cases a stirrup hanging from the handle is useful in that a foot can open the latch. Electric plugs with loop handles for gripping are easy to insert and pull out, and large electric rocker switches can be worked by the elbow of someone whose fingers are disabled.
'Lazy tongs' or long-handled grips can greatly extend a person's reach.
If the hand cannot hold a pencil, thicken the pencil for an easier grip. Sleeve it with a rubber tube which is inserted through a small perforated ball.
A knitting aid, fixed by suction cups, or a slotted board to hold playing cards, will help those who cannot use both hands. The long-handled dustpan makes domestic work easier.
For the wheelchair-bound even gardening is possible if the garden bed is raised.

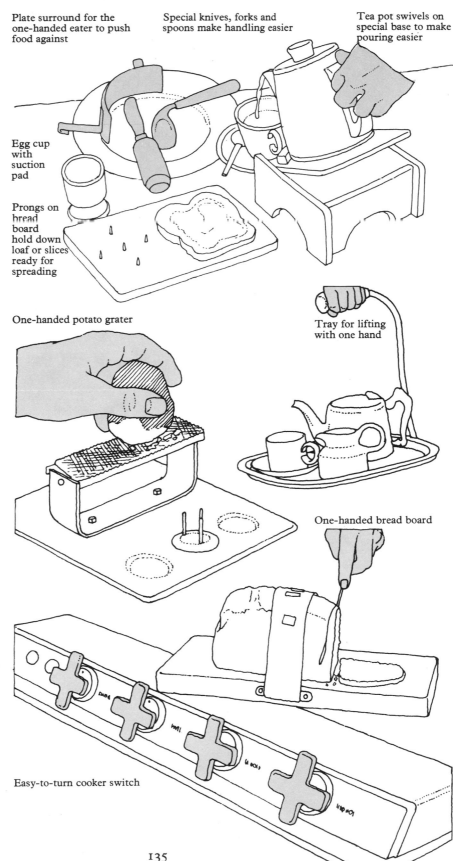

Plate surround for the one-handed eater to push food against

Special knives, forks and spoons make handling easier

Tea pot swivels on special base to make pouring easier

Egg cup with suction pad

Prongs on bread board hold down loaf or slices ready for spreading

One-handed potato grater

Tray for lifting with one hand

One-handed bread board

Easy-to-turn cooker switch

RETIREMENT

A PERSONAL LETTER TO MY FRIEND

You write with anxiety about retiring as if facing a vacuum or some dangerously unexplored territory. Why not seek guidance from one of the many Pre-Retirement Associations which exist? Or you can get information from the Citizen's Advice Bureau (look its address up in the telephone book or ask at a post office).

In the meantime you may like some ideas based on my own experience.

Science and medicine just do not confirm that the ages of sixty to sixty-five are correct ones for stopping work. Yet custom and society have chosen them, and we have to put up with it. Perhaps like so many, almost hidden to yourself, you are feeling resentment at the notion of loss of status, that of being the breadwinner, that of moving out of a job of importance where your experience counted. Remember this: you will retire merely from a job; you will not retire from being yourself. In fact the freedom may well offer you time and opportunities of better expressing your personality. Besides, would you not perhaps try to seek a part-time job? It might be for pay. It might be voluntary with, for instance, the Red Cross, in local politics or for one of the national charities.

You are thinking of moving to another town. Take care, for this does not always succeed. You may find yourself in an area, pleasant enough, but denuded of friends and personal contacts and full of strangers. I have known some who, disillusioned, have then returned to their original homes, only to find that their severed links were difficult to reunite.

If you do move do not be content just to assess the new house. Explore the surroundings. What will shopping be like? How good are the social amenities? Consider how easy of access you would be to friends or relatives who would like to visit you.

Do not take it amiss if I plead that reduced commitments should not lower your usual techniques for looking good. Remain meticulous about general grooming and appearance for the sake of those about you, as well as for yourself and your health. Watch your weight and diet. Do not let lessened activity lead to fat. Eat well and sensibly, giving yourself properly cooked meals.

And do exercise. This does not necessarily mean physical jerks. The once-a-day or once-a-week set of gymnastics is relatively less useful than repeated and frequent exertions. Cycle instead of driving; walk instead of cycling; use stairs instead of the lift; move fast up the stairs instead of plodding. Do not do your lawn with a sit-upon mower; walk with the machine. Instead of sending a messenger, do the task yourself. And develop your sports, whether they be swimming, golf or bowls.

Housework at last can be shared. Wives need to retire too! Husbands do not often catch up with the domestic expertise of women, but no special skill is required to work the vacuum cleaner or do the washing-up.

I am sure you will not neglect mental exercise. Use radio and television critically and selectively. Follow the news in local and national papers and be ready to discuss issues informatively. Chase out new books from the public library. Perhaps you will go further and enrol in the Open University.

And you will join clubs. There are many for the elderly. But are they enough for you? Older citizens have their own groups, but if you are fit and mobile beware of segregating yourself among the old. Do you not want to meet a cross-section of people? You could link these with a hobby. There are many clubs, classes and meetings that offer modelmaking, cookery, photography, sketching, embroidery, gardening and many other hobbies for all ages.

If you join an association you may be the type of person who is eventually asked to become a committee member. Do not think you are past it. You will benefit from the stimulus of the younger people around you. They will benefit from your experience.

Some thoughtless people have created an image of the Old Age Pensioner as static, senile and superfluous.

You and I know better. We'll show them!

THE ELDERLY RELATIVE IN YOUR HOME

It is often unavoidable that elderly people who need a lot of looking after have to become long-term residents in special hostels and hospitals. These places do excellent and sympathetic work but they do not offer the same background as the family home. Give much thought before deciding that an old person should not remain at home. Even though the close care and attention, and the reduction of risks cannot be of the same order as in hospital, these are well offset by the old person's sense of 'belonging'.

Some compromise can be found in temporary hospital admissions. The Day Centre of a geriatric hospital will take the patient in the daytime about once a week, giving general attention to his physical well-being (including bathing and chiropody) and providing occupational interests and a change of scene and company.

Many hospitals will admit a handicapped old person from his home for about two weeks, not for any special treatment, but to allow the relatives who have been looking after him some free time for rest and a holiday. Naturally this has to be planned well in advance.

The ideal for most elderly people is remaining in the family home. If you accept the responsibility, you must achieve the subtle and difficult compromise between looking after on the one hand and allowing privacy and independence on the other. All too often an old person may interpret these respectively as interference and neglect. Another delicate balance concerns the children in the house. To the old resident these sources of delight and interest may quickly become too much of a good thing. Gently teach the children not to obtrude too often.

More difficult sometimes is tactfully persuading your resident that you too need your own lives of privacy and independence. This can be solved delicately by working out some form of domestic routine which becomes accepted as the pattern of life in the home.

Depression is the commonest psychological ailment in the elderly. Occasionally it is caused by a chronic and not immediately obvious disease like an infection or a tumour. More often it is related to an ill-defined sense of loneliness and isolation.

The problem of *loneliness* can be solved by the company in the house. But *isolation* is a different matter. Though surrounded by others one may yet not feel part of their life and interests. With physical inactivity one may come to believe oneself unwanted or emotionally and socially discarded.

Sometimes depression lies behind a façade of contentment or sayings like 'I do not want to be a bother'. Much of it is avoidable. The knowledge that others are willing to listen, are interested in them and sympathize with them will encourage the old to discuss their feelings. In addition, some cases of depression may be eased by a doctor's prescription.

Let old people feel they are valid and valuable members of the household. Be prepared to talk with them of the day's events, national or domestic. Gossip and bring to them the outside world. Consult them. Seek their advice even if you do not really need it.

Bereavement, loss of work and loss of capabilities can take away the incentive to live. Many whose handicaps have reduced them to an existence of minimal activity ask the rhetorical question 'Why am I still alive?'—to which there are answers such as 'Because people are fond of you and value you'. Of course it is not enough just to say this. It must be demonstrated.

The formula is simple and straightforward. Old people are people who are old but, above all, they are people.

PART 3

COMMON AILMENTS

A GUIDE TO COMMON ACHES AND PAINS, HOW TO TREAT THEM, AND WHEN TO CONSULT A DOCTOR

This chapter is a guide to the common aches and pains and illnesses which most of us encounter at some time or another. The signs and symptoms are briefly discussed and some guidance given on when to seek medical help. It is not comprehensive and not meant to be; nor should it by any means take the place of your own family doctor or medical adviser. No attempt has been made to compile a dictionary of symptoms or a medical encyclopedia. The aim has been solely to inform and thus help you to distinguish between the important and the unimportant and the serious and the trivial.

When you have to seek a doctor's advice, we hope that the explanations and descriptions given here may help to make your communication with him more meaningful and useful. A better understanding of your own body and its functions should lead to a better rapport between you. An alphabetical list of illnesses has not been used, because that assumes a knowledge of disease names that you may well not have. Instead, we have taken regions or systems of the body and dealt with the common troubles that are likely to occur in that area or within that system. There are many omissions. We have included only common problems but commonness is relative; some of us seem rarely to 'catch cold' but others seem almost never to be without. The same may be said of headaches, indigestion and many other relatively common complaints. We just hope yours is included.

HEAD & NECK

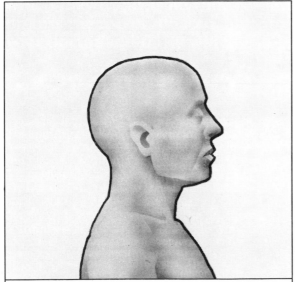

Headaches Tension headache, Migraine, Sinusitis
Vertigo
Head injuries Loss of consciousness, Concussion
Ear, nose and throat Middle ear infection, Glue ear, Earache, Common cold, Influenza, Gastric 'flu, Throat problems, Neck problems, Coughs, Choking

HEADACHES Undoubtedly the commonest of all the aches and pains we suffer is the **headache**. It takes many forms, one or two of which clearly form a recognizable pattern of disease, e.g. **sinusitis** or **migraine.** Some people never get a headache at all; some never seem to be free of them. It should be made clear at the outset that most headaches are temporary, easily relieved and innocent–innocent in the sense of being unassociated with any underlying serious disease.

Pain 'in the head' can arise either from the muscular covering of the scalp and neck, the bones of the skull itself or the actual covering (meninges) of the brain. Most headaches seem to arise from the scalp covering and are often associated with tension and anxiety. A worried, introspective, tense and anxious person is often beset by headache (or stomach ache, or chest pain or abdominal cramps), and relieving the tension and anxiety by reassurance, with or without tranquillizing drugs, will relieve the headache (or other pains) as well. The so-called 'tension headache' is a common experience, even for those who do not regard themselves as 'worrying types', and vast quantities of aspirin are consumed annually for its relief. It is rarely necessary to seek medical advice.

In general, the vaguer the location of the head pain the less likely is it to be of serious import. Feelings of 'pressure downward' or 'bursting outward' or 'all-over feelings of burning' are never symptoms of organic disease. Localized, persistent pain, particularly if accompanied by nausea or actual vomiting and unrelieved by analgesics (pain-relieving drugs), demands medical attention.

In this category is **migraine**, a special kind of headache which is responsible for much misery and time lost from work or pleasure. The word tends to be used rather loosely sometimes to describe almost any kind of severe head pain; it should be reserved for the syndrome (collection of symptoms and signs) of visual or auditory or speech disturbance accompanied by nausea and occasionally actual vomiting and then followed by severe head pain, usually one-sided, after the initial disturbances of sight, sound or speech have completely cleared. Essentially it is a headache caused by changes in the volume of blood vessels in the brain itself or in its coverings or even in the skin overlying the scalp. The precise causes elude us but effective treatment and, to some extent, prevention are now available.

The headache of **sinusitis** is usually restricted to the sinus region—the forehead (where it may be one-sided) or 'between the eyes'. A 'stuffy' nose or purulent nasal discharge may give the clue and then if simple treatment of the sinusitis does not bring relief in a few hours (inhalation or nose drops or both—your pharmacist will usually advise) then you should consult your doctor.

The brain substance itself cannot 'feel' pain. The pain of a brain tumour is due either to the local pressure on meninges or other structures in close vicinity, or to general pressure from an increase in volume of the brain substance, or to pressure of the fluid (cerebrospinal fluid) surrounding it. Brain tumours are rare and diagnosis used to depend on various uncomfortable procedures involving the injection of air into brain cavities (ventricles) or of X-ray-opaque dyes into the blood vessels of the neck. The advent of the EMI scanner, which requires no such injections, has increased the accuracy of diagnosis and made such 'invasive' procedures virtually a thing of the past.

Headaches often accompany general illness—perhaps pneumonia, food-poisoning or just a cold—and treatment of the illness usually relieves the headache. A headache is part and parcel of a hangover—and the best cure for that is prevention.

Headaches are common and are rarely the symptom of serious disease. You should treat them with simple measures—soluble aspirin or paracetamol—and deal with anything you think might be contributing, whether it be a bad cold, the 'flu or just a hangover. Eye strain is never (well, hardly ever) a cause of headache. Persistent, localized pain, unresponsive to these simple measures, accompanied by dizziness or feelings of sickness, demands medical attention.

VERTIGO Giddiness or dizziness are sensations of imbalance which are often loosely but incorrectly referred to as vertigo. Those swimmy feelings experienced by healthy people on suddenly standing up or by those with a distaste for heights on looking down from one may be properly described as dizziness or giddiness. They may also accompany a fever or overwhelm you when entering a warm room from the cold—and in the latter instance may precede a faint. True vertigo is the feeling that your surroundings are moving—either up or down, from side to side or round and round, or that your head is moving although you know that no such movement is taking place.

Like a headache, vertigo may be due to general or local causes. Of the general causes, excess intake of alcohol is probably the most common, although motion sickness runs it a close second. Vertigo is common on stepping on to *terra firma* after a rough sea crossing, or after a few minutes on the helter-skelter at the fun fair.

Of the local causes, a temporary insufficiency of blood flow to certain parts of the brain is not uncommon—particularly in the elderly when it is frequently brought on by sudden neck and head movements. The organ of balance, which is situated in the inner ear, may be affected by diseases such as Ménière's, a condition characterized by episodes of vertigo, nausea and transient difficulty in hearing. Each episode may leave a little deafness and, over the years, the deficit may become appreciable and lead to social and business problems. Tinnitus (noises in the head) is common in this condition and, like deafness, may persist after each episode of giddiness. The condition may affect both ears but commonly it is only one that develops it. Medical advice should be sought early. Indeed, episodes of true vertigo—in the absence of obvious causes already mentioned—always require investigation.

HEAD INJURIES Headache, dizziness and vertigo can, of course, follow head injury. A blow on the head, either from a fall, a mugging or a road accident can severely stun, knock out partially or completely for a matter of minutes, hours or days or, of course, kill outright. The skull may or may not be fractured; the scalp itself is very often damaged by the blow—in which case bleeding is usual and may be profuse, even from a small wound. The tiny blood vessels in the scalp cannot contract easily when they are torn or cut (the normal response to injury and an important factor in preventing blood loss) because of the special anatomical structure of the skin. For that reason bleeding continues for much longer and copiously before the clotting mechanisms finally staunch it. Pressure is usually all that is needed, although it has to be admitted that such scalp bleeds can appear quite alarming to onlookers.

Loss of consciousness is often difficult to analyse when it has been transitory –but, if in doubt, always seek medical opinion. **Concussion** is loss of consciousness due to a blow to the head and jarring of the brain. Confusion and headache after such injuries are common and a 24-hour period of rest under observation, in hospital if possible, is mandatory. In other injuries the brain itself and its covering meninges are temporarily distorted by blows to the head but the effects may not show for some hours or days–and in rare cases, weeks–after the original injury. A slowly bleeding small vein can produce a large pool of blood which clots; this in turn can produce a headache or another loss of consciousness or even a convulsion–sometimes so long after the original injury that the two may not be immediately connected. Head injury, from whatever cause, is a serious matter and medical attention is needed from the outset.

EAR, NOSE AND THROAT The ear, nose and throat are all part and parcel of what doctors refer to as 'the upper respiratory tract', and infection of one part is invariably, although not necessarily overtly, accompanied by infection of one of the others. Thus a painful, throbbing ear is a sign of **middle ear infection (otitis media)** which in turn has arisen from the nose or throat. Infection spreads up the tube which connects the cavity of the middle ear with the throat (the Eustachian tube) but, of course, not every sore throat leads to middle ear problems.

For anatomical reasons such ascending infections are much more common in babies and children. In the days before sulphonamides and all the antibiotics that followed the discovery of penicillin, treatment of otitis media very often meant surgery–the incision of the eardrum to release pus trapped in the middle ear cavity. Not uncommonly, the infection would spread to the air cells in the bony protruberance behind the ear (the mastoid process) and much of that bone also had to be surgically treated. But those are things of the past. Otitis media can usually be treated very satisfactorily with antibiotics and drugs to help restore natural drainage of the infection back down the Eustachian tube.

Repeated attacks of middle ear infection and treatment with antibiotics can lead to a chronic condition characterized by deafness because the cavity fills with a fluid which impairs the free movement of the tiny bones which transmit drum movements to the inner ear. This is the so-called **glue ear**. Again, surgery may be required–the insertion of a tiny tube (grommet) into the middle ear through the drum so that the fluid can be encouraged to drain away to the outside.

Earache, especially in children, must never be ignored–the patient won't usually let you anyway–or hopefully treated with pain-relieving drugs. Medical advice is needed without more ado.

Sinusitis has already been mentioned. Sinuses are off-shoots of the upper respiratory tract and share the same linings. Infection thus spreads very easily. The worst features of a heavy cold are due to the invasion of the already virus-infected linings by bacteria which readily produce excessive secretion of mucus or pus and spread the infection throughout the tract. Indeed, the spread may be to the lower respiratory tract, i.e. the windpipe (trachea) and its branches (bronchi) and its twigs (bronchioles). Thus tracheitis, bronchitis or bronchiolitis may follow–in other words, the cold 'goes to your chest'.

As everyone knows, the **common cold** takes a variety of forms, and as yet no truly effective prevention or treatment exists. Claims abound and need no detailing here. The common complications of a cold are otitis media, sinusitis, laryngitis and bronchitis. For all of these medical attention must be sought.

INFLUENZA Abbreviated to 'flu, this is a common viral infection and has a seasonal peak in the early months of the year. It is responsible for much loss of working time. So much so that many large concerns believe it to be economic to pay for prophylactic immunization of their workforces in the months preceding the 'flu season. There is no doubt that immunization can be effective. However, as one cannot predict with certainty just which particular sort (strain) of virus is going to be around (and the 'flu virus changes its character with remarkable fickleness) vaccination can at best bring only partial immunity against related strains of 'flu. Nevertheless, some immunity is better than none at all, and for those at particular risk in an epidemic, e.g. patients with chronic bronchitis or any similar illness which a new, generalized infection could worsen, the 'flu jab can be a wise precaution.

Most people know what influenza is like. The classic picture is that of a sudden rise in temperature, preceded perhaps by some hours of generally feeling unwell, with aching, shivering, headache, a dry cough and often a sore throat as well. It is self-limiting and no specific treatment is available. The order of the day is symptomatic treatment–either aspirin or paracetamol and bedrest. All achings, shiverings and general feelings of being unwell are, of course, not necessarily 'flu; but if you think you might have 'flu and yet the symptoms don't abate in the usual two to three days you should call a doctor. It is particularly important to seek early medical advice for the elderly patient, even if it's 'only a bit of "flu"'.

The so-called **gastric 'flu** is a 'flu-like illness accompanied by nausea, often with vomiting and probably diarrhoea, or both. It may be a variant of 'flu but is much more likely to be food poisoning. Two or three days should see it through – but if in doubt, see your doctor. It is particularly important not to ignore 'flu-like symptoms or gastric 'flu in infants; indeed *any* infant who has diarrhoea and vomiting for 12 hours or more must be seen by a doctor. Especially in the very young, diarrhoea and vomiting ('D & V') leads all too readily to dehydration which is a potentially life-threatening condition. Sometimes it can be due to conditions like ear infections which a doctor can treat.

THROAT PROBLEMS The **throat**, whether guarded by its tonsillar pair or not, is a frequent site of initial infections, be they of the common cold virus, the 'flu virus or that once-serious invader, the streptococcus. The throat, as has been discussed in other sections, should be considered as having three parts – the **pharynx** (the 'curtain' with central uvula, most readily seen with tonsils or their denuded beds in the wings), the **naso-pharynx** (the back wall of which is seen behind that curtain) which continues upwards with the nasal passages and downwards with the last part of the throat, and the **larynx** or voice box.

The point to make here is that pharyngeal infections can be readily seen and treated, either by using throat paints or sucking lozenges. Gargling is a waste of time. The gargle does not reach the pharyngeal tissues unless it is swallowed – and most proprietary gargles cannot be. Most sore throats clear within a matter of days whether lozenges are sucked or not. If lumps can be felt or seen in the neck – indicating a spread of infection to the lymph glands which surround the pharynx – whether or not such enlargements are accompanied by fever, medical advice should be sought. The streptococcus, a bacterium at one time a relatively common cause of acute pharyngitis or tonsillitis, no longer has the virulence it once had and the diphtheria bacillus is almost unknown in the UK. Nevertheless, if treatment does not clear the initial infection, a laboratory test may be needed.

The **naso-pharynx** is frequently infected by 'back-tracking' from the nasal passages, particularly during a common cold. Looking beyond the 'curtain' of the pharynx (easily done by saying 'aaaah' in front of a mirror) may show streaks of pus or blood on the back wall. This in itself is nothing to worry about as such secretions harmlessly find their way into the stomach (not the lungs – the cough reflex sees to that) where they are neutralized and dealt with in the same way as is food. It may not be a pleasant thought, but it is true. However, much visible discharge is a sign of nasal infection, with or without sinusitis, and if it persists after the cold or 'flu has gone, certainly needs attention. Neither gargling nor throat lozenges will do anything for this type of infection.

Lastly, there is the **larynx**. Usually the first sign of infection is a change in voice sound which may be a slight huskiness or 'wetness' and a feeling that you want to clear your throat. Occasionally, sudden, total voice loss occurs, or this may come on gradually. Gargling or lozenges are useless. The inhalation of Friar's Balsam or a creosote tincture may relieve your discomfort but, in general, laryngeal infections do not respond to such local measures and some systemic treatment (i.e. medicine given by mouth or by injection) is usually required if the condition persists. It is self-limiting, and only if the symptoms persist for more than a few days do you need to seek advice. Occasionally a voice change may be noticed in the total absence of a cold, 'flu or generalized sore throat. While occasionally this *may* be due to generalized disease such as subnormal activity of the thyroid gland, when the deepening or coarsening of the voice pattern may in fact be so slow as to be almost imperceptible, more commonly it is due to the development of nodules on the vocal cords (the so-called 'singers' nodes') which can and should be treated.

NECK PROBLEMS The neck itself is a highly muscular structure, permitting head movement in infinite variety. A stiff neck may simply be due to localized muscle spasm, particularly if it is held to one side by some apparently invisible force (the so-called 'wry neck' or spasmodic torticollis), or to the pain of swollen lymph glands in the neck tissues (as, for example, in glandular fever or acute pharyngitis) or, more rarely, to degeneration of the small joints of the vertebrae making up the cervical part of the back bone. It is possible to have disc degeneration in the neck just as in the lower part of the back (the so-called 'slipped disc') with consequent pain, usually radiating down the shoulder or arm and a feeling of neck stiffness and pain localized to one, possibly two, vertebrae. Neck stiffness may also occur in more general body disease – but this is usually something the physician finds rather than the patient complains of.

Warmth and gentle movement will ease most 'stiff necks', but the fixed wry neck or acute disc prolapse will need expert medical attention. Manipulation is sometimes effective but should never be undertaken by the unqualified.

COUGHS The cough is a survival reflex. Our air passages are designed to cope with air and nothing else. A foreign body—be it a drop of water, a pea, a noxious gas or particles of smoke —will trigger a neuro-muscular reflex with such force as can effectively shoot the offending substance many feet away.

A cough is perhaps as common a symptom as a headache—and is only a symptom, not a disease in itself. A cough can be expected if the common cold 'goes to the chest', in some types of 'flu, in bronchitis, pneumonia and pleurisy. Coughs are of two main types—dry or producing sputum. There is also a 'nervous' cough and the cough accompanying bronchial spasm, as in asthma. Since the cough is a symptom, it is essential to identify the cause. If none is apparent, seek medical advice. The chest cold may last as long as two or three weeks but if it still persists you should see your doctor. A cough accompanied by fever, with or without chest pain, should also have medical attention. A cough accompanied by an apparent increase in breathing rate or unusual shortness of breath or difficulty in getting one's breath also needs the doctor. And the cough that produces excessive mucus or pus, or a mixture of both, or contains obvious blood, also needs medical attention.

Never treat a persistent cough with proprietary remedies, particularly of a suppressant type which can be readily bought over the counter. And remember the now almost forgotten health adage that 'coughs and sneezes spread diseases'. Use paper tissues for your cold and your productive bronchitis and burn them or flush them down the lavatory. Don't keep the germs in a handkerchief in your pocket to be shaken out next time you look for a clean portion for your next cough.

Sometimes the foreign body is large and the cough reflex is, as it were, caught napping. A cough needs an initial intake of air with which to perform its explosive expulsion— but a bolus of food wedged in the upper part of the windpipe can prevent this happening and the result is **choking**. This is an emergency and not infrequent at the meal table, particularly the celebration banquet. It demands prompt action to clear the airway. Try to dislodge the object by giving four sharp blows with the flat of the hand between the patient's shoulder blades. If this measure does not bring up the object into his mouth, or expel it altogether, then apply abdominal pressure—see page 181 for details and illustrations, also for instructions on how to deal with children and what to do if the patient becomes unconscious.

SKIN

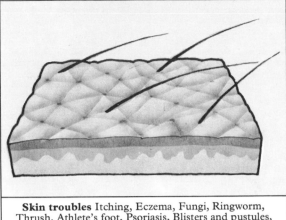

Skin troubles Itching, Eczema, Fungi, Ringworm, Thrush, Athlete's foot, Psoriasis, Blisters and pustules, Boils and carbuncles, Warts and verrucae
Skin colour Bruises, Suntan, Sunburn, Pallor through shock

The skin is a complex structure made of two parts—an upper protective water-resistant layer (the epidermis) and a lower more functional portion (the dermis). Both parts may be afflicted by diseases peculiar to the skin itself and both can reflect the presence of disease in other organs elsewhere in the body. The epidermis reacts to external onslaughts such as irritant substances, injury, heat, light and cold in various ways—by itching, redness, scaling, peeling, blistering, pimpling and so forth.

The commonest symptom is the **itch** —a symptom difficult to describe but common enough not to need it. Among the most common causes of itch are insect bites (your pets being the most likely source, however well you think you groom them), irritant solutions or powders (domestic cleaning materials and some foods) and allergies (reactions to clothes, fur, dust, pollen and the metals used in fastenings are well-known). Persistent itching and the inevitable scratching for relief may lead to the condition known as **eczema**, a very common skin reaction.

It is often not possible to identify the cause but unless that can be done the condition is likely to run a prolonged course or, at best, desist and recur at intervals. Treatment is removal of the cause, if possible, and this may be achieved by applying lotions or ointments which usually contain steroids; some of the older remedies like coal-tar may be just as effective. Steroid lotions and ointments can only be obtained on prescription in the UK but until expert advice can be obtained a simple preparation like calamine lotion will usually suffice to allay itching and inflammation. Avoid anti-histamine preparations which in themselves can sensitize the skin and make matters worse.

Contact dermatitis is the name given to the eczematous reaction which some individuals can receive from contact with certain materials, both natural and synthetic. Of the natural materials, flowers (especially the primula), animal fur and wool may be the culprits; of the synthetic, washing powders, nylon and cosmetics are not uncommon causes. Certain materials used in industry may cause dermatitis, and compensation may be awarded in cases where such conditions have been statutorily recognized.

The skin has an inbuilt and very efficient anti-bacterial defence system and unbroken skin is resistant to nearly all disease-causing bacteria; if it were not we should be made very miserable for the skin is in constant contact with germs. **Fungi** are in a different category for they can get a foothold on unbroken skin. **Ringworm** and **thrush** are common invaders and in themselves can produce eczematous reactions, sometimes in other parts of the body. The classic example is **athlete's foot**, an infection which settles in between the toes and may go unnoticed or even regarded as a normal state of affairs before an eczematous reaction on the palm of the hands (rejoicing in the name of **cheiropompholyx**) sends the patient to the doctor who is then alerted to search elsewhere for fungal infection. Treatment of the hands alone will do virtually nothing; removal of the prime cause is essential.

Psoriasis is a common but relatively non-itchy condition which in its severer forms is very difficult to treat. The cause is unknown but the predisposition to it is undoubtedly inherited. It is a scaling condition, one of a group of skin diseases characterized by a disorder of keratinization—the name given to the formation of the outer layers of the epidermis, a process which is constantly at work to replace outer skin cells as they are lost through the normal 'wear and tear' of daily living. All except the mildest cases of psoriasis need medical advice in the first instance. The number of effective drugs is limited although there are some promising compounds, derived from vitamin A, which may soon become available for the moderate to severe forms.

Blisters are the result of chafing, pressure, heat, cold or chemicals. They may also be the sign of generalized disease. A blister is essentially a local accumulation of tissue fluid from cell damage. The affected portion of skin becomes 'walled-off' by healthy cells, leaving the typical vesicle, or pocket containing clear fluid. Infection of the fluid gives rise to a **pustule**. Invasion of the dermis by an infecting organism, usually in a sweat gland or a hair follicle produces a **boil** (furuncle). Large boils, usually with multiple compartments, are known as **carbuncles**. A boil affecting the pulp of the finger or thumb is known as a **whitlow** (or felon).

Blisters and pustules respond to home remedies—protect the former, particularly if it bursts, and soak the latter in a hot saline solution or water. Boils, carbuncles and whitlows need expert treatment usually, if they do not respond to applications of dry or wet heat. The danger is in the possible spread of the infection. This complication may be indicated by the appearance of red streaks up the arm and painful swellings in the armpit if the trouble is arising from the hand or fingers or wrist, and by similar signs in the leg and groin if the ankle or foot is the prime site. Antibiotic treatment is frequently necessary and you should not delay getting medical advice.

Warts are of many types but they are all, or nearly all, due to infection by a virus. The interesting thing about warts is their propensity for disappearing as mysteriously as they appear. On this phenomenon has been built a veritable cornucopia of cures—from rubbing the affected part with the skin of a live toad (preferably when there is a full moon) to the simple wearing of a wart 'charm'. However, some warts do persist for months or even years and may need more positive treatment either with a cautery or with solid carbon dioxide ('snow'), i.e. either by burning or freezing.

The **plantar wart** is particularly painful for it appears, as its name implies, only on the sole (the plantar surface) of the foot. The swimming bath or the shared domestic bathmat are the places most likely to conceal the virus of this particular wart and many public swimming baths provide medicated foot-baths the use of which may be compulsory both before entering and when leaving the pool area. The medical name for the plantar wart is the **verruca**—but it is a wart, just the same (see page 156 for treatment).

SKIN COLOUR The normal skin changes colour, within a limited range, from various internal and external causes and from exposure to light in particular. Sun*tan* is familiar to everyone, as is the itching, redness and sometimes blistering which results from actual sun*burn*. The **bruise**, resulting from bleeding from minute, contused blood vessels in the dermis or the underlying tissue, is the cause of *local* colour change which may, however, be quite extensive. Spontaneous appearance of bruising without any apparent trauma raises the suspicion of a blood disorder and needs a medical opinion; likewise the appearance of bruising after only the slightest of physical injury.

Skin colour may also reflect disease elsewhere, for example, the yellowing of jaundice, the orange-yellow from chronic over-indulgence in carrot juice and the bronzing from a rare kind of diabetes.

Shock, whether emotional or true surgical (see page 176) is accompanied by a pallor which may indeed be 'deathly white'. There is also the pink of carbon monoxide poisoning and the blue of oxygen lack (cyanosis). Transient skin colour changes are not important. However, a gradual yellowing of the skin (perhaps first noticed in the white of the eye) may be the early indication of liver or gallbladder disease and no time should be lost in seeking medical advice.

CHEST

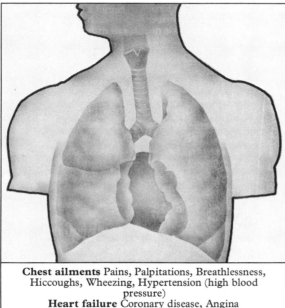

Chest ailments Pains, Palpitations, Breathlessness, Hiccoughs, Wheezing, Hypertension (high blood pressure)
Heart failure Coronary disease, Angina

The 'thoracic cage' (ribs, backbone and breastbone) protects the heart and lungs. Pain, discomfort and tightness are common symptoms and, because they occur in this area of vital organs, especially the heart, worry people more than symptoms felt anywhere else in the body. We can feel pain only in organs provided with the appropriate 'pain sensors'. Thus, no pain can be felt in the lungs and the bronchial tubes, nor in the blood vessels supplying heart or lungs. Pain can be felt in the lining membranes of the lungs and heart and in the heart muscle itself. Pain can also be felt in the ribs and in the muscles between the ribs. The location of the pain is not always at the site of the trouble. Pain in the tip of the shoulder may arise from inflammation of the lung lining (pleura) in the lower part of the chest, for example. Pain behind the breastbone may arise from a gastric or duodenal ulcer, from a diseased heart muscle or from an inflammation of the gullet.

The nature of the pain—whether it is like a stabbing or an ache, whether it throbs or

sickens, or is dull or sharp—is less important than its relationship to other things. A chest pain starting after a meal may be from the heart, but it is more likely to be from the gullet, stomach or, unusually, the duodenum. A pain felt on exertion or in anger or after a cigarette is more likely to come from the heart. A pain in the side of the chest, made worse on breathing more deeply, may be due to pleurisy (inflammation of the lung or chest-wall lining) or simply a broken rib. All pains in the chest should be taken seriously and medical advice sought. But remember that chest pain itself does not mean heart disease. You can help your doctor by trying to describe not only the kind of pain, but whether it is associated with anything you do, what times of the day or night it occurs, what seems to relieve it and what makes it worse. Indeed, that is a general rule about any kind of pain, not just chest pain.

Sensations in the chest other than pain are numerous. **Palpitation** is the commonest of these but is rarely associated with disease. Described variously as a fluttering, pounding or jumping, usually in the left side, palpitations arise from the temporary irregularity of the heart beat which all of us experience at some time or other. The heat beat is essentially an electro-chemical phenomenon and the circuits can get 'bugged'. The 'extra beat' is common, but it is the pause in the rhythm which follows it which probably gives the sensation of a 'missed beat'. This pause is quite normal and the rhythm is restored after a fraction of a second. The missed beat is a not uncommon occurrence at the end of the day, or when we are just getting off to sleep. Fatigue, both physical and mental, may be a contributory factor. It is nothing to worry about. Persistent palpitation may indicate a more important disorder of rhythm, and medical advice should be sought.

BREATHING PROBLEMS Breathlessness is natural after or during moderate exertion in some people but only after or during severe exertion in others, and it is only when breathlessness seems out of proportion to the degree of exertion that medical attention is indicated. Breathlessness is not to be confused with that state of affairs which some describe as 'being unable to breathe' or 'get my breath', nor with the difficulty that asthmatics have in emptying the lungs. The sufferer from breathlessness pants for breath, just as a dog does on a hot day, or after a chase. It is a normal phenomenon, a way of paying off the debt of oxygen that has been incurred by a spate of unaccustomed exercise. Roger Bannister was breathless after his less-than-four-minute mile— but he was not unfit. The trained athlete can increase his ability to exert himself without the handicap of breathlessness to a point far beyond that reached by the untrained.

Undue or inappropriate breathlessness therefore demands medical attention. The cause may be simply **anaemia**– which impairs the blood's oxygen-carrying capacity, and which increased oxygenation by accelerated breathing tries to make up for–or it may be in the lungs themselves. If so, it may indicate the collapse or partial collapse of a lung lobe, pneumonia, acute or chronic bronchitis. The cause may lie in the heart, one or both sides of which may become ineffective in terms of moving oxygenated blood around the body. Breathlessness from all these causes is usually of gradual onset.

A sudden bout of breathlessness, often painless, follows the collapse or partial collapse of a lung. This is called 'spontaneous pneumothorax', and may occur in apparently healthy people, usually men, between the ages of 20 and 40. It is uncomfortable, but harmless and the lung usually reinflates itself over a period of weeks or months. Medical advice is necessary for the cause and the extent of the collapse must be sought, although in nine cases out of ten it is a benign condition resulting from the rupture of the small surface cyst which communicates with the air passages (bronchi).

It must be remembered that, while our breathing is totally automatic, that is, is under the control of the autonomic nervous system, it is very readily disturbed by emotional factors. The gasp of delight or horror is typical, the held breath of fright and the overbreathing of anger or emotion are common and such phenomena do not need a doctor's attention. But when they occur without the accompanying delight, horror or anger and in totally inappropriate places, or situations, they may become a source of anxiety to the victim. Anxiety itself compounds the situation and sets up a vicious circle. Reassurance, with or without the help of mild sedation, is usually all that is necessary on these occasions.

Hiccoughs are rarely the sign of serious disease. One of medicine's unsolved physiological mysteries, the hiccough sometimes hits the headlines when a victim is afflicted for days on end but the episode is usually shortlived, often associated with excessive alcohol intake, occasionally with indigestion and, more often than not, with nothing at all. It seems to arise from the diaphragm, that sheet of muscle which separates our bellies from our chests. The diaphragm is important in breathing, and the hiccough is produced by the sudden onset of its rhythmical contraction which causes a sharp intake of air at an inappropriate time in the normal breathing cycle–hence the 'hic'. 'Remedies' abound, from drinking upside down, to holding the breath firmly with nose pinched and mouth covered

and stuffing the left hand firmly into the right side of the lower rib cage or vice-versa.

The only other common breathing problem is the **wheeze**. While it is usually associated with bronchial asthma, some asthmatics never wheeze and wheezers do not necessarily have asthma. Wheezing hardly needs description. It can often be imitated by forcefully expiring air with the mouth open. Any noisy accompaniment to breathing can with justification be described as a wheeze, whether it is just a faint whistling, or loud enough to be heard some feet away. Wheezing is produced when air is forced out and the air passages are, for some reason or other, partially blocked by excess mucus or by chronic inflammation which thickens the lining, or by constriction. Constriction is caused by spasm of the muscles which surround the bronchial tubes and is commonly an allergic phenomenon. The hay fever subject may wheeze at the height of his hay fever symptoms, or wheezing itself may be all he has. The occasional wheeze can be ignored. Persistent wheezing, unless clearly associated with hay fever or asthma, cannot be ignored and should be identified and treated.

HYPERTENSION This is the medical name for **high blood pressure,** about which there is a lot of misunderstanding. As has been described, the heart is a pump with the job of ensuring that blood gets to the remotest parts of the body's system. It cannot do this without having a forcible contraction which expels blood into the main arterial trunk (the aorta) and thence by a highly complex series of smaller vessels into capillary networks and then by the extensive venous network of vessels until the heart is reached again. The force produced can be estimated by measuring the pressure needed to prevent the blood from moving in the main artery of the arm; this is the *systolic* reading. The walls of the blood vessels are elastic and expand with each heart beat. This is felt as a pulse in many places, not only at the wrist, and the elasticity is responsible for maintaining the blood pressure when the heart relaxes between each beat. This again can be judged by measurement around the arm and gives the *diastolic* reading. Thus the measurement of blood pressure is always of two readings, the systolic and diastolic, and is expressed as the height of a column of mercury which could be supported by those pressures. The systolic is written first: thus 120/80 mm Hg although in practice the 'mm Hg' (millimeters of mercury) is usually omitted.

There is no such thing as a 'normal' blood pressure. There is a range of readings within which pressures measured in a majority of healthy people would fall, depending mainly on age. In general, as we age, arteries lose some of their elasticity and the measured blood pressure tends to rise—both the systolic and the diastolic. Patients whose blood pressure readings are found to be higher than the upper limit of the normal range are said to be hypertensive or to have hypertension. This may be lasting or transient—many normal activities increase the blood pressure, e.g. driving a car, flying a plane, sitting an examination or going for an interview. If the high blood pressure is lasting, it may be undetected until it is discovered at a routine medical examination, for hypertension is not usually associated with any symptoms. Headache is not a symptom of high blood pressure. Nor are dizziness, vertigo, palpitation or chest pain.

What does it mean if you are told you have hypertension? In the first place, it is important to know if there is any detectable cause which can be remedied. In most instances, no cause can be found (for example, kidney disease or certain rather rare but benign tumours) and the condition is referred to as 'essential' or 'benign' hypertension. Does this kind of benign hypertension need to be treated at all? There is some debate among doctors as to whether mild or moderate hypertension needs treatment, but where the readings are high, then a certain proportion of such patients will develop complications sooner or later and treatment is certainly a wise precaution. It is quite beyond the scope of this book to deal with these but, in essence, continued untreated hypertension can damage the heart or kidneys, accelerate the development of arteriosclerosis and may be responsible for thrombosis or haemorrhage into the brain (stroke).

Much publicity has been given in recent years to the effect of the stresses and strains of modern living on blood pressure. There is no doubt that anxiety, tension and strain can of themselves produce rises in blood pressure and it is conceivable that a persistence of such states could bring about permanent change. There is no evidence that this happens. However, some claim that once hypertension is established yoga is as good as drugs in normalizing pressure. Other factors contribute to maintaining the hypertensive state—such as smoking and obesity—but these are usually remediable.

As there are no symptoms of high blood pressure—except those related to advanced, untreated disease—the condition will, as we have said, only be discovered during the course of a routine medical examination or 'screening'. In recent months, DIY machines have been installed in at least one London store where for 50p you can record your own blood pressure. Having done so, what next? The range of normal for age and sex is stated on the machine; if your blood pressure is clearly raised then you must firstly have it confirmed by your doctor (or his consulting room nurse) because self-measurement, even with an automated sphygmomanometer (the name given to any device that measures blood pressure) is not reliable, particularly in the hustle and bustle of a West End department store. Only when diagnosis is confirmed by a doctor should the question of treatment or no treatment be discussed. Untreated moderate high blood pressure may not lead to any complications at all; trials are presently under way to determine if drug treatment of uncomplicated essential moderate hypertension does confer benefit in terms of protection from cardiac or vascular complications. What if your random department store reading is *lower* than the normal range? Do nothing. Forget it.

HEART FAILURE This is a general term for a defect, usually temporary, in heart function. The heart, as we have seen, is a pump on the efficiency of which we depend totally for the gift of life. Many things can impair that efficiency—heart disease itself, disease of the vascular network through which blood is being pumped, disease of the blood, lungs or liver, or generalized infection or infection of the heart itself or its serous coverings. It is beyond the scope of this book to deal with all these. Suffice it to say that a diagnosis of 'heart failure' is *not* a sentence of death.

The common type of failure is due to an intrinsic defect in the heart's ability to cope with the blood going through it and is known as 'congestive heart failure'. The blood returning to the right side of the heart from the large veins (on which the heart depends for its forceful beat) piles up, as it were, and causes a kind of motorway tailback of blood which interferes with the function of other organs like the liver and lungs. This slowing up of the returning blood to the heart is sometimes detectable (by a doctor) as dilated veins in the neck or as enlargement of the liver or as a collection of fluid in the tissues round the ankles or at the base of the spine. This type of heart failure is the heart failure of old age, of acute infection such as broncho-pneumonia and of some kinds of valve disease—for example, that associated with rheumatic fever. It is treated with digitalis (digoxin) and/or diuretics*—and rest. The underlying cause has to be sought and dealt with. The symptoms are usually breathlessness, swollen ankles, a cough and usually a rapid, perhaps irregular pulse. Medical attention is, of course, mandatory.

Coronary disease can cause heart failure of this kind. The coronary arteries supply blood to the heart itself and are the first branches to leave the main blood vessel, the

---

*A diuretic is a drug used to stimulate the kidneys and cause an increased output of urine. This in turn leads to a lessening of the accumulation of fluid in the tissues (oedema).

aorta. Impairment of blood flow through these arteries and their numerous branches and capillaries leads initially to ischaemia (relative bloodlessness) of the heart muscle.

The heart muscle is of a special kind, with a high oxygen consumption compared with muscles of the limbs, for it has to do an enormous amount of work in a short time. Starved of oxygen, it reacts with pain sensations—as will any bodily muscle—and the pain is usually felt behind the breastbone and is of a gripping, penetrating and stabbing nature relieved by rest, alcohol and certain drugs. This is the pain of **angina pectoris** or, simply, angina, a word derived from the Latin and meaning strangling or choking. Indeed, the pain of angina can be described as a tightening, choking sensation (though as all pain sensations are subjective, descriptions vary greatly from one person to another).

Pain in the chest of an anginal type may also be associated with emotional stress or neurosis. True angina too can be triggered by emotion as much as by physical effort or even a heavy meal, and it is often difficult for doctors to be certain whether pain in the chest is true angina or not. It may need an electrocardiogram taken before, during and after exercise (the exercise tolerance test) to clinch a diagnosis.

The pain of angina is transient, fading when the triggering factor goes. The pain of a heart attack—when the fall of oxygen supplied to the muscle is so great or lasts so long that part of the muscle tissue actually dies—does not ease up and indeed may become steadily worse. Sometimes the pain is minimal and the general effects predominate—the victim may lose consciousness, falling to the ground or slumping forward on to a table.

This is an emergency, for the heart has stopped or at least become so irregular in its beat that it is totally ineffective as a supplier of blood to the brain and its vital centres. Artificial respiration (see page 177) should be started immediately and medical aid sent for. Some ambulances are now equipped with electrical devices for restarting the failed heart and the attendants are skilled at such resuscitatory measures. This is the loosely termed 'coronary'. It may be of the silent type which can strike a man down in the street or in his place of work without any premonition or warning whatever by way of breathlessness or chest pain. The silent coronary can also occur without the patient being aware of anything more than an overwhelming fatigue or total loss of energy. No pain is felt and diagnosis has to be made by the electrocardiogram.

Much has been written about the present-day epidemic of coronary heart disease—and it *is* an epidemic—and how to reduce its incidence. This is not the chapter for detailed discussion of the pros and cons of jogging, of eating only vegetable fats and giving up smoking. Let it only be said that it is a disease of the male much more than the female and it is associated with (and that is not the same thing as saying it is caused by) five physical characteristics. These are:

1 Overweight.
2 Smoking.
3 High blood pressure.
4 Raised levels of certain types of fat in the blood stream.
5 The sedentary way of life.

Something can be done about all these although the *proof* that correction of any one of them actually reduces the chances of a heart attack is, at present, lacking. However, while we await proof of causation, the associations are very clear. We have been warned!

DIGESTIVE SYSTEM

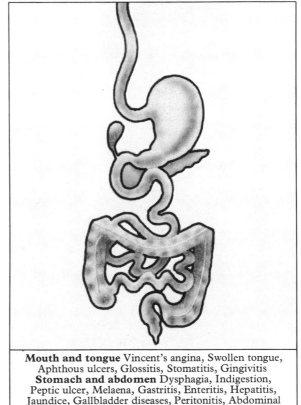

Mouth and tongue Vincent's angina, Swollen tongue, Aphthous ulcers, Glossitis, Stomatitis, Gingivitis **Stomach and abdomen** Dysphagia, Indigestion, Peptic ulcer, Melaena, Gastritis, Enteritis, Hepatitis, Jaundice, Gallbladder diseases, Peritonitis, Abdominal pains, Constipation, Piles

Digestion is an intricate biochemical process under exquisite nervous control, and it should be no surprise that it can be readily upset by anything that disturbs the normal healthy equilibrium of the autonomic nervous system. The stomach lining flushes and pales just as readily as the face; small wonder then that unpleasant experiences or their anticipation can put us off our food. Thus today, when we seem to have more than our fair share of anxiety and stress, disorders of the alimentary tract are very common. That is not to say all digestive upsets are stress-generated but many undoubtedly are.

MOUTH AND TONGUE Disorders of the mouth itself are uncommon—although dryness is often a sign of emotion—anxiety, fear or anger. Infections, bacterial or viral, are common and usually affect the linings of the pharynx and naso-pharynx (q.v.). The mouth lining and tongue covering may themselves be rarely affected by particular bacteria which produce an overwhelming infection of gums and tongue known as **Vincent's angina**. It responds dramatically to penicillin.

The tongue, a totally muscular organ, has a complex covering with highly specialized cells which form the visible taste buds on its upper surface. We are more conscious of the appearance of the surface than we are of most parts of the body; indeed to some people the early morning tongue inspection is more important than cleaning the teeth. But putting one's tongue out to the mirror each day is not as revealing, as an indicator of health, as is usually believed. A furred tongue means nothing and although colour changes may be significant, they are subtle in themselves and only uncommonly associated with general disease. Certain changes do occur in vitamin deficiencies, for example, but are only really obvious when the disease has progressed so much as to be readily diagnosed by other signs and symptoms.

Swelling of the tongue may have a number of causes. A sudden swelling, with a feeling of lumpiness in the throat and difficulty in swallowing (dysphagia, q.v.) may occur as an acute allergic reaction (angio-neurotic oedema) and this is a medical emergency, albeit an uncommon one. It may follow a wasp-sting, in the mouth or elsewhere.

The tongue surface, its edges and the mouth lining are prone to develop minute pearly-looking ulcers in some individuals. These are very painful, and if multiple, as they often are, may well cause difficulty in chewing and swallowing food. They are **aphthous ulcers** (aphthous meaning 'pearl-like') and are probably viral infections, the virus lying dormant in the cells and only becoming active through the interplay of some other factor or factors; we just don't know. Remedies abound, but there is only one reliable treatment: small steroid pellets, left to dissolve slowly in contact with the ulcers, will relieve the intense irritation and usually clear the ulcer in 24–48 hours. Although an infection, the condition does not seem to be contagious.

Glossitis is inflammation of the tongue itself. **Stomatitis** is inflammation of the whole mouth and **gingivitis** is inflammation of the gums. Although gingivitis may be a sign of some general illnesses or a reaction to certain drugs, it is more commonly a purely dental problem. Gingivitis, with bleeding of the gums, occurs in scurvy, a vitamin C deficiency disease which is probably rare today—except in the elderly.

STOMACH AND ABDOMEN Throat ailments have been dealt with under 'Head and Neck' (q.v.). The gullet (oesophagus) leads from the throat to the stomach and is muscularly equipped (as is all the alimentary canal, or gut) to deal exclusively with the movement of food, either downwards or upwards. No absorption of nutrients takes place in the gullet.

The bolus (chewed ball) of food, when swallowed, stimulates the rhythmic muscular movements which are characteristic of the gut in general (peristalsis) and it is rapidly passed into the stomach. The sword-swallower and the man in the pub who can down a pint in one gulp have learnt to inhibit oesophageal peristalsis and the sword, or the beer, can literally drop through what is then a lax tube. At the join with the stomach—the oesophageal sphincter—the peristaltic wave relaxes the opening and the food passes through. The sphincter is normally tightly closed, especially when the stomach is full. Sometimes the control of this first part of the process of digesting food goes wrong and the bolus either takes a long time to get through the gullet or even sticks half-way; indeed, even in the absence of a bolus, spasm of the gullet muscles may generate a feeling of something 'half-way down'. Thus in moments of great stress or emotion we feel 'a lump in the throat'.

The feeling of food not going down is termed **dysphagia** (literally, difficulty in swallowing). While often it is simply a nervous phenomenon—it may occur in anxiety states—it does have some potentially serious organic causes and should always be investigated. The oesophageal sphincter referred to earlier becomes less efficient with age and may allow some stomach contents to reach the gullet, the lining of which reacts with inflammation and consequent pain which is usually felt in the chest, behind the breastbone (sternum).

These symptoms may be rather lightly dismissed as 'heartburn' and treated with antacids which will relieve the discomfort but leave the cause undiagnosed. Healing may well take place but so may scarring and contraction of the gullet itself, leading to a **stricture**. This is one of the important organic causes of dysphagia. Dysphagia, fortunately, is readily investigated by X-ray and by the use of the endoscope, an instrument allowing direct vision down the gullet, into the stomach and even the duodenum. Initially, the 'barium swallow' is taken. A drink of X-ray-opaque barium sulphate is treated by the gullet as if it were a bolus and the peristaltic wave can be observed by the radiologist as it happens. Endoscopy not only allows direct vision of any obstructing lesion but enables a sample of the tissue to be 'snipped' for microscopical examination (the biopsy).

Indigestion is a broad term covering a variety of symptoms for which there are many, many local descriptive terms: fullness of the stomach, bloating, nausea, flatulence, burning, heaving, heartburn, acidity, and so on. The one thing common to all is that they are usually, but not always, associated with eating or drinking – although when symptoms arise some hours after food the association may not be immediately apparent. Minor gastric discomforts due to over-indulgence are usually of no consequence. Of course, persistent discomfort or pain in the abdomen or lower part of the chest occurring after food – either soon after or up to one or even two hours later – needs investigation. So, too, does pain arising in the night or at any time when the stomach is empty; such pain suggests stomach or duodenal ulceration.

The term **peptic ulcer** is also a broad one describing ulcerative lesions of the mucous lining of the lower gullet, stomach or duodenum. By investigation the precise site can be located and the correct term applied – gastric, duodenal or oesophageal ulcer. Peptic ulcers are common in Western societies and much more common in men than women. They are regarded as manifestations of stress and typically associated with the busy, lunch-entertaining, hard-working, obsessional, cigarette-addicted, middle-management or top executive man.

Treatment has been revolutionized in recent years. New drugs seem to have done away with the need for bed-rest, strict diet and lengthy medical supervision; the drugs are powerful, effective remedies but should never be self-prescribed. Accurate diagnosis is essential before treatment. The malignant lesion may appear to respond and if treated 'blind' can lead to endless problems later. Ideally all medically treated peptic ulcers need post-treatment assessments by X-ray or endoscope, but such a counsel of perfection seems likely to lead to overloading the already burdened NHS. However, accurate diagnosis before treatment is more important, and at present this seems a perfectly practical proposition.

Peptic ulcers may be the cause of chronic or acute bleeding. If a small vessel in the ulcer itself has been eroded by the ulcer process a slow trickle of blood may start and this will either be vomited or carried along with the food being digested, pass through the small and large intestines and be passed with the faeces. If it is vomited it is seen either as red blood or as dark granules, rather like coarse coffee grounds, depending on how long the blood has been in contact with the acid stomach secretions. If it is passed on down the gut then other digestive processes change the blood pigments and the effect is to colour the faeces to a total black – tarry black is the usual description. This is **melaena**. The passing of one melaena stool may go unnoticed and indeed such stools may be passed for days before being so noticed – and, even then, put down to a change in diet. Iron tablets, which can be bought over the counter, can also produce stools which are black. Needless to say, the occurrence of even one melaena stool means that medical advice is imperative.

Sometimes the blood vessel eroded in an ulcer is a large one and leads to copious bleeding which is always, or nearly always, immediately vomited. The appearance is of pure blood; it is a serious medical emergency and the patient should be made to lie down on his right side and the ambulance and doctor called. Nothing at all should be given by mouth.

Gastritis means, in its strict sense, stomach inflammation. Coupled with **enteritis** (inflammation of the small intestine) it is used to describe a number of specific bacterial or viral conditions characterized by sickness and diarrhoea which may be described as 'gastric 'flu'. It is seldom that any one part of the gut is affected in isolation although the involvement of other parts may not be overtly symptomatic. Gastritis can arise in itself, a common cause being over-indulgence in alcohol. The vomiting and belly pain which rapidly follows an excess of alcohol is alcoholic gastritis. Sometimes the rest of the gut is involved, when diarrhoea and central abdominal pain will occur. Gastritis may also accompany actual stomach ulceration and, of course, true 'food poisoning' – the infection of the gut with micro-organisms or their toxins from ingested foodstuffs.

Simple gastro-enteritis, following over-indulgence with unsuitable foods (re-heated meats or tinned food opened and eaten over a matter of days, for example) is usually self-limiting, and lasts only a day or so. Treatment should be: nothing by mouth other than water until the appetite returns. Most moderate 'tummy upsets' will resolve in this way, usually in 24 to 48 hours, and there is no need to rush either for the bottle of kaolin, the chlorodyne mixture or the doctor. Some pain or discomfort is usual, but analgesics and purgatives are best avoided. If there is no lessening of symptoms after 24 or 36 hours, then you should call your doctor. If the diarrhoea is bloody, or the vomit is seen to have the 'coffee ground' appearance referred to above then medical attention is imperative and urgent.

The **liver** is much maligned by food abusers and others. Any 'off-colour' feeling—especially first thing in the morning or if accompanied by nausea, unpleasant mouth tastes and the like—is referred to as 'feeling liverish' and, by implication, impugns that organ. Fortunes have been made on promotions of over-the-counter medicines which are claimed to stimulate the liver, mend its errant ways and cure it and you of 'liver problems'. Liver salts and spa waters of one sort or another have *no* direct or specific action on the liver nor indeed on any other digestive organs and mostly simply act as aperients.

We have seen in Part 1 that the liver is the body's chemical factory, producing substances essential for the proper digestion of food. It works hand in hand with the **pancreas** and has its own storage space in the shape of the **gall-bladder**, which nestles closely to its under-surface.

One of the liver's jobs is to deal chemically with not only certain foodstuffs (glucose for example) but with noxious substances such as drugs and certain poisons, which it can render harmless. One such drug (or poison) is alcohol and the overburdening of the liver through excessive alcohol intake may be a factor in causing **hangover**. All nutrient material (i.e. substances derived from food and absorbed by the gut) is carried first to the liver where various chemical changes take place. Every drop of alcohol we consume passes through the liver. Its capacity to cope with vast quantities—either in a short burst in a matter of hours, or a steady intake over months or years—is truly astonishing. Some livers cannot cope, and we don't know why. In the susceptible, chronic alcohol intake above a defined level (20 grammes per day according to some researchers—equivalent to four double whiskies or four pints of beer) can lead to permanent damage after anything from five to twenty years.

Hepatitis is the name given to liver disorders generally whether or not these are infections. Thus we speak of alcoholic hepatitis, infective hepatitis, toxic hepatitis and so on. Hepatitis may or may not be accompanied by **jaundice**. This is the yellow appearance of the skin and whites of the eyes due to the excess of bile in the blood stream which is commonly found in certain types of the disease. The urine is darkened and the stools lightened. Bile, manufactured by the liver, is normally excreted thence via tiny bile ducts to the gall-bladder where it is stored and squirted as required, particularly after a fatty meal, into the duodenum. In hepatitis it cannot escape from the liver and is absorbed into the blood stream to a greater or lesser extent. When the amount

in the blood stream is higher than a certain level, then jaundice appears. Some of the excess bile is extracted from the blood by the kidney and appears in the urine—hence its darkening—and as there is little or none in the gut, the stool loses its typically brown colour and becomes rather like light clay.

Jaundice is not a disease in itself (although loosely described as such) but a sign of certain diseases and requires investigation. The commonest cause of jaundice in the young adult is **infective hepatitis** which is a viral infection of the liver. It was very common among troops in the Middle East during the last war and occasional sporadic outbreaks occur in this country. However, one form of viral hepatitis is more serious than the others and all patients with these types of hepatitis must have blood tests to identify the responsible organism. Virus 'A' is the common type and causes a relatively benign condition which, although resulting in a fairly prolonged illness, during the early days of which the victim can feel quite unwell, usually leads to no complications and full recovery. There are exceptions, however, and bed-rest until the jaundice begins to subside is essential. Alcohol can damage the liver and you will be told to avoid it totally during the disease and for six months to a year after recovery.

Virus 'B' is the other type and we believe the mode of infection is quite different. Whereas Virus 'A' infections are probably airborne, Virus 'B' requires direct contact with another infected person or with something the other person has used. Commonly, this is a shared syringe; the occurrence of Virus 'B' hepatitis may even give rise to suspicion that the patient is, or has been, a drug addict. It is a potentially lethal condition and patients must be nursed in isolation. Healthy people can carry the infection and be a source of danger to others, but such carriers can be identified by blood tests and are usually totally prohibited from working in or being anywhere near hospitals where renal dialysis units are situated. There is a great danger that the virus can get into the dialysis equipment with disastrous consequences.

Gall-bladder diseases are common among the developed, so-called civilized sections of the world. In the United States it is estimated that at any one time some 30 million people suffer from them. There are many varieties of disease of this organ from simple inflammation (cholecystitis) to frank gallstones (cholelithiasis). The gall is bile—a mixture of chemicals needed for the proper absorption of fat. The bladder contains roughly 25–50 grammes at any time and its activity is directly related to the amount of fat present in the meal just eaten. We can live quite happily without our gall-bladders, and they are very frequently removed when they have become diseased. The commonest reason for the operation is the presence of gall-stones, which have irritated and set up inflammation, causing a lot of pain.

Gall-bladder disease may make itself known either by starting an attack of jaundice or causing severe pain–or both. Gall-bladder pain is typically right-sided or central in the abdomen and tends to go through to the back. It may mimic the pain of a peptic ulcer (q.v.) because of its relationship to meals, but it can and does occur frequently between meals. Gall-bladder disease is commoner among women than men–especially in the over-35s and in the overweight rather than the slender. The older physicians would say that the typical gall-bladder patient would be 'fair, fat and forty'.

When you consult your General Practitioner about belly pain he depends very much on your history, i.e. the story of your illness, the kind of pain, when it occurs, what alleviates and what aggravates it, to decide whether you are likely to have a peptic ulcer or gall-bladder disease. If the former, he will probably arrange for a barium meal X-ray, and if the latter, a special kind of X-ray called a cholecystogram which shows up the gall-bladder by making it fill up with and excrete a special substance which can be visualized when X-rays are passed through the abdomen.

If you are found to have a gall-stone how will it be treated? In recent years, advances have been made in the medical treatment of certain gall-stones and the need for surgery is eliminated. The medical treatment of such stones is time-consuming and not all that pleasant (concentrated mixtures of bile acids have to be taken three or four times a day) but many patients would prefer this to the prospect of an operation. Not all gall-stones are by any means treatable in this way; they have to be not too large, their composition must be of a certain type and they must not have been in the gall-bladder so long that a chalky shell has been built up round them. The nature of many stones can be judged by careful radiological examinations, and the best treatment decided.

Gall-stones form in the gall-bladder itself; like kidney-stones, however, they may move and cause trouble elsewhere. A stone may get lodged in one of the ducts through which the bile normally comes from the liver or through which it goes on its route to the duodenum. In certain circumstances, this results in an emergency which requires immediate surgery. There is no place for medical treatment when stones are obstructing the bile passages.

The abdomen itself contains, as we have seen, not only the organs of digestion–liver and pancreas–but the digestive tract itself. This comprises the stomach, duodenum, small bowel (jejunum and ileum), the large bowel and rectum. All these abdominal organs are collectively known as the **viscera** and are all protected by a specialized sheet of tissue which is intimately associated with the organs and forms also the lining of the abdominal cavity. Some organs such as the kidneys, uterus and bladder are outside this lining membrane, which is known as the **peritoneum.** Because of its intimate contact with the viscera, it can become involved with disease affecting any of the organs with which it is associated.

Inflammation of the peritoneum is known as **peritonitis**, once a very common sequel to operations, notably on the appendix. Peritonitis is nearly always a complication of some intra-abdominal condition. Peritonitis due to tuberculous activity, which affects the glands in the abdomen, is not uncommon among Asian immigrants in the UK. It causes generalized abdominal pain, with constipation and sometimes retention of urine. It is always accompanied by a generalized upset such as a fever, nausea, weakness and sometimes collapse.

Abdominal pain must always be treated seriously and urgently investigated; attempts at self-diagnosis are foolish. Some pain is, of course, physiological, that is to say, associated with the normal functioning of the abdominal contents. Discomfort amounting to pain will occur with an overfull rectum and will be relieved by defaecation. Likewise an overfull bladder! An overfull stomach can cause discomfort, not pain. The small bowel typically produces pain which is felt in the middle of the belly just around the umbilicus and is referred to as griping or 'the gripes'. Food-poisoning will often be preceded by this sort of pain which is likened to the green apple pain many of us experienced during childhood after an illicit visit to the orchard.

It is always of great help to the doctor for a patient to be able to describe his pain carefully, although let it be said that a patient doubled up in agony with knees drawn up to his chest, doesn't need to say anything. The localizing of abdominal pain is particularly difficult but it is helpful if you can indicate where the pain appeared to begin. The time scale is also important–its relationship to meals, to urination, to defaecation, to day and to night.

The pain of **appendicitis** typically begins in the centre of the belly and only later tends to move and be felt in the right side of the lower abdomen. The pain of **enteritis** is central and griping. The pain of **colitis** may be on the left or on the right but more generally is felt all over. That of **proctitis** is felt deep in the pelvic area and rectum. The pains of a **peptic ulcer** are felt in the upper mid-abdomen and in the angle formed by the lower end of the breast bone and ribs. The pain of **gall-bladder stone** may be right-sided or centrally in the back. The pain of **kidney-stone** may be in the right or left lower abdomen and typically goes down into the groin. Both gall-bladder pain and kidney pain due to stones are typically colicky in nature, i.e. they are spasmodic and sharp and knife-like in their intensity. The liver and spleen are insensitive organs and although the liver may feel tender when it is felt by the examining doctor (and it can only usually be felt when it is enlarged or swollen by disease because normally the lower ribs cover it) it is never the site of real pain. Likewise, the spleen, which can grow to an enormous size as a result of some diseases, e.g. malaria and certain blood disorders, without producing any symptoms at all.

Not so the pancreas, the organ which snuggles close to the duodenum and stomach and is intimately concerned with digestion. It produces many enzymes required for assimilating protein, fat and carbohydrate and also, from certain of its glands, insulin for the adequate utilization of sugar. **Pancreatitis** is uncommon but the pain it produces is one of the worst, if not *the* worst, that can be experienced in the abdomen.

It is appropriate to end this section on the gut with the **rectum** and **anus**. The rectum is a chamber leading off the large bowel, the transit camp where faecal material awaits its turn for evacuation. Water tends to be absorbed here and the faeces gradually become dry and hard. If evacuation does not soon take place, then certainly discomfort, if not actual pain, will ensue; the passage of hard faecal material may in itself abrade the bowel lining and cause bleeding. The blood, because there are no digestive juices there to water it, remains bright red and perhaps adheres to the faeces. Sometimes pure blood seems to be passed (usually painlessly) and this is most likely due to piles (haemorrhoids). The occasional streak of blood, particularly if associated with **constipation**, is not to be worried about. Nor is constipation itself unless it is causing a great deal of discomfort or pain. It is *not* necessary to have a daily evacuation; the rectum need only be emptied when it feels full. No 'poisonous substances' are absorbed back into the body from faeces held in the rectum. Laxatives and aperients should never be necessary. Sufficient dietary roughage, sufficient fluid intake, sufficient healthy exercise and a mind focused away from the abdomen are the ingredients of regular, painless, healthy evacuation, be that daily, every other day, every two or three days, weekly or even monthly. Due probably to over-indulgence by worried mothers, mindful of the supposed importance of the daily potty in childhood, many adults have been brought up

on laxatives and now cannot do without them. The baby 'born constipated' is a myth. The problem—if ever there was one—is compounded by further abuse of aperients in childhood and into adult life.

Lastly in this section: **piles**. Again, it is probably a disease of civilized living and certainly related to our two-legged attitude. Cats and dogs don't get them. What are they? At one time they were thought simply to be varicose veins in the lower part of the rectum. But we now know that their anatomy is a little more complex than that. Minor degrees of piles leading to very little discomfort, occasional bleeding, soreness and itching round the anus are quite common. Symptoms can be simply and effectively dealt with by local application of soothing ointments or pessaries which any pharmacy will advise you about. When the condition becomes more seriously inconveniencing—when, for example, after defaecation, some of the rectal lining feels as if it is projecting through the anus (it can be pushed back with a finger)—then expert advice is needed, for piles are an eminently treatable condition and can be dealt with by the surgeon in an out-patients department. Piles making their first appearance in middle-age, whether mildly symptomatic or not, must always have the attention of your physician. Persistent bleeding, the appearance of a discharge and particularly a change in bowel habits, even without anything else, must never be ignored.

URINARY SYSTEM

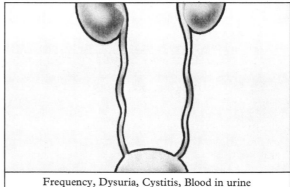

Frequency, Dysuria, Cystitis, Blood in urine

Normally, passing water is a painless, relatively quick procedure which is semi-automatic in the sense that when the bladder is full signals penetrate the consciousness and urine is then released—if the circumstances are appropriate. Micturition (the act of passing urine) is always under the conscious will—at least up to a point. In childhood that control is usually excellent; as we grow older that control, especially among men, becomes less effective. Many things can go wrong with the 'water works', from bed-wetting in childhood to bed-wetting in old age. We will here deal only with the common disorders in adult life; there are specialized books dealing with disorders in childhood, particularly the common problem of bed-wetting which is rarely due to anatomical or physiological defects of the bladder mechanism itself.

The urine tells much about the general condition of the body. For example, the presence of sugar may indicate diabetes; that of protein, kidney disease, and of blood, either local infections, bladder tumours or other kinds of kidney disease. The commonest urinary symptom by far is **frequency** – by which is meant simply having to pass water more often than usual. There is often a nervous cause for this, such as the imminence of an exam or an interview, the excitement of an anniversary and so on. But frequency can also result from infection of the urethra or bladder itself, although frequency on its own is uncommon as a symptom of urinary tract infection. Some **dysuria** (painful or difficult urination) is common. It is often accompanied by burning, which is felt while the urine passes down the urethra. Some infections also cause slight bleeding, tingeing the urine the colour of port wine.

For anatomical reasons, urinary infection is much commoner in women than men. It is usually of the bladder and is called **cystitis.** If you think you have cystitis there is no need to seek urgent medical attention. The commonest bacteria to cause the condition does not thrive well in alkaline urine and very often copious fruit drinks, especially lemon or orange barley water, will be sufficient to clear up the condition.

However, expert attention should be sought if the infection persists more than a day or two, if the urine appears blood-stained or if you are feverish. **Blood in the urine** in the absence of pain or frequency or irritation on micturition should be treated as seriously as you would treat blood in the vomit or in the stools. No time should be lost before seeing a doctor. Take a sample with you or be prepared to pass one at the time of the consultation. As has been mentioned, the appearance of very dark brown urine may herald the beginning of jaundice and hepatitis, particularly if the stool in the meantime is becoming pale. As the common cause of this is infective hepatitis, at least in the younger age groups, it is better to call your doctor in rather than go to him.

Urine very frequently goes cloudy while standing or may appear cloudy while being passed. Such changes usually mean nothing more than the appearance of harmless mineral salts and only if the cloudiness persists or you are able to see beadlets of pus in the urine, need you seek advice. Needless to say, any discharge or appearance of blood when *not* micturating also needs urgent investigation.

Frequency in older males, particularly if there is difficulty in stopping or starting the act of urination, or if there is dribbling or if the urine cannot be held for long when the bladder is full, usually indicates underlying prostatic disease. This is most commonly just a benign enlargement which occurs in a large number of males over the age of 60, but all such symptoms should be totally investigated to exclude malignancy. Very often a simple clinical examination is all that is necessary, perhaps followed by a blood test and an X-ray.

THE LIMBS

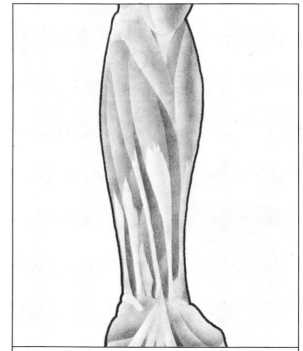

Arms and shoulders Cramps, Arthritis, Tennis elbow, Fractures and dislocations
Legs and feet Arthritis, Fractures and dislocations, Gout, Athlete's foot, Verrucae, Flat feet, Ankle injuries

The **arms** and **shoulders** are made up of wonderfully complex joints which permit an almost infinite variety of movement, but like joints anywhere else are prone to disease in certain individuals. The mechanism of muscular co-ordination of joint movement is controlled through a network of nerve trunks and fibres all of which originate in the spinal cord at neck and upper chest level. Consequently neck problems – and to some extent chest problems as well –

can cause pain in the arms. Changes in the shape of the small neck vertebrae can irritate or compress nerve roots as they emerge from their bone-encircled exits and give rise not only to pain but also to impaired arm movements and, if prolonged, to muscle wasting.

The nerve trunks of the arm run deep in the under-surface of the arm and are easily compressed without our realizing it. The typical instance is the armchair snooze, with the arms flopped over the sides of the chair. This can result in a virtual, fortunately temporary, paralysis of the upper limbs; permanent injury could occur if the position were maintained for a long time – as it could easily be if the armchair 'flop' is that of a stuporous, drunken man. It usually affects one arm, and is sometimes referred to as 'Saturday night palsy'.

Cramps of the arm muscles are rare, but common enough in the legs and feet. Cramps are difficult to treat; doctors don't know the cause. Quinine is often prescribed and does help in many cases. Recently a new, preventive treatment has been described which appears to be successful in many instances. Basically it is a muscle-stretching routine concentrating on calf and foot muscles. It is carried out in bare feet, standing facing a wall about one metre away and with arms outstretched and hands flat against it. The angle of lean towards the wall is increased by bending the elbows but keeping the feet absolutely flat on the floor until a 'pulling' sensation is felt in the backs of the legs. This angle is maintained for five to ten seconds or so and then repeated twice after a rest. The whole exercise should be done two or three times a day until the night cramps have disappeared.

Osteo-arthritis, the degenerative arthritis of age, is more likely in shoulder joints than elbows but more common in knees and hips. On the other hand the arthritis of the **rheumatoid** type is more likely to affect the small joints of the fingers, hands and wrists. The **elbow** has its own problems – in particular one that gives intense pain on certain movements, the so-called **tennis elbow**. Like **housemaid's knee**, by no means confined to housemaids, tennis elbow afflicts other sportsmen than tennis players and indeed non-sporty types as well. It is not a form of arthritis, does not spread to other parts, and if treated early and not neglected will usually respond to simple local treatments, principally an injection of steroid hormone at the site of maximum tenderness (generally the outer edge of the elbow joint).

Arm injuries are, of course, very common. A fall on an outstretched hand, on the elbow itself or on the shoulder is likely to cause **fractures** or **dislocations**. The collar-bone (clavicle) is also at risk, as every soccer or rugby player knows. Pain is the cardinal symptom of a broken bone or dislocated joint. Pain, with inability to move the painful part and obvious (but often not so obvious) deformity, means a fracture.

Never 'test' for a fracture – use your eyes alone and let the doctor in the Accident and Emergency Department do the testing. Sometimes the deformity is very obvious. The typical 'broken wrist' (Colles' fracture) produces a shape not unlike a table fork, the outer aspect of the wrist being humped up with the rest of the hand slightly flexed and motionless; once seen, not forgotten.

Occasionally the ends of bones extrude through the skin – the **open fracture**. The danger here is damage to blood vessels and thus rapid haemorrhage, and infection. The aim should be complete immobilization and a covering of the wound with a sterile 'field dressing' before transit to hospital (see page 184).

Children in pubescent years are prone to a particular kind of fracture, called 'greenstick' (because that is just what it's like). The breaks tend to be longitudinal, not across the bone – in fact just what happens when you try and 'snap' soft wood. A common site is the wrist and lower part of the arm. Treatment is just as important as with other types of fracture.

Much of what has been written about the arm and wrist goes for the leg and foot, too. Again, the common site for osteo-arthritis is the hip joint and for the rheumatoid variety, the knee and ankle. The big toe, usually the second joint from the nail, is the commonest site of **gout**, that peculiarly male-favouring disease associated in the minds of many with alcohol excess and good living, unjustifiably so.

The **foot** is heir to many common ailments from **athlete's foot** (tinea pedis) to **plantar warts** (verrucae, q.v.). Athlete's foot has little or nothing to do with sport but a lot to do with hygiene (see also page 104). It is a fungal infection which affects mainly the between-toe skin and is certainly more likely to attack the sweaty and infrequently washed foot than the cool, well looked-after one. Oddly enough the first clue to this disease may come from the appearance of a scaly, eczematous eruption on the sides of the fingers and the palms of the hands, with blistering and much itching (cheiropompholyx). It is a sensitivity reaction to infection elsewhere – usually athlete's foot – and clears when the distant infection clears, although the hand condition may need treatment at the same time (of a soothing nature, no anti-fungal lotions are necessary). Athlete's foot tends to be an intractable condition; there are many proprietary remedies but in the first instance see your doctor to be certain that it is tinea and not some other condition. But good foot care is the best preventive medicine.

The other common infection of the feet is the **verruca** (plural verrucae) or plantar wart. It is not a fungal infection but a localized viral one. Plantar warts are painful, often multiple and tend to occur just in those parts of the sole of the foot most in contact with the ground – the ball of the foot and the heel. They are *contagious* and are commonly passed from one member of the household to another or from one user of a public swimming pool to others. There are many proprietary treatments; verrucae sometimes need curetting (gouging out) under local anaesthetic or freezing with carbon dioxide 'snow'. Like all warts, they often go as mysteriously and as quickly as they came, a fact made use of by many claiming to be wart charmers. However, if they don't disappear and are particularly persistent and painful you will have to see your doctor. It is better not to use a proprietary remedy as some of these are not only painful to use but can damage the surrounding skin.

Flat feet ('fallen arches') may be congenital or acquired. Home diagnosis is easily made in the bathroom; the footprint on the bath mat should be

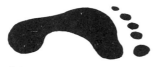

and not like this

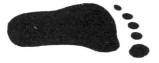

In the middle-aged the condition is common and may only require supports in the shoes. Avoid proprietary remedies until medical or chiropodal advice has been sought. In the young it is especially important to seek expert advice because remedial exercises may prevent trouble later on in life.

The **ankle** is a complex joint and prone to injury. Uneven ground is the usual culprit: the foot may be twisted inward or outward, the former being much commoner. The sudden movement causes intense pain and quite rapid swelling and discoloration of the upper part of the foot; this can look quite alarming but does not of itself indicate broken bones. This is the classic sprained ankle and requires no more treatment than rest (cold sponging can be most soothing). But if the pain continues for more than twelve hours or so, or rapidly worsens or the blue discoloration (which is due to the spread of blood from small ruptured veins in the soft tissue under the skin) spreads widely, then fracture is a possibility.

In its severest and crippling form this type of inversion (i.e. turning inward) injury is called a Pott's fracture (Pott was a famous 18th-century Guy's Hospital surgeon). The lower end of the tibia is wholly or partially split away from the main shaft of bone and the injury may need reduction (the realignment of the bone parts involved) under anaesthetic.

There is no need for all ankle injuries to be X-rayed because most of them produced in the way described are simple sprains. If in doubt, you must consult your doctor or go to the nearest hospital Accident and Emergency Department. Colles' and Pott's fractures are common in the elderly following trips and falls and the idea of sprain must not be entertained; X-rays are mandatory.

THE BACK

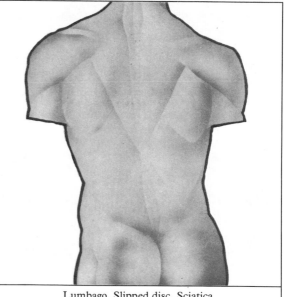

Lumbago, Slipped disc, Sciatica

Back strain, low back pain, lumbago, sciatica, 'slipped disc' and vertebral osteo-arthritis are the happy hunting ground of chiropractors, osteopaths, physical therapists, faith healers and of bed and corset manufacturers. Had man not adopted the upright posture, walking on two legs, bone setters and manipulators would be hard put to it to find work. Animals, unless specially bred, like racehorses, long back bacon pigs and dachshunds, don't seem to have back trouble at all. The spinal column is a highly complex structure apparently well adapted for use in the vertical position. The strength of the column is due to the ligamentous attachments of one vertebra to another and to the coordinated operation of stabilizing musculature. It follows that while we seem unable to do anything about strengthening ligaments or improving the quality of the bone of each individual vertebra, we can and should do something to keep the supporting muscles in good trim. Poor sitting and standing positions (the ladies in finishing schools who made their pupils walk with books balanced on their heads knew a thing or two) allow muscles to dodge the work they are designed to do, and become less efficient when called on to do the proper job. That is, of course, an over-simplification of the case, for the total study of spinal anatomy and physiology is complicated and cannot concern us here.

The back is not a rigid rod. It has natural curves, both forwards and backwards but should have no sideways bends. The neck part is slightly convex forward, the chest very slightly backward and the lumbar region (the loin area) has a much more pronounced forward convexity. The whole structure sits straight and wedge-like into the bony pelvic girdle, from which the tail remnant (the coccyx) curves gently forward again. This is what your back should look like when standing naturally, not strictly at attention and not stooping. The books-on-the-head position is best.

LUMBAGO Spinal troubles occur in two areas—the lumbo-sacral region (the 'small' of the back and the adjoining pelvic area) and the cervical or neck area. The first is the commoner site by far and the classic **lumbago** (which just means back pain) afflicts young and old, though more frequently the latter. The pain is usually lumbo-sacral, tends not to move from the small of the back position, can be relieved by lying supine (i.e. flat on back) on a firm surface or by sitting with a very firm support pressing into the painful area. The pain is most likely muscular in origin, comes on gradually and usually requires nothing more than mild analgesics, perhaps local heat, a firm mattress and a faith in the healing power of nature. It may be precipitated by bouts of gardening, unaccustomed positions of working such as getting under the car or painting the ceiling and, of course, by lifting. Proprietary remedies abound—liniments, various local heat-producing creams and 'back ache pills'—and consultations with chiropractors and physical therapists are very popular.

Simple lumbago always gets better whatever you do although it may be helped by the measures indicated above. Low back pain which seems to be unassociated with posture and is not relieved or aggravated by movement or changes in position of the back may be indicative of disease in the pelvic region, such as the bowel, bladder and so on. In such cases medical advice should always be sought, and early.

A variant of simple lumbago is that commonly known as the **'slipped disc'** or 'putting the back out'. This usually has a much more acute onset which may or may not be associated with unusual movements or exercise. The pain may remain localized or often is felt in one buttock or another or down the back of the thigh, or even as far as the foot. This particular aspect of the pain is known as **sciatica** because it follows the path of the sciatic nerve which is the main nerve trunk of the leg. It was an Australian who first defined this type of back problem which he identified as being due to the prolapse of one or more of the discs which separate the bony vertebrae. Although this is referred to as a 'slipped disc' it is a purely lay term which is now widely used— a matter of regret for such an occurrence is an anatomical impossibility.

The intervertebral discs are not slippery pads of jelly-like material which separate each vertebra up and down the back bone, but are firm pieces of cartilaginous material (although elastic to some extent), enclosed by ligaments which are themselves attached to the bony vertebrae and which completely encase them and prevent all movement other than compression. What happens in 'slipped disc' is that for various reasons, not all of which are completely understood, a portion of one of the discs protrudes through its ligamentous sheath, rather like an inner tyre tube might protrude through the outer cover if the latter were split, and while pressure is maintained from above or below, it cannot readily return to its former position. When the pressure is off—with the spine horizontal for example—the protruding portion may slip back and frequently does. Thus *rest* is the first requisite in treatment of the condition of prolapsed intervertebral disc.

Immediate manipulation may help but requires not only accurate diagnosis but the services of a skilled medical manipulator or osteopath. One way to take off the pressure on the disc is by traction, which again allows the gaps between vertebrae to be widened slightly and the pressure between them to fall. The simplest way to achieve traction is hanging by the hands from the top of a door jamb or a convenient part of the landing floor, reached from a few steps up the stairs if you have that kind of house. Two or three times a day for a few minutes may be all that is required. On the other hand, traction may need the services of a trained physiotherapist.

Acute back pain may well respond to such treatments—primarily rest in the position which gives most obvious relief and intermittent but regular stretching. In this situation, the surrounding vertebral muscles stiffen (go into spasm) to help minimize movement of the vertebrae at that point. This itself is a protective mechanism but is thought to be the main cause of the pain. Thus local warmth (electric blanket or hot water bottle) and mild analgesics (aspirin or paracetamol) may also be needed.

The condition quite often becomes chronic and intractable, and surgery may be required in a few instances. This is usually the case if the prolapse of the disc is sufficiently large to irritate the roots of the sciatic nerve (which emerge between some of the lumbar vertebrae). This not only causes acute buttock and leg pain but may interfere with the proper functioning of leg muscles and cause weakness and, in extreme cases, paralysis. Continuing muscular weakness in turn leads to muscle wasting and difficulty in walking.

If surgery is needed, part of the bony arch of the vertebrae against which the nerve roots are being compressed has to be removed. This is the operation of laminectomy. This may have to be combined with spinal fusion, which is an operation to graft bone (usually taken from a leg or hip) to two or three vertebrae to fix them so they cannot move in any direction, particularly up and down so that pressure on the weak disc is avoided.

An alternative way of 'fixing' the lumbar vertebrae is to have a specially designed corset or belt which is made to measure and gives very firm support where it is needed. Never buy such corsets 'off the peg'; if a belt is needed then it must be obtained through a qualified surgical appliance fitter (the service is available on the NHS through orthopaedic consultants) and it will need to be fitted by him and then checked periodically. Needless to say, an ill-fitting belt is worse than useless.

MENTAL DISORDERS

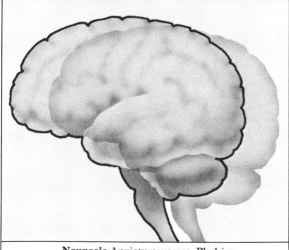

Neurosis Anxiety neuroses, Phobias
Psychosis Manic-depressive psychosis, Schizophrenia

This term covers a very wide range of minor and major illnesses from the relatively simple and common **anxiety neurosis** right through to **depression, dementia** and **schizophrenia**. The term neurosis and neurotic, psychosis and psychotic are in general not well understood by the layman. At the outset let it be said that neurosis and neurotic tendencies are very common indeed and this section will be mainly confined to them. Psychosis and psychotic states are not as common and only passing reference need be made.

Neuroses or neurotic states can be defined as exaggerated responses to common situations; while in this state the subject is relatively unamenable to reason. To be anxious, i.e. apprehensive of an outcome, for example, about passing an examination, meeting a stranger or seeing a doctor is a quite normal and healthy reaction. If the anxiety is deeper than the reason for it might indicate, and if simple reassurance seems not to modify it, or if it continues after the reason for it ceases, then it is right to call it a neurosis. The subject *knows* he is anxious and even realizes that his anxiety is much more than it need be; nevertheless he has difficulty in 'pulling himself together', cannot be reassured and may suffer from physical effects such as headache, abdominal discomfort or even pain, diarrhoea, nausea, frequency of passing urine, palpitations and so on. He may not connect his physical symptoms with his mental state and ultimately his awareness of anxiety may diminish and of his physical symptoms increase. He may then be anxious about his palpitations or his abdominal pain and so a kind of vicious circle may be set up which is difficult to break.

ANXIETY NEUROSES of one sort or another are the commonest neurotic illnesses we know. This is not the place to go into the reasons for them, but it is appropriate to note that these neuroses are very common, that patients can rarely respond to pull-yourself-together appeals, that tranquillizers (including alcohol) may alleviate but do not cure, and that the condition is pretty well self-limiting although it has to be admitted that it can very easily become chronic. Tranquillizing drugs are a tremendous help in that alleviation can be achieved while the causes are sorted out and, hopefully, eliminated.

An anxiety neurosis is subtle in that the only symptom complained of may be vague abdominal pain, headache or loss of appetite. The patient may not be aware of any underlying worry. He may have been initially but usually, once some bodily function gets disarranged, it becomes a convenient whipping boy and a focus of attention. Thus a patient with abdominal pain occurring after food may think he has indigestion, may therefore buy one of the many advertised indigestion remedies (which usually in this situation have very little effect) and see his doctor because he thinks he may have an ulcer. His original anxiety will have become submerged by the newer anxiety about his stomach ulcer–which perhaps he may fear will be a cancer.

There are many other kinds of neurosis and in an ideal world the patient with a neurosis should be treated with psychotherapy. But it is not an ideal world and most neurotics have to learn to live with their problems or at least dampen the symptoms by the use of tranquillizers and sedatives.

PHOBIAS A phobia is a fear–a very normal human (and animal) reaction. As children, most of us were afraid of the dark, but only exceptionally do such fears persist into adulthood. A fear-reaction out of proportion to the cause is a neurosis and, according to the triggering factor, many phobias are recognized. Thus we have claustrophobia, xenophobia, agoraphobia and so on. These are all neuroses, not psychoses.

Phobias are particularly resistant to psychotherapy, hypnotherapy or aversion techniques and the social disadvantage that some of these conditions confer can be lifelong and psychologically very crippling.

PSYCHOSIS This is a true mental disorder. The neurotic may have seemingly odd ideas (the obsessional neurotic may, for example, wash his hands *before* as well as *after* using the lavatory) and he knows he does and will have what is to him a rational explanation. Nevertheless, he can be dissuaded by argument and discussion even though he may not stop doing whatever it is his obsession compels him to do. The psychotic, on the other hand, does not know that what he is doing or thinking is regarded by others as abnormal. Psychosis is 'madness' in the old sense of the term. We tend to use the word too lightly these days–'Oh, he's mad'–when we probably only mean he is neurotic.

The difference is readily apparent to some but confusion is still very common. It may help to say that both the neurotic and the psychotic build castles in the air, but it is only the psychotic who believes he lives in them (paying a rent, the cynical add, to the psychiatrist). The psychotic is not open to reason but the neurotic usually is.

The commonest psychosis is probably **manic-depressive psychosis**; the next commonest is probably **schizophrenia**. Depressive illness is very common but it is not often part of the manic-depressive psychosis. Depression–whether endogenous (i.e. arising without any obvious cause) or exogenous (i.e. apparently due to some outward event, such as a bereavement)–is, in fact, a neurosis although the depressive patient is not always as amenable

to reason as, for example, the patient with 'simple' anxiety neurosis. In recent years there have been considerable advances in the treatment of the various depressive illnesses by drugs, although these are much more useful in the endogenous types of depression than the exogenous or 'reactive' depressions.

True manic-depressive psychosis is relatively uncommon and is a psychosis not a neurosis. In the 'manic' phase a patient with this disorder often displays super-human effort and can achieve much in the days, months and sometimes years for which such states may last. Such people seem to have boundless energy, need very little sleep, are full of ideas and very talkative. This state may abruptly or slowly revert to the total opposite–inactivity, both mental and physical, black moods of despair and total lack of personal caring.

Psychosis may have an underlying organic cause–the delirium of high fever is an example of such a psychosis. The classic organic psychosis was the dementia resulting from untreated syphilis, the so-called GPI (General Paralysis of the Insane) from which probably at least one British monarch suffered. Today syphilis rarely goes untreated and GPI has been replaced by other organic dementias such as those resulting from the abuse of alcohol or addictive drugs.

GENERAL AILMENTS

Allergies, Anaemia, Diabetes, Epilepsy, Insomnia

In the preceding pages complaints relevant to a particular part or system of the body have been touched on. In this section we shall cover some common complaints that do not readily fit into a system based on anatomical or physiological considerations. For convenience, they will be discussed alphabetically.

ALLERGY An allergy can be described as the body's abnormal response to 'foreign matter'. In nine persons out of ten, a wasp or bee sting will produce an unpleasant, but purely local reaction to the foreign matter–that is, the material injected through the sting (in the case of the bee, the sting is left behind too). A red, painful swelling, which goes down in an hour or two or a day or two, soon follows but generally that is all. The tenth person will be less fortunate.

He will be allergic to the sting and in addition to the local swelling will have signs and symptoms which range from a generalized itchy rash (urticaria or 'hives') to a state of collapse, with a fall in blood pressure, wheezing, running nose and eyes and, rarely, heart arrest.

Allergies to many things have been identified, and the things are always proteins (complex molecules of organic matter) like, for example, grass pollen, house dust and animal fur and, of course, the stings of bee, hornet and wasp, also snake venoms. The allergen, i.e. the foreign material, doesn't have to be injected like the insect stings: it need only be *on* the skin, *on* the mucous lining of the nose or mouth or bronchial tubes, or *in* the food we eat.

Once identified the allergen can usually be avoided and in some cases used to prepare vaccines for desensitization. Such preparations are much used for hay fever sufferers and a course of desensitization can be obtained through the National Health Service. These materials are not truly vaccines but solutions of the allergen in varying concentrations which are used to 'educate' the body's immunological defence system to 'recognize' the allergen as a friend, not a foe, and react more peaceably towards it. With many hay fever sufferers this treatment works, although for them the body's immunological education is short-lived and a course of desensitization has to be gone through each year.

Food allergies have become of considerable interest in recent years and it is now known that gluten sensitivity (a disorder of the small intestine induced by a protein part of flour which can be totally corrected if gluten is excluded from the diet) is only one of many food intolerance syndromes that by a careful process can be diagnosed and treated. **Lactose intolerance** (lactose is a milk protein) is being increasingly recognized and indeed is widespread, almost universal among certain immigrant groups in the UK. There are a number of allergy treatments if the prime allergen cannot be avoided or if a course of densensitization is ineffective.

A relatively recent advance which has been most useful in the symptomatic treatment of **allergic rhinitis** (hay fever) and **asthma** is a drug which suppresses the abnormal response which is giving rise to the symptoms. The drug may be sprayed into the nose, inhaled or swallowed.

The investigation of allergic states is a job for the expert, but the field of food allergies has become a happy hunting ground for the food crank and dietary faddist. Allergy is capable of sound scientific rational investigation and its elucidation in a particular instance, although time-consuming, is rewarding because prevention is so much better than cure.

ANAEMIA This is a common condition with a variety of causes. Pallor does not necessarily mean anaemia although if the paleness is of the normally pink-looking membranes – the inside of the eyelid, the sides of the cheeks, the tongue –

then abnormal paleness may indicate anaemia. The condition is simply one of insufficient blood redness to give the skin and the mucous linings their normal healthy pink/red colour. But before this is noticed, other symptoms may become apparent such as tiredness, shortness of breath, rapid heart beat, palpitation and so on and medical advice may well be sought for these. Passing pallor – after a fright for instance – means no more than a decreased blood flow through the skin, a normal reflex to maximize the amount of blood going through heart, lungs and so on, in preparation for the emergency situation. The pallor following true shock, i.e. loss of blood from injury, is, of course, serious (see page 176).

If you think you are anaemic or your friends or relatives think you are, then a simple blood test will confirm or refute. If anaemia is confirmed, then it is essential to ascertain the precise cause. You may not be getting enough iron in your diet (or there may be enough but you have lost some of the capacity to absorb it or, if you absorb it, to utilize it to form haemoglobin, the pigment that gives you your healthy pink colour). Alternatively you may be bleeding slowly, but insidiously, from an ulcer in the alimentary tract, from piles, from polyps, or a growth. Again, hospital tests can usually pinpoint the problem and thus the right remedy be applied. Don't just go to your chemist and tell him you think you need iron. If there is slow bleeding and thus loss from the gut, adding more to the diet by a proprietary medicine or tablet would improve the anaemia temporarily but leave the underlying cause unchecked.

Iron preparations should never be taken except by prescription because serious disease can be masked in that way. It is essential to have a proper diagnosis made in this really quite common condition.

There are forms of anaemia which do not require iron at all, but special vitamins. **Pernicious anaemia** is one of these. It is a relatively common disease for which injections of vitamin B12 are the proper treatment; there is usually sufficient iron in the diet to make further iron supplement unnecessary.

DIABETES There are two general types of this disease, the full name for which is diabetes mellitus (a 'running through of sweetness'). One type affects the young; the other affects the middle-aged. In both the fault is one of failure of the body to utilize sugar for energy. Carbohydrates (that is, the starchy parts of the food we eat, including cane and other sugars) are large molecules which require chemically breaking down to smaller and simpler chemical compounds before they can be utilized to provide energy for all the body processes, such as growing, breathing, using muscles, and so on.

One of these simple chemicals is glucose. Glucose can be used immediately as an energy fuel or stashed away as a substance called glycogen which is a storage form of energy. Utilization of glucose, whether derived from glycogen or immediately from ingested foodstuff, requires insulin, a hormone (chemical messenger substance) and it is this hormone that the person with diabetes lacks, or of which he has a relatively low supply.

Diabetes is diagnosed by the finding of the special form of sugar (glucose) in the urine – a simple test which takes only seconds of the doctor's time and which can be carried out in the surgery. (Incidentally, the ancients who named the disease could only have discovered any sugar by actually tasting the urine of their patients.) If sugar is found in the urine, then a special investigation is carried out which follows the fate of a measured amount of sugar given by mouth as it is taken up and circulated in the blood stream. This is the glucose tolerance test, which requires attendance at a hospital or clinic so that blood samples can be taken and analysed at set intervals, usually hourly, for a matter of four to six hours. The normal person shows an initial rise of sugar level in the early blood samples which then falls rapidly as the sugar is picked up and stored in the liver. Levels fall to normal in three to four hours. In diabetes, the blood sugar level remains high, falling only very slowly during the time of the test.

Young, untreated diabetics lose weight, usually have an excessive thirst, pass a lot of urine, have a sweetish smell to the breath and may rapidly become seriously ill, falling into coma. Before the discovery of insulin in 1922, the disease was invariably fatal. Now, with daily or twice-daily injections of insulin, such patients can live virtually normal lives. Insulin does not cure the disease – indeed none of the many complications of it seem to be significantly affected – but replacing the failed hormone does avoid the weight loss, the excessive thirst and many other troubles. The patient's diet has to be more or less strictly controlled, matching the carbohydrate intake to the body's requirements for growth and activity and giving enough insulin to make proper use of the dietary intake of such foods. Crises can occur, nonetheless, and emergency advice is given on page 182.

The other form of diabetes is not associated with weight loss but usually with weight gain – this is the so-called **maturity-onset diabetes**, a disease, as the name suggests, of middle age or maturity. This type of diabetes does not usually require that the patient has injections of insulin for its control. All that is necessary for most patients is for them to diet under medical supervision. Some may need in addition anti-diabetic drugs which fortunately can be taken by mouth and need only be taken once or twice, rarely thrice, daily.

EPILEPSY The 'falling sickness' has been known for centuries. It is a disease characterized by fits which vary between brief moments of partial unconsciousness (which to the onlooker seem to be 'daydreaming') and episodes of quite violent limb, face and jaw twitchings during which the victim may injure himself or others and may also micturate or defaecate.

The 'daydreaming' type of episode is known as *Petit Mal* (the little sickness) and the more severe types of fit episode are known as *Grand Mal* attacks. The difference is probably only one of degree. The brain is very complex electrically, with many interdependent and interlocking circuits. In epilepsy the pattern of brain-waves as picked up by the sensitive device known as the electroencephalogram (EEG) is totally awry. Whether this is cause or effect brain physiologists are not sure. The prime upset may be a biochemical one and the disordered electrical activity may merely reflect those changes. For our purposes it doesn't matter, for the end result is the same.

A fit seen for the first time can be frightening for the onlooker. The patient is totally unaware of what is happening to him although he may have an 'aura' just before an attack. This is a warning signal which can be in the form of a visual disturbance, an unpleasant taste in the mouth or a peculiar smell which only the patient notices. After the attack, when the patient will have been totally oblivious of what is happening to him, he will usually be very exhausted and want to sleep. In fact, some attacks merge into normal sleep without an intervening period of wakening. Attacks can even occur at night during sleep and the only evidence in the morning may be a wet bed, a bitten tongue or objects knocked to the floor from a bedside table. For advice on what to do if you see a person having a fit, turn to page 183.

The cause of epilepsy remains a mystery. However, occasionally a fit may be a sign of a brain tumour or of an addiction to alcohol. The latter is a more common cause of fits than brain tumours. Epilepsy is one of the few medical conditions for which the barbiturate series of drugs is the treatment of choice. Of that series, phenobarbitone has been used for epilepsy for nearly seventy years or more. New anti-convulsant drugs have come along – phenytoin, for example – and these are sometimes used together with phenobarbitone or other barbiturates. If fits can be controlled by drugs (and they usually can) then the epileptic can live a normal useful life and even drive a car. A few patients have major severe and frequent fits and may need institutional care. The minor form of the disease *(Petit Mal)* is not uncommon in children and very often disappears in adolescence. Occasionally, the minor form becomes major in adult life.

INSOMNIA Like anaemia, insomnia is a symptom or sign, not a disease in itself – although it may became part and parccl of an anxiety neurosis or depressive illness. A vast amount of hypnotic drugs is consumed annually, most of which is probably quite unnecessary. Anxiety is a prime cause of insomnia and with so many anti-anxiety drugs at the doctor's disposal it is not surprising that these are prescribed in place of time-consuming consultations which are needed to identify, analyse and then eliminate the causes of the anxiety and thus relieve insomnia.

Myths about sleep abound. The eight-hour stint beloved of folklore is one of them. Some people do need eight hours, some more, many less. The waking hours may seem endless, but in the morning the insomniac, so-called, may feel absolutely fit and not in the least tired. The brain itself seems – unlike the body – not to need complete inactivity after all; in dreams it is very active, free-wheeling if you like, but nevertheless active. Bodily fatigue is conducive to sleep and it may be useful, if you have a sedentary occupation, to tire your body before retiring by means of a brisk walk, with or without the dog.

Sleep is a matter of habit, like defaecation. A warm, familiar bed (with a warm, familiar spouse) are the essentials; many people find that a strange bed, in hotels for instance, is not conducive to sleep unless fatigue is overwhelming. The use of sleeping tablets is widespread but some distinction must be made between the true hypnotics, i.e. the sleep producers, and the minor tranquillizers, i.e. the sleep inducers. In the former class are the barbiturates and similar drugs (chlorphenazone, chloral itself, and so on). Their action is virtually anaesthetic, their effect is cumulative, and in general they are habit-forming and potentially addictive. These drugs have very largely been supplanted by the tranquillizers, particularly of the benzodiazepine class of which Valium is the best known. These are not anaesthetic drugs in the doses used, may be habit-forming but are much less likely to induce true addiction than the barbiturates.

The occasional use of such drugs as nitrazepam (Mogadon), flunitrazepam (Dalmane) and dichloralphenazone (Welldorm) is acceptable; a sleep habit pattern broken by bereavement, anxiety or other stress may be helped to restoration in this way and the drugs can be discontinued eventually. In older patients these drugs may cause, or appear to cause, excessive dreaming not always of a pleasant nature. For such patients a small warm milk drink, with or without the added benefit of alcohol in the form of whisky or brandy, may be much better. Older people seem to need less sleep in any case and should be encouraged not to go to bed too early.

Don't rush to your doctor if you cannot sleep or seem not to be waking fully refreshed. Try and eliminate all the obvious and less obvious causes first – and try the non-drug methods first. Warmth, both outside and in (the hot drink, or a modicum of alcohol), restful music from a bedside radio, a good book read until it falls from your hands – all should be tried before getting a prescription for sleeping tablets.

CHILDREN'S ILLNESSES

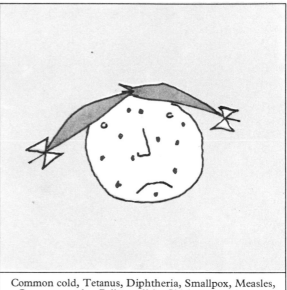

Common cold, Tetanus, Diphtheria, Smallpox, Measles, German measles, Poliomyelitis, Chickenpox, Mumps, Scarlet fever, Weight problems, Growth, Nervous problems

In terms of bacterial and viral threats, babies and young children are exposed to the same environmental hazards as adults, but because their mechanisms for developing immunity are relatively untested at such tender ages, their reactions to infection are very variable and, to some extent, unpredictable. Furthermore, they will meet specific viruses and bacteria for the first time, develop a typical disease and, if the immune functions *are* working properly, will develop virtually life-long immunity. Further contact with the particular germ responsible for the initial illness will be totally innocuous. The common childhood infections to which most adults are therefore immune are: chickenpox (varicella), measles (morbilli), german measles (rubella), whooping cough (pertussis) and poliomyelitis. We wish we could add to that list the common cold; let's deal with it first.

COMMON COLD Babies and young children are as prone as adults to infection with the common cold viruses, although the temporary immunity that one attack confers seems to last a little longer than in adults. Because the nasal air passages are not fully developed in the infant, sinus infections (usually caused by other bacteria which 'cash in' on the poor state of the nasal mucous membranes brought about by the cold viruses) are rare. However, the little tube which connects the middle ear to the throat (Eustachian tube) is not at this young age as effective a safety valve for the middle ear cavity as it is in adult life, and infections of the middle ear (otitis media) are very frequent complications of the common cold in infants.

Colds in young babies must not be ignored or shrugged off as 'just a head cold'. A fever, with or without a 'wet cough', is a common concomitant of the head cold and if the baby is feeding well and sleeping, can safely be ignored at least for a day or two. If in doubt, seek your doctor's advice.

Resist the temptation to give an antibiotic that happens to have been left in the medicine cupboard from some other time. Avoid cough remedies bought over the counter. Most babies most of the time get over colds very quickly.

Continued feverishness, loss of appetite, restlessness, crying, persistent cough, obvious breathing difficulty and poor colour are all signs that say: 'Get the doctor'. Don't let symptoms go on—the young patient can so soon become very ill. It is sensible to protect any infant when family colds are raging; protection doesn't mean coddling, but fresh air, good ventilation, avoiding sleeping in the same room, and mother—if she has a cold—wearing a mask when feeding, changing or bathing.

TETANUS, DIPHTHERIA AND SMALLPOX In addition to the list of common infections mentioned above, which confer immunity, we must add three that are rarely seen because prophylactic immunization has almost eliminated them. Indeed one *has* been eliminated. They are tetanus, diphtheria and smallpox. The first two are bacterial infections, the last viral. Tetanus and diphtheria vaccines have been in use for many years and both the diseases are now very rare. Not all the credit for the very low incidence of tetanus should go to the vaccine because improved hygiene, and the increased awareness of the danger of the soiled contaminated wound, have both played a part. (For further information about tetanus, see below.) As far as diphtheria is concerned, perhaps all the credit should go to the vaccine, although like the streptococcus, the diphtheria bacillus has lost some of its old-time virulence.

Diphtheria is still about, however, and immunization is recommended. It is a disease caused by a specific bacterium which attacks the throat and mucous linings of the nose and lungs, forming a tenacious membrane of mucus, dead bacteria and cells which coats the tissue and eventually chokes the victim to death. It was one of the earliest vaccines to be produced and its planned and widespread use has now virtually eliminated this dire disease from the UK and many other parts of the world.

Smallpox has been eradicated worldwide.* Indeed the World Health Organization has offered a monetary reward for anyone that can produce documented evidence of a single case. Nevertheless, such a deadly virus could make an unwelcome reappearance and vaccination is still a requirement for entry into many countries. Indeed visas for some countries will not be issued unless a valid certificate of vaccination is produced at the time. It is no longer official policy to vaccinate infants in the UK.

MEASLES A viral infection attacking the linings of the respiratory tract, it brings typically the symptoms of the common cold, followed rapidly by fever, cough and rash. Complications may occur, particularly otitis media (q.v.) and pneumonia. Vaccine is now available and is 80 per cent effective. There is no specific drug treatment and the routine use of antibiotics has not been shown to have any appreciable effect on the incidence of complications. The latter should be treated by a doctor when and if they arise.

GERMAN MEASLES This is another common viral infection which, although a very mild upset in itself, often only appearing as a rash with the very slightest of general malaise and therefore often missed, is capable of damaging an unborn baby if its mother has the misfortune to contract it early in her pregnancy. Fortunately, vaccination is now available and it is vital for every young girl who for certain has not had rubella in childhood to be vaccinated and thus protect her unborn children. Indeed, as one can never be absolutely sure whether the disease has occurred or not, unless there are documented medical records, it is best to be safe and vaccinate all girls in their early teens.

Although tests are available to detect rubella antibodies in the blood of young girls— and where there is doubt about a childhood episode this clearly must be done for any young women contemplating marriage or cohabitation —it is the duty of any parent of girl infants to make sure that any suspicious rubella-like rash is seen by a doctor and confirmed or refuted. No girl should reach child-bearing age without her being sure that rubella has been contracted or that immunization has, or will be, undertaken.

---

*That is to say, the virus does not seem to be around any more—except in special research laboratories, from one of which it recently escaped with tragic consequences.

POLIOMYELITIS A vigorous campaign of immunization, first with an injectable vaccine and then with an oral one, started in the late 1950s after the epidemics of the '40s and early '50s, and this virtually eliminated poliomyelitis ('polio') from the UK. Occasional cases still occur, the infection having been picked up when abroad.

The disease shows itself in many ways—headache, fever, breathing difficulties, photophobia (turning away from the light) and aching in the limbs which may become difficult to move. Diagnosis can usually be clinched by an examination of a sample of spinal fluid, obtained by lumbar puncture. The after-effects may vary from the permanent weakness or total paralysis of part of a limb to total paralysis of all four limbs or a paralysis of the muscles of respiration which will necessitate mechanical respiratory aid for life. There have been several epidemics, principally those of the 1940s and '50s, and some of the casualties from those periods still require mechanical ventilatory aids and live in 'Drinker' respirators (iron lungs). Self-styled 'responauts', such people cope marvellously well with their appalling handicap and are able with the aid of highly ingenious electronic gadgetry to live useful lives.

The disease is endemic (that is, is still around) in some countries and immunization is available to the traveller through the NHS.

TETANUS Tetanus (lockjaw) is a serious bacterial infection which can, like poliomyelitis, affect nerves and kill. The bacterium is found in many types of soil, particularly where horses and certain farm animals are to be found. It requires not just broken skin to get infected, but a wound which penetrates the deeper layers.

Lacerations, stab and gunshot wounds and open fractures are the common types of wound which favour the entry and multiplication of the tetanus bacillus. Children are no more prone to the disease than adults, but it is included in this section because, like diphtheria, tetanus immunization given in infancy has done much to reduce the incidence of this very unpleasant disease.

Tetanus must not be confused with tetany, which is a symptom characterized by muscle spasms of a very different type, due not to bacterial or viral infection but to a number of diseases which change the balance of minerals, particularly calcium, circulating in the blood stream.

WHOOPING COUGH This is a bacterial disease which is still common, although reasonably effective immunization is available. Spasmodic cough, with a rapid intake of air between spasms (which cause the 'whoop') during a feverish illness should immediately raise the parent's suspicions. For the young infant, the disease is fraught with complications such as pneumonia, which can lead to some degree of permanent lung damage and consequent disability. Unfortunately, the uptake of immunization has fallen off in recent years because of the adverse publicity this vaccine has had through its rare association with brain damage.

If your baby has not been protected and develops whooping cough, it is imperative to have the doctor in, however mild the symptoms appear to be. Some infants don't develop the classical whoop, but vomiting with a cough is a further indication. Infants under the age of about six months are particularly vulnerable to the infection and it is in them that complications may readily occur.

CHICKENPOX is caused by the same virus as that associated with shingles (herpes zoster). Primary infection with the chickenpox virus at any age causes chickenpox; reactivation at some later stage of the virus, which may have lain dormant in the body since childhood, produces shingles. If an adult who has never had shingles, and did not have chickenpox as a child, comes into contact with a child with chickenpox (or an adult with shingles), he is much more likely to get chickenpox than shingles.

Chickenpox is usually a mild infection although the rash is irritating and scratching can easily produce secondary infection. Complications are rare. Soothing lotion such as calamine may be useful, and cortisone preparations, taken by mouth, are sometimes prescribed. Don't be tempted to use anti-histamine creams (see section on Skin). Adults who contract chickenpox often have a pretty bad time—the general effects can be most uncomfortable and the patient can become quite ill.

MUMPS Another virus infection, mumps, shows itself by enlargement of the parotid glands (just below the ear, over the jaw joint, in front of the bony protruberance known as the mastoid process) which can become quite gross. The appearance is that of a swollen face and neck, and it is painful. There is no treatment; the disease is self-limiting but it is infectious until the swellings have gone down.

There are two important complications of mumps—orchitis and encephalitis. Orchitis—swelling of one or both testicles—is the commoner complication and requires that the child (or indeed adult) be kept at rest in bed. Occasionally, mumps orchitis leads to sterility. Encephalitis is very uncommon but nevertheless a very serious complication if it does occur. High fever, headache, delirium, unconsciousness or partial loss of awareness are worrying signs. A doctor must be called in.

SCARLET FEVER is included because of its historical interest. The particular germ responsible is a species of streptococcus which has apparently lost its virulence over the years. Scarlet fever produces a typical all-over rash, high fever and headache. Before sulphonamides, penicillin and the later antibiotics, this illness was serious, for complications – usually in the form of nephritis (infection of the kidneys) – were common. Fortunately, the other streptococcal-associated diseases – erysipelas, rheumatic fever and the 'strep' throat – have virtually all disappeared.

WEIGHT PROBLEMS There is no doubt that patterns of obesity are laid down in early childhood. The fat podgy toddler rarely turns into a slim adult, but the skinny, spare child may become obese in his teens. Overweight is more unwelcome from a health point of view than underweight. How can we stop our children getting fat? Here are four courses of action.

1 When weaning, don't overdo the cereal. All the pre-packed, almost-ready-to-serve baby cereals are so convenient, but so fattening. A balanced diet is as important for the baby as it is for the toddler, the infant and the schoolchild as it is for all of us. For the meaning of a 'balanced diet' see Part 2(a) 'Eating Well'.

2 Get them out of the 'sweet habit'. The occasional reward is OK but more than that is not. Some might protest that it's easier said than done – but is it? The parent sets the behaviour of the child. Non-smoking parents rarely have trouble in dissuading their children from taking up the habit. Likewise the non-sweet-eating, non-stodge-stacking, non-gannet parents will find their children will follow suit without badgering.

3 Look to your own diet pattern and the child's will be less likely to be abnormal. Indeed, look to your own weight, you may have a problem anyway. Starch and sugar are the arch enemies of the slim. The sweet-toothed child is easily bred. Encourage an appreciation of the less sweet, the more savoury. Do not reward good behaviour with a promise of cake for tea or a bag of sweets tomorrow. If you don't eat cake, or sweets, or take an excessive amount of biscuits, then neither will your child want to do so.

4 Encourage physical activity. For the toddler, encouragement is probably not necessary, for the healthy ones never seem to be still. But at school, encourage participation in sport; it helps too if the parents take part. The garden football with dad, the family swim or cycle ride – all are some of the essential ingredients of healthy living. The others are (and we make no apology for reiteration) a balanced diet and a reasonable amount of sleep.

What if, in spite of everything you try, your child is podgy, fat and idle? Don't shrug your shoulders and say, 'It's all glands anyway'. Seek advice. Much research has gone into the causes of child obesity in recent years and there are many centres with clinics for just such problems. Treatment can be long and difficult, but is utterly worth it in the long run.

The skinny child, other things being equal (that is to say, no recent obvious weight loss and an apparently normal appetite) is best left alone, teased though he may be at school or by fussing relatives. As with adults, the thin are usually much, much fitter than the fat – although to inexperienced eyes they don't always look it.

GROWTH is a different matter. Whether thin or fat, if you think your child is small for his age, it is as well to check. Doctors have tables which have been laboriously compiled over many years from measurements of thousands of children in all age groups from birth to 18. Such tables set the pattern of the 'normal range', and the growth rate to be expected at any age. Weight and height increase do not run in a straight-line gradient from birth to manhood. The initial weight gain is rapid (a baby normally doubles its weight within five months) and if that rate were maintained we should not be able to move at all by the age of 10. By one year, the weight is only about three times the birth weight. The baby's height (usually referred to as length) doesn't increase so drastically. At five months it will have increased by about a third but then at a year it is only about half as much again as its birth length. This is why the one-year-old looks so chubby.

Weight and height increase fairly evenly during infancy and early childhood, but this phase is followed by a fairly sharp increase of rate at puberty – the so-called 'adolescent spurt'. It is a matter of common observation, and it has been confirmed by the painstaking and methodical observations referred to above. This increase in weight and height is also shown in diagram form on the facing page.

The black lines show the mean height or weight for any given age; the shaded areas demonstrate the range of normal around that mean figure. Statistically, the limits of what can be termed normal range can be calculated and are used to determine whether this or that weight/height is 'abnormal'. Observations made over months or years can thus determine the normality or otherwise of actual growth.

The first thing to establish therefore is whether weight or height seems to lie outside the ranges indicated. This decision can be left to your doctor although it is not difficult to use the charts provided you can weigh and measure your infant fairly accurately. The bathroom scales are notoriously unreliable; conversely, the time-honoured carving knife notch in the door, planted carefully therein after being slid horizontally across the top of the head while the child is standing bare-footed with his back to

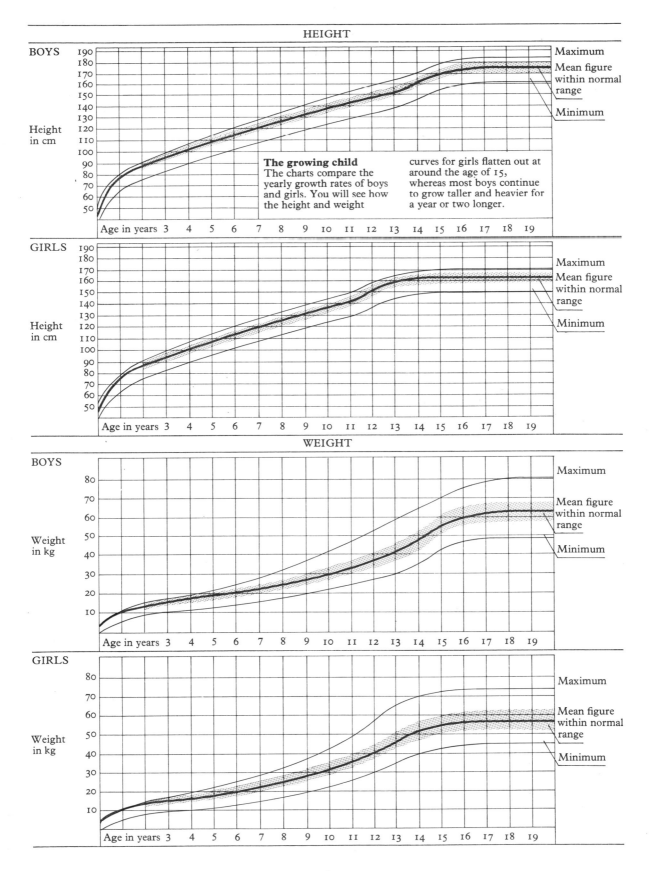

HEIGHT

BOYS

Height in cm

Age in years 3 4 5 6 7 8 9 10 11 12 13 14 15 16 17 18 19

Maximum

Mean figure within normal range

Minimum

The growing child
The charts compare the yearly growth rates of boys and girls. You will see how the height and weight curves for girls flatten out at around the age of 15, whereas most boys continue to grow taller and heavier for a year or two longer.

GIRLS

Height in cm

Age in years 3 4 5 6 7 8 9 10 11 12 13 14 15 16 17 18 19

Maximum

Mean figure within normal range

Minimum

WEIGHT

BOYS

Weight in kg

Age in years 3 4 5 6 7 8 9 10 11 12 13 14 15 16 17 18 19

Maximum

Mean figure within normal range

Minimum

GIRLS

Weight in kg

Age in years 3 4 5 6 7 8 9 10 11 12 13 14 15 16 17 18 19

Maximum

Mean figure within normal range

Minimum

the door, has much to recommend it,
particularly if dates are scratched alongside the
various levels. Father may take a dim view of
the trauma to his paintwork, but the resulting
record is of value and interest, especially to a
large family.

Graphs like those shown are available
through any good medical bookseller. Parents
can then document their children's growth *and*
compare it with standard patterns.

NERVOUS PROBLEMS As every parent
knows, children are highly sensitive to
atmosphere. Only rarely does one find an
unhappy child in a happy home, practically
never a happy child in an unhappy home.
Before rushing to the doctor because Johnny is
not sleeping, not eating, biting his fingernails,
wetting the bed, crying at the slightest thing,
not playing with toys, showing aggressive
trends, withdrawing into himself, not talking –
indeed showing any signs of 'abnormal'
behaviour – look to the family relationships,
between you and your husband, him and the
child (or other children), you and the child (or
other children), and anyone else (like Granny)
who is sharing the home with you.

Children of all ages need to feel
secure. Anything which appears to threaten
that security will be a threat to the child. A
father who is never seen by his children because
he is a beaver, rushing here and there in the
world, working late, leaving early before the
children are awake and being just a weekend
dad, is a threat, willy-nilly, to that child's very
important need to know that he has a mum and
a dad; and he desperately needs both. The
single-parent child may know no better, but
when aware that his friends have a mum and a
dad, he too will feel deprived and insecure.

Children are as subject to neuroses
(q.v.) as are their parents, although the
manifestations of depression, anxiety and fear
are rather different. Behavioural problems can
be very complex and occasionally will need the
professional attentions of a child psychiatrist or
of the Child Guidance Clinic. See your doctor
first; it is important not to allow abnormal
patterns of behaviour to continue, although
many are self-limiting.

One of the most common is bed
wetting. By the age of three, most children
have achieved adequate control over their
bladders; nearly 90 per cent are totally
continent by about the age of four and a half,
and at least 95 per cent are so by the age of
seven. Occasionally, bed-wetting is due to some
organic cause (urethral stricture and some
congenital abdominal deformities), but 90 per
cent of cases are psychological. Medical advice
should always be sought if your child is not dry
at night most of the time by the age of five or
six.

MALE DISORDERS

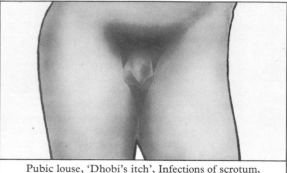

Pubic louse, 'Dhobi's itch', Infections of scrotum,
Blockage of urinal passage

The male genitalia, being almost wholly
external, are very vulnerable as every schoolboy
soon learns. A blow on the testicles from a ball
or the toe of a football boot (or, usually later in
life, the well-aimed knee of a threatened
woman) is excruciatingly painful and can be
incapacitating for hours, if not days. Apart from
trauma – from which, of course, the organs can
be protected – the other threat is that of
infection. The skin covering the genitals is just
as prone to bacterial and fungal infection as the
rest of the body. The pubic hair in both sexes is
as prone to infestation by the louse as is the
head or axillary hair; the creatures differ slightly
(although their effects are similar). The head
and axillary louse are known as *pediculis capitis*
and *pediculis corporis* respectively and the one
with a preference for the pubes is the *pediculis
pubis*. They all (that is, the female of the species)
lay eggs on the hairs to which they are firmly
stuck with an insect-world adhesive which is
pretty resistant to water. One way to be rid of
such creatures and their eggs is to shave the hair
completely and burn it. Another is to apply
preparations at regular intervals that kill the
insects and also catch the newly hatched ones
before they can lay eggs. In spite of the
generally better hygienic habits of the civilized
world the head, body and pubic louse are still
about, although such infestations are usually
only associated with overcrowding in poor
surroundings and with inadequate laundering
of bedclothes.

There is a fungus, too, with a
predilection for that area – *tinea cruris*, which
finds warmth and comfort on the skin of the
thighs and to some extent on the scrotal skin as
well. This is the so-called 'dhobi's itch' – in the
days of the Raj, the sahibs' ill-laundered pants
would come back from the dhobi, or laundry
boy, with a quota of tinea ready for invading
that delicate white skin. Treatment of louse
infestation and of fungal infection is a matter for

expert attention although there are proprietary anti-fungals readily available. In general, all skin irritations, lesions and rashes affecting the external genitals in both sexes should not be left for your or a friend to treat; always consult a doctor.

The contents of the scrotum—the testes and their appendages—are, apart from being prone to trauma, also very prone to infection. If the scrotum itself or the testes seem swollen and painful, don't try and decide for yourself whether it is the testicle itself, or fluid in the scrotum or a rupture—see your doctor as soon as possible.

Cystitis is uncommon in the male but frequency and pain on micturition or the passage of blood or mucus demand immediate attention. Prostatitis or prostatism are common over the age of 55 or so. This affects the prostate gland which lies below the male bladder. The early signs indicate partial obstruction of the urethra, the urinary passage which runs from the bladder to the outside world. Thus a poor stream, dribbling, difficulty in starting, overlong micturition, frequency and getting up at night are all signs of enlargement of the gland which call for advice. Very occasionally total obstruction to the passage of urine occurs. The bladder extends enormously, making the patient more and more uncomfortable, but yet no urine can be passed. This is an emergency and a doctor must be called. If there is a delay some comfort can be had from lying or sitting the patient in a warm bath; indeed, not infrequently this has the effect of allowing urine to be passed, although without emptying the bladder. It does not mean that the doctor is after all not necessary. No man should ever experience more than one attack of acute retention, which is what this particular episode is called.

FEMALE PROBLEMS

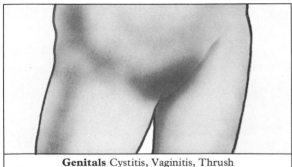

Genitals Cystitis, Vaginitis, Thrush
Reproductive tract Menstruation pains, Premenstrual tension
Pregnancy Nutritional problems, Home/hospital delivery
Breasts Lumps, Breast cancer

Women carry not only our children but the burden of a complex reproductory system which, like any other complex system, has an infinite capacity for going wrong. There are no physicians or surgeons specializing in disorders peculiar to men, only to women—gynaecologists and obstetricians. The male reproductive organs seldom give much trouble. Furthermore, once the male has embarked on his reproductive life he stays on it more or less until he drops; the female, once entered, undergoes all the changes peculiar to pregnancy, and then has to go through a fundamental change at the end of her reproductive life—the menopause. It is no wonder that there are doctors who spend their professional lifetimes looking after women.

Here we are committed only to the common problems. These are best classed as problems related to the genital organs themselves, the reproductive tract (the uterus and its appendages) and the breasts.

GENITALS The external genitals of the female are obviously less vulnerable than the male's, at least to trauma. However, the female urethra—the outlet from the bladder—is much shorter than the male and this makes her more prone to bouts of **cystitis** than him. Bacteria can very easily ascend the relatively short tube from the outside world and gain access to the bladder where they multiply and infect the bladder linings. The commonest organism to do this is the *bacillus coli* that normally lives in the lower bowel and rectum, causing no disturbance and certainly no infection. However, the journey from anus to urethral opening is not long and faulty hygiene would help to make that journey easier. Cystitis not infrequently follows sexual intercourse and in the days when couples were more commonly celibate before marriage than they are now, cystitis was a not infrequent occurrence in the first few days after the ceremony; indeed it was, and still is, termed 'honeymoon cystitis'.

The symptoms of cystitis, whatever the cause, are frequency, painful passing of urine and occasional bleeding. If drinking copious bland fluids—fruit drinks, mineral waters and the like—doesn't cure the problem then you should see your doctor. Prevention means good vulval hygiene and good sense with tights and pants. Nylon seems an almost inevitable choice for both of these but remember that nylon doesn't 'breathe'. Keep warm but not sweaty; change frequently. Repeated attacks of cystitis can be very troublesome and you should seek advice. There is a world-wide association for sufferers of cystitis and other urinary and vaginal disorders. This is the U and I Club, 9e Compton Road, Islington, London, N1. Advice and information, particularly on how to avoid the infection, can be obtained from this organization.

Vaginitis is also common. The symptoms are irritation and a discharge. There is always some secretion from a healthy vagina – its internal surfaces are in contact and have to be lubricated by a mucus secretion – which in some women can be quite copious. That's normal. An offensive discharge, a frothy white or a creamy yellow one spells infection with bacteria or, much more commonly, with a fungus or with a minute single-celled parasite. The fungus is usually *candida albicans* or *monilia* – known as **thrush**. Thrush infections occur elsewhere in the body, such as the mouth and anus. A frothy white discharge is typical of thrush but it is essential to have a proper diagnosis. See your doctor, who may well send you to a gynaecological clinic where there are, of course, special facilities for rapid, accurate diagnosis. Treatment is straightforward. Don't buy pessaries or any other self-treatment remedies. Thrush tends to recur and can become quite difficult to treat; the earlier you are seen, the better.

The parasite – really a protozoon, a primitive animal – is the *trichomonas vaginalis*. It is now known that both monilial and trichomonal infection can be classed among the sexually transmitted diseases although the infection can and does frequently occur in the absence of any sexual activity. A creamy discharge is an indicator of trichomonal infection and, as with any vaginal infection, accurate diagnosis is important. You must get expert advice and have the correct treatment. Both these common vaginal infections can now be treated with oral medicines – the messy douches, the gentian violet paintings and the pessaries are more or less things of the past although they may have to be used in addition.

REPRODUCTIVE TRACT In the natural biological order of things, a woman would probably never menstruate because she would always either be pregnant or breast-feeding her children. However, we are far removed from the natural biological order of things, women have fewer children and they are spaced out, with years of menstruation sandwiched between pregnancies. True, menstruation in a woman not taking the oral contraceptive pill is natural enough, but in the pill-taker the 'period' is nothing more than 'withdrawal bleeding' – the result of lowering the blood level of the hormones that the pill provides for the best part of the month.

Dysmenorrhoea – painful menstruation – is a common gynaecological complaint but the widespread use of the oral contraceptive pill has reduced its incidence quite markedly. **Premenstrual tension** (or premenstrual syndrome, as most gynaecologists prefer to call it) is also a common complaint, but, again, use of the contraceptive pill very often ameliorates the condition or even dispenses with it altogether. So, for the benefit of readers not familiar with the oral contraceptive, we include a summary of these two conditions.

Dysmenorrhoea is typically a pain in the lower abdomen which occurs during menstruation and often just before it as well. The end of the period sees the end of the dysmenorrhoea. The pain can be severe, and a day in bed once a month is quite normal for some young girls. The cause is unknown but there is undoubtedly a psychological element in most instances. Dysmenorrhoea is not common among married women or in those who are living with a boyfriend or at least 'sleeping around'; in each case sexual activity seems to be active therapy and the birth of the first child cures nine cases out of ten. However, not everyone is agreed that sexual activity should be prescribed for dysmenorrhoea and one has to fall back on simple measures which do not require the assistance of a partner.

Perhaps the most important of these is to minimize the attention usually paid to the monthly inconvenience; much dysmenorrhoea seems to be the direct result of wrong maternal attitudes. Homely remedies abound – the hot bath, laxatives, alcohol and total bed-rest. Simple analgesics such as paracetamol and aspirin may be all that is required, but some patients may need a specialist's opinion to decide whether there is an abnormality (such as a congenital defect) which needs a surgical operation or whether a simple treatment to stretch the neck of the womb, the procedure known as 'dilation and curettage', or 'D & C', will be all that is necessary.

Premenstrual tension consists of a variety of symptoms (but very few signs) which arise in the few days before the period and are relieved by the appearance of the menstrual flow. The symptoms may be just of bloating, swollen ankles, tender breasts, headache, nausea, actual vomiting, irritability and depression (but seldom, if ever, tears), insomnia and loss of libido. There is usually a heightened tension and impatience with the rest of the family, who may suffer as much as the sufferer herself.

Much has been written about premenstrual tension in recent years and at least one London teaching hospital has a special clinic for patients referred by their GP. The condition is quite successfully treated, either by small doses of oral diuretic (a drug which helps to rid the body of excess water), hormones, vitamin B6 and, least successful of all, tranquillizers. The symptoms are thought to be due to an imbalance of the hormones concerned with initiating the menstrual cycle and, to some extent, to a mild degree of oedema (water retention in tissue).

Depression is a not uncommon part of this syndrome. Recent research has implicated a disorder of the metabolism of vitamin B6 in some patients which seems to be corrected by giving that vitamin in moderate doses by mouth daily from mid-cycle to the onset of menstruation. Although married life and having children has put paid to some of the gynaecological problems of the unmarried and childless, pregnancy itself, the child-bearing years and the menopause are often associated with troubles, both minor and major. A few are discussed here.

PREGNANCY Once pregnancy is confirmed, good ante-natal care is essential if the mother's health, the actual birth and the health of the infant are to be trouble-free. In no other branch of medicine is prevention of such importance. Ante-natal care is directed towards monitoring both the mother's general health and the infant's development *in utero*.

As far as the mother's general health is concerned, perhaps the most important single factor is nutrition. The developing foetus is a parasite and as such has first call on the food supply which, of course, it can only get from its mother. If the mother herself is on a marginal intake of nutrients it is she who will suffer malnutrition, not the baby. The first common problem of pregnancy is a nutritional one and the commonest dietary constituent which the mother may go short of is iron. Measurement of the amount of iron circulating in the blood is one of the most important things done with that first specimen of blood which is taken at the ante-natal clinic or by your doctor on his confirmation of pregnancy. Many women start their pregnancies in a state of relative iron deficiency and the prescription of oral iron tablets (almost universal during the war years) is most important.

It is a common fallacy that it is necessary to eat for two when pregnant but it is essential to eat the right things. It is well known that, especially in earlier pregnancy, some women develop odd tastes and cravings, and if these are for the starchy foods it is all too easy to put on more weight than is appropriate during pregnancy. Some weight gain (over and above that due to the steady growth of the 3.5–4 kg of new life within the mother to be) is inevitable, but obesity must be avoided. Appetite often increases and the extra intake that naturally follows should be 'across the board' of a good mixed diet (see also page 60). If in doubt, don't hesitate to talk to your doctor about it.

The development of the foetus is traditionally monitored by manual estimation of the growth of the uterus and its comparison with the foetal age of its contents, as calculated from the known date of the last menstrual period. In this way, underdevelopment can be detected ('small for dates') and also overdevelopment – which usually means not a bigger-than-expected baby but a multiple pregnancy, in most cases twins.

Towards the end of pregnancy ante-natal examination should be more frequent, in the hope of thus avoiding complications in the labour. There have been many advances in techniques of pre-natal diagnosis; indeed pre-natal paediatrics has become a sub-speciality. The pre-natal paediatrician will normally work closely with the obstetrician responsible for overseeing the delivery.

Some congenital abnormalities can be detected by examination of a sample of the amniotic fluid – the liquid that surrounds the foetus in its placental sac in the uterus. This can be obtained in the latter weeks without disturbing the pregnancy. Ultrasound examination can be used instead of X-rays to confirm the suspicion of multiple birth.

The 'home versus hospital' debate for the actual birth continues but the choice remains a personal one, guided by your doctor. In very general terms, it is better to have your first baby in a hospital or nursing home, and if that turns out to be straightforward then you can certainly consider home for the next. Much depends on what emergency facilities are available in your area and what your own doctor thinks will be best for you and the baby. Having a baby at home is usually less upsetting for the rest of the family, allows them to enjoy the event and feel that having a baby is not an illness to be treated in hospital. If the birth is straightforward, what better place to be than in your own bed and home?

But there are no hard and fast rules and one cannot generalize. Unless there are cogent medical reasons for being in the maternity wing of a hospital, then plump for home if your doctor is prepared to be present at the birth. But remember not all general practitioners in the NHS are on what is known as the 'obstetric list'. To remain on that list a doctor must be experienced in midwifery, have continuing experience and be up to date with developments in obstetrics.

BREASTS The female breast is very responsive to the regular hormonal changes of the menstrual cycle and it is a matter of common observation that enlargement occurs and tenderness is felt in the few days before a normal menstrual period. Note the word 'normal'. If you are taking oral contraceptives then the period is not normal and you will not notice those breast changes. Note too that breast enlargement and tenderness, with or without a feeling of warmth or tingling, are also early signs of pregnancy, and if such feelings in any month are *not* followed by a period then probably you are pregnant. However, the sign is unreliable and, of course, if a period is missed you must have a urine test to be sure if you are pregnant or not.

Lumpiness of the breast, which may be discovered while bathing or on regular or casual self-examination, is common in women who have had children or who are overweight. This is usually 'chronic mastitis', which is not a malignant condition. The finding of a single lump in the breast is always alarming but remember that by no means all lumps are malignant—that is, are cancers. Obviously, if you find a lump you must go to your doctor because if it is cancer then the earlier it is treated the better. In recent years there have been significant advances in the early detection of breast cancers by special forms of X-ray examination (mammography), and in some areas clinics specialize in screening for breast cancer in this way.

A skilled surgeon can usually say whether a particular lump is likely to be malignant or not, but when there is doubt, both in the doctor's mind or on mammographic examination, the assumption has to be that it is malignant and surgical treatment must be advised. This does not mean automatically that the breast must be removed (mastectomy) and there are other options. A biopsy may be taken (a biopsy is the removal of a piece of tissue for microscopical examination) and examined immediately while the patient is still in the operating theatre and the decision taken there and then about treatment. This would either be to leave well alone, to remove the lump from the breast (lumpectomy), to remove the breast alone (simple mastectomy), or to remove it together with its surrounding lymph glands and the underlying muscle of the chest wall (radical mastectomy). While treatment of breast cancer remains predominantly surgical, other methods such as deep X-ray and anti-cancer drugs are used, usually after surgery to treat any tissue adjacent to the removed breast in which there might be dormant cancer cells. As with any cancer anywhere in the body, early detection and treatment are of vital importance.

VENEREAL DISEASES

Syphilis, Gonorrhoea, Non- specific urethritis (NSU)

Venereal disease is now very common—the new morality (a euphemism for promiscuity) has seen to that. There are three common diseases—syphilis, gonorrhoea and non-specific urethritis (NSU); as a group they are often referred to as the sexually transmitted diseases or STD. For advice on sexual hygiene, see page 106.

Syphilis begins, usually, as a small ulcerating type of lesion which may occur anywhere on the body, not necessarily on the penis, the vulva or in the vagina—although these latter sites are by far the most common. It is a painless lesion and feels bigger than it looks. It is called the primary chancre. Left to itself the chancre will usually appear to get better in one or two months although it always leaves a scar. It was this character of the chancre which made syphilis such a menace before widespread awareness of its dangers became known through propaganda and health campaigns. The healing of the chancre meant nothing more than that the bacteria had left that site for other parts of the body, invading blood vessels, nerves and brain, and the disease would last anything from five to twenty years or more.

This is not the place to detail the stages of this disease; in any case the majority of patients who contract it get treated early and are cured. Rarely does the disease go untreated and pursue its relentless course. Forty or more years ago many beds in our mental hospitals were taken up by patients suffering from the final psychoneurological form of the illness—general paralysis of the insane (GPI).

The treatment is penicillin. In the first early infectious stage—the primary lesion—one massive dose by injection will usually suffice with perhaps a repeat dose after a couple of weeks.

Never, never attempt to treat yourself with penicillin or anything else. First of all accurate diagnosis is essential, and secondly, once a diagnosis has been made and the correct treatment applied, a follow-up examination and blood test are essential to be sure that the disease has been totally eradicated.

Gonorrhoea is much commoner than syphilis but is a more difficult disease to identify and to eradicate. Two-thirds of women with the disease have no symptoms at all, or at most quite trivial ones which may be passed off as cystitis or as an apparently harmless vaginal discharge. One woman can infect many men. In the male the usual symptom is a discharge from the tip of the penis, although in either sex it may be confined to the rectum. Like syphilis, treatment if begun early is totally curative, and again penicillin is the drug usually employed.

The importance of early advice when a sexually transmitted disease is suspected cannot be overemphasized. It is also vital to return for tests both in syphilis and in gonorrhoea to ensure cure. Neglected gonorrhoea can lead to endless troubles and misery and, in women especially, permanent sterility. The male and female urethra can also be infected during intercourse with viruses and bacteria other than the specific bacterium causing gonorrhoea (gonococcus). These agents give rise to what in these days is probably the commonest form of STD, a group of diseases clumped together for want of a better name as non-specific urethritis (NSU) or non-gonococcal urethritis (NGU). Treatment is in general rather unsatisfactory and relapses are very common.

There are a number of other sexually transmitted diseases but these need not be discussed here. The message should be clear—any suspicious lesion or discharge occurring at any time from two to ten days (for gonorrhoea) or three to four weeks (for syphilis) after intercourse needs serious attention and a visit to your doctor or to any of the special clinics held in most major cities in the UK. The sentence 'delay can be dangerous' is *not* an overstatement.

HOME MEDICINE CUPBOARD

Wherever you decide to keep your bottles of aspirin or paracetamol—the bathroom cupboard is the usual, but the *worst* possible place—make sure that if there are young children in the house they can't reach it or, if they can, that it cannot be opened. Do not forget that the humble aspirin is a poisonous drug if taken in quantity and it is especially poisonous to children. We apologize for the reiteration—but **PLEASE, PLEASE KEEP ALL MEDICINES SAFELY OUT OF CHILDREN'S WAY.**

Why is the bathroom cupboard a bad place? Quite apart from accessibility to children, as a storage area it is unsuitable because it is warm and damp. Heat and moisture are damaging to tablets and medicines however well you think they are corked up. Your bedroom or your landing are the best places—but the cupboard must be lockable wherever it is, or in some other way be made child-proof.

What to keep in it? More accidents occur in the home than anywhere else, so obviously the first items are those you'll need for **first aid** (see page 189 for a reasonable list). You can't possibly cater for every emergency. The commonest accidents in the home are burns, scalds and cuts—so a reasonable stock of clean dressings makes sense for a start.

For the rest, you need to be able to treat minor illnesses without rushing to the telephone to ask your doctor's advice. What are these minor illnesses likely to be? Here is a list alongside which are the simplest home remedies which are worth keeping. Remember always that whatever you are treating you are doing so

on a temporary basis, and if improvement doesn't occur in a reasonable time then, of course, you must seek your doctor's advice.

Headache
Aspirin tablets (soluble are the best). Paracetamol tablets (you can also get the soluble variety).

Coughs and Colds
Gee's Linctus (only a palliative, but a safe one). Aspirin and paracetamol (listed above), and perhaps one of the proprietary cold remedies, e.g. Coldrex, which if used sensibly according to the manufacturer's instructions can give quite good relief from the early symptoms of the common cold.

Indigestion
Antacid tablets or mixtures, e.g. Milk of Magnesia. There are many brands of antacid tablet and your pharmacist will advise you about these.

Tummy Upsets
Kaolin mixture (without the 'morph'). A mild aperient, e.g. Eno's or Andrew's.

And that is really about all. Please note—no antibiotics, no anti-histamine creams or tablets. As a general rule if any prescribed medicine is not totally used up it should be thrown out or returned to the pharmacist. Never give prescribed medicines to anyone other than the person for whom they were originally prescribed even though you know, or think you know, that his or her symptoms are the same and therefore the medicine or tablets will do just as well.

In general, don't keep tablets or medicines more than two years from the original date of purchase. Some proprietary medicines carry an expiry date on the label. If not, then it makes sense to write on the date when you buy it.

TAKING TEMPERATURES You can if you wish keep a **clinical thermometer** in the cupboard. It is a precision instrument for registering body temperature and has a constriction in the fine glass tube to stop the mercury going down as soon as you take it from the patient's mouth; it has to be shaken down each time it is used—which is how most get broken.

Cheap, convenient and unbreakable **temperature strips** are now available from pharmacies and are really all you need. Placed on the patient's brow, the strip gives a clear 'read-out' after a few seconds—either the letter 'N' (for Normal) appears or actual figures, usually in centigrade. They cost less than £1 (in 1980), can be used many times and are accurate enough for home use. Unless you already have a clinical thermometer we suggest you buy a temperature strip. Remember though, it is far better to try and judge the degree of illness than the degree of fever.

PART 4

ACCIDENTS

AND

FIRST AID

A-Z REFERENCE GUIDE

In this section the conditions needing first aid are given in alphabetical order for quick reference. However, the avoidance of shock heads the list, and should be read before any of the individual conditions, since it applies to all severe injuries.

Note that *first* aid aims to stop your patient's condition from worsening and perhaps to save life. It is not treatment proper, which is *second* aid and a matter for a nurse or doctor.

In this book there is room only for an outline of the important measures, and it is not feasible here to try and teach the complexities of, for example, cardiac massage. For a more detailed grounding in first aid it is well worthwhile that at least one member of every family learn the subject thoroughly by attending one of the many easy and interesting courses organized in the UK by the St John's Ambulance Association, the British Red Cross or (in Scotland) the St Andrew's Association. Your telephone book will give the address of the nearest branch or you can contact their headquarters for further information. The address of each is listed in the Summary on page 207.

Please now read and learn the following sections: Artificial Respiration, Bleeding, Choking, Electric Shock and Poisoning. All these are emergencies with which you should be ready to cope immediately at any time, without having to look them up.

AVOIDING SHOCK

All major injuries like bleeding, wounds, burns and fractures can bring about shock. In medicine this word does not mean simply emotional upset. It is a very definite physical condition in which the heart and circulation progressively lose power. The patient, whose system at first may seem to be weathering the situation, and who may even show signs of restlessness, gradually becomes pale and cold, drowsy, perhaps comatose or even unconscious. The speed of this collapse varies very much with the severity of the damage.

Whenever someone has been badly injured you must, as well as giving specific help, apply measures to arrest or to reduce the shock process. They are extremely simple, but do not let the fact that they are easy to remember mask their importance.

1 **Move the patient as little as possible.** Unless it is dangerous to do this (e.g. a house on fire) attend to him on the spot, and keep him there until help (doctor or ambulance) arrives.

2 **Position him** lying down so that his head is kept low and his feet are raised. This helps the circulation to favour his heart, lungs and brain. Naturally you will have to use judgment and (by far the lesser of two evils) avoid shifting the position of any part which may be fractured. See also the description of the Recovery Position on page 188.

3 **Loosen any tight clothing** such as braces, belt, collar, corset. This not only improves comfort, but eases breathing.

4 **Keep him warm** by laying a blanket, coat or other available cover loosely over him. Should he be lying on a cold surface, have protection under him as well. But *never* use hot water bottles; added heat would draw blood to the skin surface, denying it to the deeper organs which need it.

5 **Let him be reassured** by your attitude of sympathy and confidence, by your calm and methodical way of treating him. If he appears unconscious remember that he may yet be able to hear unfavourable comments or that you are whispering.

6 **Give nothing by mouth.** Alcohol is a false stimulant. Drinks of water, tea or coffee may be vomited, and the vomit may flow into the windpipe and choke him. Also any food or drink taken may complicate matters in hospital should it then be found that he needs an anaesthetic.

ABDOMINAL WOUNDS

Have the victim on his back. To reduce the pull on the abdominal wall muscles have his thighs bent a little upwards at the hips by means of cushions or blankets under the knees. Loosen clothing. Make your dressing amply large and your bandaging wide.

If any abdominal contents protrude from the wound do not try to replace them. See they are well covered and that the bandages do not press too hard.

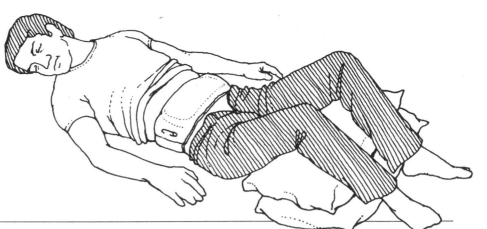

ARTIFICIAL RESPIRATION

Give this when breathing has stopped; never try it if the patient is still breathing. The technique is not difficult but it is far better to learn it from a class demonstration and practise on a manikin, as provided by the St John's, Red Cross and St Andrew's organizations. Work very fast, with no delays.

1 Get the patient on his back. Bend the head fully backwards (which gets his airway open). Quickly scoop your finger round his mouth to clear away any obstruction like mud, vomit or loosened dentures.

2 Pinch his nose shut with thumb and forefinger; the heel of the same hand on his forehead helps to keep his head bent back. With the fingers of the other hand pull the jaw to keep the mouth open; do not let them overlap across his lips.

3 Take a deep breath in.

4 Seal you own lips well over his mouth and breathe out steadily and smoothly. Your air will pass into his chest which should rise. Do not blow hard.

5 Lift your mouth off. Turn your head to one side to let you see that indeed the chest has risen, and is now falling as the air comes out. Take another deep breath in.

6 As soon as the chest has fallen repeat steps 4 and 5. You should give the *first three breaths* very fast to make sure that his lungs receive a great deal of air at the start. After that you time yourself by the natural rise and fall of his chest.

Some extra notes:

(a) In the case of children you need not pinch the nose, but let your lips seal over the patient's nose and mouth. Breathe gently, just enough to get the chest moving. For very small babies only small puffs are sufficient.

(b) If the patient vomits turn his head to one side; let the vomit flow out and with your finger scoop any residue from his mouth. Resume artificial respiration now (or after any other interruption) with three quick breaths.

(c) Continue artificial respiration until a doctor or ambulance expert takes over.

(d) When there is no improvement in colour, no pulse and the pupils remain dilated, cardiac massage is needed. This is a difficult skill that must be learned by going to a class.

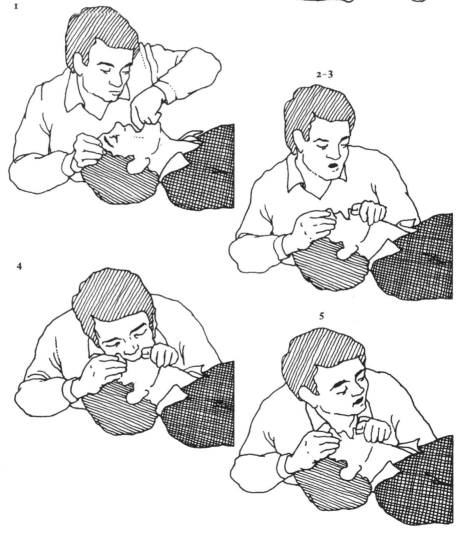

177

ASTHMA

Has the patient any tablets or inhaler prescribed for the emergency? If so let him use this, but make certain he does not exceed the advised doses; he may already have tried them. Other points are:

1 Get his clothes loose. Open the window, but do not let him get cold.
2 Calm and confidence help a lot to get the patient relaxed, which is very important. Physical or mental tension worsens the asthmatic tightness.
3 Tell the patient to go quite loose, except for his back which he keeps straight.
4 Tell him to make his breathing efforts not from the uppermost but from the lowest part of his chest, and to make a special effort to breathe *out*.
5 A drink of warm (not too hot) strong coffee can sometimes help.
6 Do not hesitate to call a doctor if the attack does not ease.

BLEEDING

Bleeding will generally stop if you apply firm pressure, which allows clotting to occur. Mild bleeding can be controlled if treated as a Wound (see page 188). What follows here concerns severe bleeding.

1 **Immediately press hard** on the wound, either pinching together its edges with thumb and finger or using the palm of your hand. Even if your hands are dirty act at once.
2 **Raise a bleeding limb,** maintaining pressure all the time. However, if circumstances suggest a fracture, leave this part out.
3 **Get the patient lying down,** unless you think the movement would seriously disturb a fracture.
4 **Slip a thick pad** on to the wound, under your hand or fingers, maintaining pressure all the while. For the pad use anything handy; a handkerchief, towel or scarf will serve.
5 **Bandage the pad, very firmly.** A necktie, towel, belt or stocking can be the bandage. Do not let the pressure go until bandaging is complete.
6 **Apply anti-shock measures** and get medical help or an ambulance.
7 **Keep a watch on the bandage.** If bloodstaining oozes through, then the control has been insufficient. Do *not* remove anything but apply another pad and firm bandaging over the stain. Move the injured part as little as possible, so as not to disturb clotting.

See also Ear Bleeding (page 182); Nose Bleeding (page 187), and Tooth Socket Bleeding (page 187).

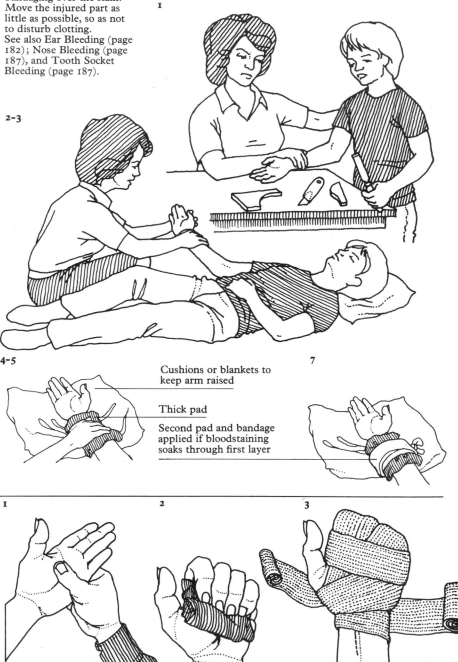

1

2-3

4-5

7

Cushions or blankets to keep arm raised

Thick pad

Second pad and bandage applied if bloodstaining soaks through first layer

CUT PALM OF HAND

1 This can bleed quite severely. **At once press on to the palm,** using your thumb and hand. Elevate the patient's arm. Maintain pressure until bleeding eases.
2 **Fit a thick pad into the palm;** fold the patient's fingers over this; if he has the power, let him make a tight fist.
3 **Bandage up the whole hand very firmly,** leaving the thumb outside. The knot should be made at the wrist.

1

2

3

BLISTERS

Blisters are best left alone to look after themselves and be slowly absorbed under a protective pad and bandaging. However, there are times when their very bulk makes this impracticable. Then, and only then, can you pierce them.

Boil a long needle in water for 10 minutes. Pour away the water, without touching the needle which you allow to cool in its container. Meanwhile, after washing your hands, carefully clean the blister and its surrounding skin with soap and water, using clean cotton wool or linen.

Handle the needle only by its blunt end; do not let the sharp end touch anything but the area you have cleaned on the patient. Pierce the base of the blister at two diametrically opposite points. Press the blister down through a pad of clean material to squeeze out the fluid. Put on a generously sized clean dressing as for Wounds (see page 188) and bandage. Dealing with the blister this way is not likely to work if it is a day or two old, for then the fluid could have become thick and jelly-like.

If a blister becomes painful, red and turbid, it probably has become infected, and you should get a doctor's advice.

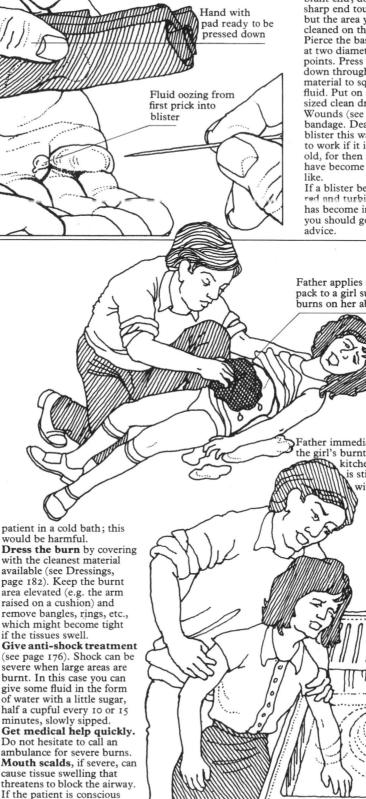

Hand with pad ready to be pressed down

Fluid oozing from first prick into blister

BURNS

The key to dealing with burns is to cool the area as soon as possible. Severe as may be the surface burn, it is the heat retained deep in the tissues which does the grave damage. For information on Chemical Burns, see page 180.

If clothes are on fire put them out at once by water or by smothering them with the nearest available thick cloth, rug, blanket, towel or even your jacket. Wrap this closely over the burning area to exclude air. Pull off any material which is left smouldering, and stamp on it (or throw it into a safe place like a sink). Do not tear off burnt material which is stuck to the skin.

Cooling the burn. Immediately apply cold water. Either plunge a burnt limb into a basin or sink of water. Or, for other parts (e.g. face or abdomen), apply a large thick pad soaked in cold water. Just pouring on water is insufficient (though a burnt finger-tip can be dealt with by being held under a running tap). Keep this cooling going for at least 10 minutes. If the pain has not eased considerably by then, repeat for another 10 minutes. A wet pack, taking up the heat, may dry and warm up and need renewing during this time.

It is worth doing this cooling even if you begin treatment up to half an hour after the accident. Please note:

1 Do not use iced water; ordinary water from the tap is right.

2 Do not plunge the whole patient in a cold bath; this would be harmful.

Dress the burn by covering with the cleanest material available (see Dressings, page 182). Keep the burnt area elevated (e.g. the arm raised on a cushion) and remove bangles, rings, etc., which might become tight if the tissues swell.

Give anti-shock treatment (see page 176). Shock can be severe when large areas are burnt. In this case you can give some fluid in the form of water with a little sugar, half a cupful every 10 or 15 minutes, slowly sipped.

Get medical help quickly. Do not hesitate to call an ambulance for severe burns.

Mouth scalds, if severe, can cause tissue swelling that threatens to block the airway. If the patient is conscious give him ice to suck.

Father applies a thick wet pack to a girl suffering from burns on her abdomen.

Father immediately plunges the girl's burnt arm into the kitchen sink while it is still filling up with water.

CAR ACCIDENTS

If you come across a road smash and the rescue services are on the spot, move slowly past and do not interfere.

If you have to give help stop your car safely so that it is not at risk from passing traffic and will not make it difficult for ambulance or fire service cars to get close to the injured. Then act in this order:

1 Look for and attend to any urgent life-saving work needed to control bleeding (see page 178) or to ensure a clear airway (see page 181). Leave victims in the car unless there is danger there, e.g. from fire or gas.

2 Look for the not-uncommon event: accident victims thrown over a side hedge or low wall.

3 Switch off ignition and lights of any car involved. If there is smouldering from the engine use your fire extinguisher. Forbid smoking. Make certain the brakes are on. If they are defective and the car is on a slope, get the wheels blocked by an object like a box or a car seat.

4 Set bystanders or warning triangle signals 100 metres or more ahead of and behind the scene to warn and slow down other drivers. Otherwise they may run into you.

5 Call the ambulance (via 999 telephone dialling)

through a bystander. Write down his message which will include exactly where you are, and the number of victims and their apparent injuries.

6 Treat any other victims as best you can as they are in the car. Do not be tempted to pull them out, for this may worsen their injuries, especially if the car body is deformed. Wait for the rescue services.

See page 189 for advice on a First Aid Kit for the car.

CHEMICAL BURNS

At once wash the area very copiously with running water or water poured repeatedly from a jug. Keep at it until no more chemical is likely to remain. Remove any contaminated clothes. Then apply a clean dressing.

If chemicals have entered the eye the patient will be screwing his eyelids together from pain, and you may have to prise them open gently. Try to tilt him so that the water runs off without passing over the unaffected side of his face.

Get medical help.

CHILDBIRTH

In an emergency where someone unexpectedly goes into labour and you await help from a doctor or midwife, be comforted by the fact that these fast labours are generally easy, normal ones without great complications.

Get the mother on a bed and see that the upper part of her body is covered and warm. Wash your hands thoroughly, and prepare towels in which to wrap the baby and also clean cloth pads or handkerchiefs.

Ask the mother to relax as much as she can and let nature take its course without interference. At some time the membranes surrounding the baby will rupture, releasing fluid; this is normal.

As the baby nears expulsion the mother will be feeling quite strong contractions ('pains') at fairly short intervals, e.g. every two to five minutes. Let her then be on her back with her legs apart and her knees bent. When the baby's head appears it will distend the vulva and eventually, during a contraction, emerge from it. Just as it seems about to emerge prevent it doing so too rapidly by gently cupping your hand over it to control it. Ask the mother to take quick panting breaths at that moment, for this reduces the force of expulsion.

When the baby's head is well out there is a small possibility that the umbilical cord will be wrapped round its neck, where it would interfere with the rest of the delivery. With your finger feel carefully and, if you find the cord thus, gently try

to loop it over the head or shoulder so that it lies free. Wait now for the next contractions, which will get the baby's two shoulders out. Then firmly hold the baby under its armpits and gently lift it out. Hold him with his head low to let any fluid in the mouth and nose drain out. He is very wet and slippery so you must be careful. Also avoid moving him any way which will pull on the umbilical cord which has partly emerged from the vulva. Lie the baby on his side, by the mother and wrap towels round him. The next contractions should deliver the placenta ('afterbirth') and you encourage the mother to bear down with each of them. Once the placenta is out, cover it too with a clean towel.

If there is much bleeding, slowly and gently but firmly, rub the mother's abdomen over where you feel the upper end of the bulk of the womb: this will be at about the level of the navel. Put a clean cloth or sanitary pad over the vulva. Should the placenta not come out, put a clean pad over the length of the umbilical cord which has been exposed.

If the baby does not cry within two minutes of birth give Artificial Respiration, but do this gently with small puffs (see page 177).

CHEST INJURIES

Any wound which makes a penetrating hole in the chest can dangerously draw air into the chest space and compress the lung.

At once close the hole with your fingers or by the pressure of your hand (see illustration). Keep this up until you can replace the hand by a thick and large pad of material which you hold and then bandage or strap on to make it as airtight as possible.

Have the patient lie *tilted towards the wound side*. This reduces the likelihood of any blood flowing through the air tubes into his good side.

If he develops breathing difficulties have him propped up on cushions, coats or blankets, half-sitting, half-lying towards the injured side; this eases the mechanics of breathing.

1 The hand pressed firmly on wound should follow the curve of the patient's chest.

2 Bandaging is placed firmly over a large pad.

3 The patient lies in the half-propped position; this gives relief if he develops breathing difficulties.

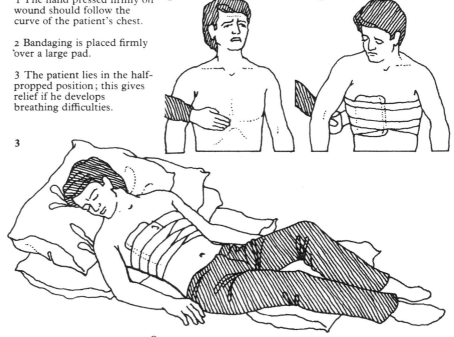

CHOKING

1 **If the victim is coughing,** he is making his own rescue efforts—do not interfere.

2 **If he cannot cough or speak,** then:
(a) Give four hard sharp blows with the flat of your hand between his shoulder blades. Try to have his head low. You can support a child hung over your bent knee, or a baby on your thigh, as in the illustrations.
This may dislodge the object choking him. If it does not, follow at once with

(b) abdominal pressure to try to force air and the object out of his airway. Stand behind the patient and encircle him with your arms. Make a fist with one hand and place it firmly (thumb side first) in the soft space between the lower end of the breast bone and the level of the navel. Cup the other hand over this. Now give a hard sharp thrust inwards and upwards. Repeat up to a total of four thrusts if necessary. If you are successful the object may shoot out of the mouth.

Or it may come into the mouth from where you will have quickly to scoop it out lest he take a big breath and aspirates it down again.
You can do this with your patient either standing or sitting. Should he have fallen to the ground, then you will have to turn him on his back and kneel across his thighs. Pressure is done with the heels of your two hands overlapping. A very small baby can be treated held lying face up on your thigh. Press with two fingers only.

If these measures fail continue the alternating treatment of four back blows and four abdominal pressures.

3 **If the patient becomes unconscious,** begin Artificial Respiration (see page 177). This may let your air filter past the obstruction sufficiently to keep him alive until medical help arrives.
The abdominal thrusts can occasionally cause internal injuries. The calculated risk is justified to save a life. The patient must be checked by a doctor as soon as possible after he recovers.

Four ways to administer four hard slaps with the flat of the hand. Choose your method according to the size and position of the patient.

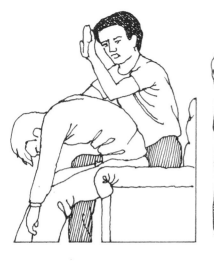

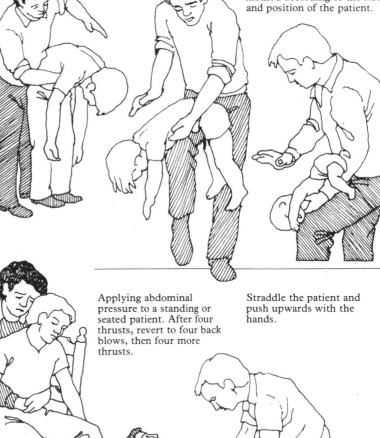

Applying abdominal pressure to a standing or seated patient. After four thrusts, revert to four back blows, then four more thrusts.

Straddle the patient and push upwards with the hands.

COLD

See Hypothermia, page 186.

CRAMP

Generally cramped muscles can be eased quickly by stretching.

1 Front of the arm. Pull the arm right back with the elbow straight.

2 Back of the thigh. Swing the leg forward as far as it will go, and straighten the knee.

3 Front of the thigh. Throw the leg back and bend the knee as far as possible.

4 Calf. With the leg straight, bend the foot up at the ankle. Some cramps all over the body can be the result of great loss of fluid and body salts, as with abnormally heavy sweating or severe diarrhoea and vomiting. You can help by giving suitable drinks like Oxo, Marmite or Bovril. These must be taken tepid and in slow sips, so as not to provoke further stomach upsets.

DIABETES

Someone on treatment with insulin for diabetes may, by over-exertion, erroneously large insulin dose, missed meal or mischance suddenly develop a condition of too low a sugar level in his blood.

He may be pale, sweating, trembling and with uncoordinated movements or slurred speech. He may become mentally vague or behave unreasonably. He may rapidly become unconscious.

If you suspect this state give two lumps or two teaspoonfuls of sugar or glucose in water. Failing these, use any sweet food available (jam, honey, chocolate, cake). After about ten minutes repeat the dose. Rarely, the altered mental state makes him refuse help and even fight or shout: throwing handfuls of granulated sugar into his mouth is an inelegant but effective solution. The dose of sugar is not critical; it is wiser to give too much than too little.

If he is unconscious (see page 188) you must give nothing by mouth. Get a doctor quickly.

DRESSINGS

On page 189 you will find advice on a First Aid Kit for the home.

There are many times when an emergency forces one to improvise dressings from everyday material. A pocket handkerchief, or a small smooth towel makes a very good dressing, but you should not apply it as you find it. Picking it up by its corners let it fall open and still handling only by the corners refold it so that what was its inside surface is now on the outside and can go, untouched by hand, on to the wound.

Soft pads over the dressing can be made from clean towels, socks, scarves, stockings, or thick folded handkerchiefs.

For bandages use stockings, scarves, towels or neckties. The two main errors made in putting on dressings is to have them too small and too loose. Extend your dressing well beyond the area of the wound, and take care to have the bandage as smooth as possible and well tied, firmly (but not tightly) in position. There are three ready-made dressings which are useful.

PREPARED STERILE DRESSING

This consists of sterilized gauze, pad and bandage in one. Get it carefully out of its pack so that you do not touch the gauze surface which goes on the wound. The smaller bandage length at one end is wound first and then the longer from the other end. Use the medium and large sizes.

ADHESIVE DRESSING STRIP

This long ribbon of slightly padded gauze is flanked by adhesive strapping. Cut off a suitable length and pull the covering off the adhesive parts to put the gauze on small wounds. The 5 cm and 7½ cm widths are the most useful ones.

PERFORATED FILM ADHESIVE DRESSING (PFA)

Each sterile dressing is individually packed. After opening its envelope handle it carefully only by the plain gauze back. The smooth shiny surface goes on the wound. Available sizes are 5 × 5 cm (rather too small for general use), 10 × 10 cm and 10 × 20 cm.

Applying a prepared sterile dressing.

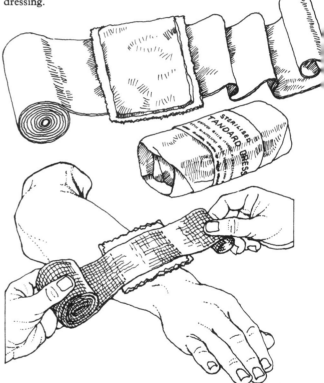

EAR BLEEDING

Any bleeding from within the ear is likely to be small in amount and not dangerous in itself. But when it follows a blow on the head one must be very guarded and suspect a fracture within the skull— a dangerous situation needing medical attention at once.

In such a case have the patient lie down towards the side of the injury to allow the blood to flow out. (If it remains in the ear canal it could form the seat of an infection which might affect the brain through the fracture.) Then bandage a clean pad over the ear to protect it from dirt.

EAR: OBJECT IN

An object stuck in the ear might perhaps fall out if the head is tilted well over to that side. Do not try to probe it out: you might not only push it deeper but also injure the ear drum.

If an insect or small piece of vegetation is suspected inside the ear canal, have the patient lie on his side with the ear uppermost. Gently pour in a little cool water or olive oil: the object might float to the top and could then be mopped away. But do *not* pour anything in if the ear is painful or if the ear drum might have some injury or perforation, for then the fluid could enter and damage the deeper part of the ear.

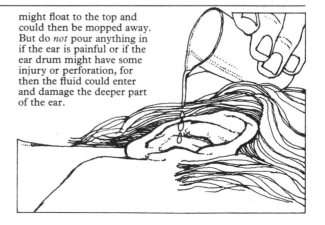

ELECTROCUTION

1 Domestic Currents
Immediately switch off or disconnect the electricity, and do not touch the victim until this has been done. If for some reason you cannot disconnect the electricity and the victim is still in contact with a live part you must try to knock him from it using *dry*, non-conducting material, like a wooden stick, a wooden chair or rope. You must not risk becoming electrocuted yourself. In an absolute emergency, when nothing else is available, you can pull the victim through dry, thick material like a rug. The diagram shows how to handle it.

As a result of electrocution the patient may have stopped breathing and need Artificial Respiration (see page 177). He may have had Fractures (page 184), or Burns (page 179). He may collapse some minutes or hours after the rescue and so must be at rest and under observation.

2 High power currents
The current of extremely high voltage found in some factories or from electric pylons is a very different matter. It can reach out and kill as one approaches. Do not try to rescue the victim, but stay at least six metres away until the right authorities confirm that the current has been cut off.

Using dry thick material to move the patient away from contact with the electric current.

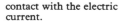

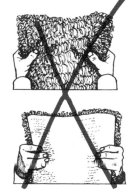

Right method

Wrong method

Rear view

Front view

EPILEPSY

In a fit the victim will fall and be unconscious. For a short while he is immobile, rigid, and then he may start jerking his limbs before being quiet again, and eventually recovering consciousness. While unconscious he may froth at the mouth, bite his tongue and he may be incontinent and wet himself. The pattern of attacks varies greatly from patient to patient.

Do not try to restrain the jerking. Rather make sure he does not hurt his limbs; quickly pull furniture away from him or put soft buffering things (e.g. cushions) against any wall or unmoveable furniture near him.

Mop away froth from his mouth, so that it does not get down his throat. You may try to protect his tongue from being bitten by putting something *soft* between his teeth at the angle of his mouth. But do not put anything hard, which might break the teeth; and do not leave something small like a gauze pad which could slip in and obstruct the throat. One end of his tie or coat lapel, or of a bunched handkerchief which you hold could do. And do not try to force the mouth open if it is firmly shut in spasm. After the jerking has stopped, place him in the Recovery Position (see page 188) until he has fully recovered. This should be followed by getting medical advice. Beware of a succession of epileptic attacks coming on in unusually close frequency on the same day. The situation may get dangerously out of hand, and you should call a doctor. For more general information about epilepsy, see page 162.

EYE INJURIES

1 Chemical in the eye See page 180.

2 Wound of the eye Do nothing more than bandaging or strapping a large dressing and pad over the whole eye. Get medical help quickly.

3 Object in the eye Begin by telling the patient not to rub the eye, which he is likely to be doing. Sit him down in a good light and stand behind him, positioning his head back so that you look down into the eye. Take a clean handkerchief and moisten and roll one corner of it into a small point. Look for the object: if it is on the front of the eyeball and on the white of the eye try to pick it off gently with the handkerchief tip. If it does not come easily do not persist—it may be embedded.

If the object is within the iris and pupil, i.e. the coloured area of the eye, *do not touch it*. Manipulation here may injure that part through which vision passes. Put a protective dressing over the eye and get medical help.

Generally the object is not immediately seen, having moved under one or other lid. As the patient looks up, pull the lower lid down. If it is not there, search under the upper lid. For this you have to evert the lid. Hold a matchstick along its upper edge with one hand. With

1 When looking for the object, stand behind the patient in a good light.

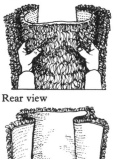

2 If the object is on the white of the eye and on the front of the eyeball, tip it out with the rolled corner of a moist handkerchief.

3 Rolling the upper lid upwards over a matchstick to reveal the foreign body.

finger and thumb of the other hand, firmly grasp the lower edge of the lid and roll it up over the matchstick while the patient looks down.

Pick the object away with the handkerchief. This is nothing like as uncomfortable to the patient as it sounds.

FAINTING

If the victim merely feels faint let him lie down. Loosen any tight clothes (collar, braces, belt), raise his legs a little with cushions or folded blankets beneath them. Cover him loosely. Tell him to take deep slow breaths. He is likely to recover soon, and is just as likely to want to get up again before he is fully better. Keep him comfortably lying down a little longer, and give him a drink of water.

Someone feeling faint under circumstances where he cannot lie down (e.g. in a theatre auditorium) should bend forward to get his head as low as possible between his knees.

For Unconsciousness, see page 188.

FEVERISH FITS

Small children sometimes have a sudden fit when an infection sends their temperature high. They go rigid and lose consciousness briefly.

Put the child in the Recovery Position (see page 188), and make sure his breathing is safe by wiping away any vomit or excess fluid from the mouth and throat.

Loosen his clothes and cover him with a light blanket. But if he is very hot, cool him by sponging his limbs with cold water. Do not overdo this; aim to get the temperature down only slightly.

Call a doctor, but keep the child under observation in case a second fit follows. If it does, repeat the procedure above.

FRACTURES

If you suspect the likelihood of a fracture (i.e. after a crush, severe blow or fall) do not hesitate: treat the case as a definite fracture. No one will blame you if the X-rays later show an intact bone.

1 Tell the patient not to move; tell others not to move him.

2 Stop any severe bleeding at once. Dress any open wound with the least disturbance of the injured part.

3 If professional help (doctor, nurse, ambulance) will soon be with you then wait and cover the patient loosely and warmly. Otherwise splint the injured part by bandaging it firmly to the most appropriate part of his body.

Immobilization follows the following principles: Unless unavoidable do not move the injured part. For example, move the good leg towards the bad one. Immobilize not only the whole area involved, but also the joint on either side. Put soft thick padding between the two parts of the body involved. This acts as a buffer and helps to keep the whole secure. Rolled up scarves, wool, socks or towels will serve.

Bandage the parts together to prevent any movement at all. Use belts, ties, towels, stockings if you have nothing else. Pass the bandaging round the areas slowly and carefully. Avoid having any bandage directly over where you think the fracture lies. Make the knots on the good side, really firmly but not tightly. With arms and legs check that toes or fingers are not going dusky because your bandaging is so tight that it interferes with the circulation.

The methods illustrated are designed to deal with likely home mishaps and may differ in detail from those of the main first aid organizations.

JAW Remove any dentures carefully. Let the victim support the jaw with a pad held in his cupped hand (or do this for him if he is not fit). Then apply the bandage. Beware of blood or other objects in the mouth which might choke him, especially if he is unconscious (see page 188).

Bandage

Soft pad

RIBS Leave the chest alone, but support the arm on the injured side in a sling.

UPPER ARM AND FOREARM Bring the limb across as slowly and gently as possible, giving complete support until the sling is in position and working.

If the elbow gives pain and therefore might be fractured, do not move it. If it lies bent then immobilize as above. If it is straight keep it so, and bandage it to the body as shown.

COLLAR BONE This fracture is almost always from a fall on to the outstretched arm; the blow travels up the limb to jerk and snap the collar bone.

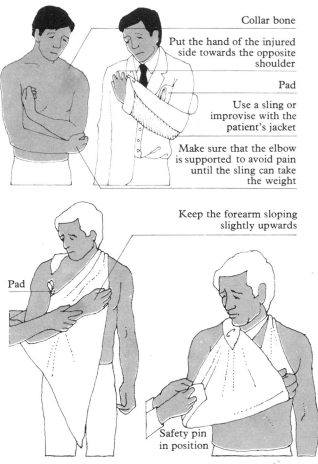

Collar bone

Put the hand of the injured side towards the opposite shoulder

Pad

Use a sling or improvise with the patient's jacket

Make sure that the elbow is supported to avoid pain until the sling can take the weight

Keep the forearm sloping slightly upwards

Pad

Safety pin in position

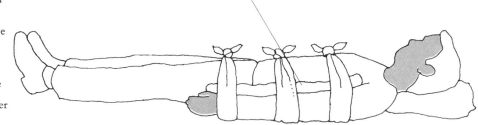

Padding between damaged arm and body

PELVIS Let the victim lie on his back and put his legs and feet in the position he finds most comfortable. He may well be eased by thick padding (blankets, coats) under his knees. (If the fracture has injured the bladder the victim may feel this as a need to pass urine. Tell him to desist as otherwise the urine might pass into the surrounding tissues and damage them. Await medical advice.)

THIGH AND LEG Bring the good leg alongside the injured one and get padding between. Bandage the legs together at the knees, and round the feet and ankles. If the leg is bent and any gentle attempt to straighten it is painful, leave it alone except to support it in its position with such things as pillows or rolled-up blankets against it.

FOOT Remove footwear gently. A cushion or thick blanket tied firmly round the foot gives very good immobilization.

NECK AND BACK
Fracture of the spine may have very grim consequences, damaging the nervous spinal cord and so causing loss of feeling or paralysis which could well be permanent. This can also happen to the as-yet-intact spinal cord if the victim is moved, especially if his trunk is bent. Never under any circumstances pick up and carry in a 'folded' position anyone, conscious or unconscious, whose injury might have fractured the vertebrae of the neck or back. Transport needs specially learnt and practised techniques and stretchers. Keep the victim quite still and warmly covered until expert help arrives.

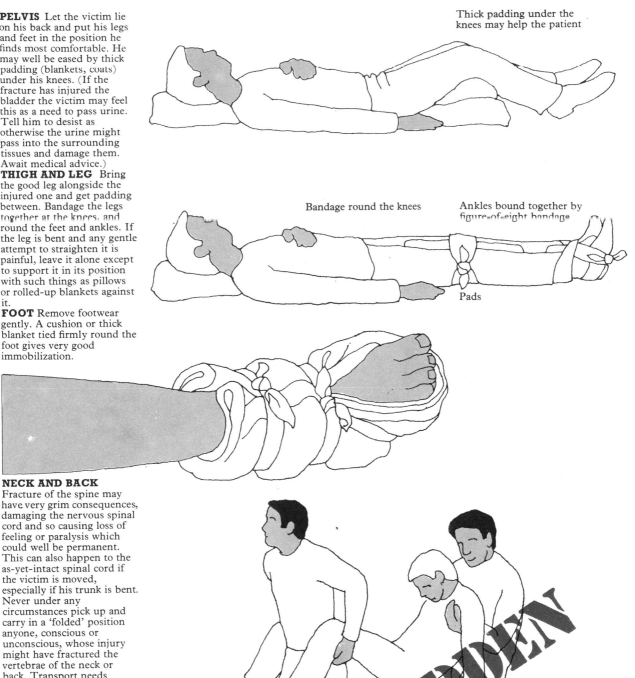

Thick padding under the knees may help the patient

Bandage round the knees

Ankles bound together by figure-of-eight bandage

Pads

FORBIDDEN

FROSTBITE

Take off any wet clothes and anything tight, such as a glove or ring. Cover the frostbitten area with something dry and warm. But do not apply anything hot, for the frostbitten area must warm slowly. You can cup the palm of a hand over an ear lobe or nose. Frostbitten fingers could be tucked into an armpit. What you must *not* do is to rub, least of all with snow. The weakened skin circulation will not stand it.

HEAD INJURY

Complications arising from a head injury often show themselves late or develop insidiously. All cases where there has been a cut, a blow or unconsciousness (however brief) or some impairment of the mental state and behaviour (however transient) should receive medical attention. **Concussion** is the immediate 'knock out' which follows a blow. Coming-to may be a matter of seconds or hours. **Compression** describes changes which develop as a result of bleeding within the skull, disturbance of brain tissue or pressure from displaced fractured bone. It takes minutes or hours to show up, and may follow after recovery from concussion. Progressive headaches, nausea, confusion, sleepiness and finally coma may be features, but one should not wait for these to appear before getting the doctor's advice.

If the victim is conscious and alert, let him rest: keep him under observation.

If he is dazed, put him in the Recovery Position (see page 188) and watch him closely.

If he is unconscious, follow the procedure described on page 188.

But remember that quite a proportion of those who have head injuries may also have damage elsewhere on the body (arm, leg, abdomen). Look for this and safeguard any part which may be fractured. Particularly dangerous is the likelihood of spine fracture in someone who has fallen. Any bending or twisting could do tragic harm. A possible fractured spine or neck must be protected should you have to correct a breathing difficulty in the unconscious victim whose head is bent forwards. Bring the head slowly and smoothly backwards *without twisting sideways* and detail someone to guard it thus. If a victim on his back is likely to vomit he must be turned on his side. This is a difficult thing to do without interfering with the neck, but it can be achieved if someone is carefully holding the head all the while and preventing rotation on the neck.

If there is bleeding from nose or ear, or bruising round an eye (however slight) this could be due to fracture within the skull and must be investigated swiftly.

HEART ATTACK

This vague term covers two major possibilities. One is the acute heart failure where a defective heart muscle suddenly loses power; the pumping action of the heart is weakened and the lungs become congested. Each breath is bubbly, making a wet sound. The patient is coughing, breathless and distressed but not in pain. The second is the coronary occlusion in which there has been sudden complete or partial blockage of one of the small vessels supplying the heart muscle. The characteristic marks of a severe attack are intense gripping pain in the centre of the chest, often radiating to neck, shoulder or arm, breathlessness, shock-like sweat and pallor or blueness, and a fast and feeble pulse. However, a coronary occlusion can happen with much slighter symptoms, which unfortunately the sufferer neglects or treats as 'a bit of indigestion'.

In either case:

1 Send for urgent medical help. The sooner the doctor reaches the patient, the sooner he can give relief and the better the outlook.

2 Loosen tight clothing. Open the windows, but keep the patient covered and warm.

3 If the patient is shocked, keep him lying down. But if his major difficulty is getting his breath, have him sitting up against banked pillows and a headrest. This last can be improvised with an upturned chair.

Emotions, like fright, do much to worsen these conditions. Sympathize fully with your patient, but convey an attitude of positive confidence that the situation, horrible as it is, will be eased. Be reassuring, but avoid crowding the patient and fussing.

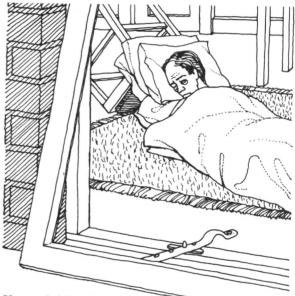

Upturned chair with pillows makes an improvised headrest

Window open to admit air; but keep the patient warm

HEAT EFFECTS

Hard work, high heat and heavy sweating may combine to produce **heat exhaustion** in which the patient may collapse, with the appearance of shock. His skin is moist and pale, his pulse fast and feeble. Because of the heat-removing action of the evaporating sweat, his temperature will be near normal. He is suffering from depletion of fluid and of minerals from the loss of sweat and the body minerals it carries with it.

Get him lying down in a cool area and let him drink freely (but, lest he vomit, slowly) either water or fruit juices to which you have added a little salt (half a teaspoonful is enough for a big tumbler).

Different is **heat stroke**, which is hardly likely to occur in domestic circumstances in the UK. His temperature rises extremely high and he can collapse very suddenly, with a red skin and a bounding pulse. This man needs rapid cooling with sponging or fanning in a cool shelter. Refer also to Feverish Fits (page 184).

HYPOTHERMIA

This is a dangerous state of extremely low body temperature to which small babies and elderly people are particularly susceptible, especially in winter where sudden frosts can produce an icy bedroom or nursery. The victim is marble-cold, even in the parts of the body under the bedclothes, with white skin. (A baby, however, may be misleadingly rosy.) He is lethargic, perhaps comatose or unconscious and pulse and breathing are slow and feeble.

This is an emergency and the doctor must be called. In the meantime get the patient into the Recovery Position (see page 188) and keep him well but loosely covered. Do not warm him directly but *warm the room*. If he is conscious give warm drinks to be taken slowly. Do not give hot drinks. Do not give alcohol.

INSECT BITES

If the sting has been left in, pull it out with tweezers. Apply them at the base, close to the skin: this avoids squeezing in toxin still left in the top of the sting.

NOSE BLEEDING

The vessel which bleeds is almost always within the soft part of the nose. It is useless to press the bony bridge.

Grasp the whole lower half of the nose between finger and thumb and maintain the pressure without interruption for at least 10 minutes.

Repeat if necessary. The patient can hold his own nose, and he should sit up, preferably with his elbow resting on a table. He must not blow his nose or sniff.

Nose bleeding after a blow to the head may be more serious. See Head Injury (page 186).

POISONING

1 If the patient is unconscious, is he breathing?

No. Begin Artificial Respiration immediately (see page 177).

Yes. Keep him in the Recovery Position (see page 188), and urgently get an ambulance. There is nothing more to do except to treat for Unconsciousness (see page 188).

2 If the patient is conscious, ask him what he has taken. Check the labels of any bottles or containers, and make sure that these go with him to hospital. Urgently summon the ambulance.

Give soothing drinks to dilute the poison and ease the stomach damage: best are water, milk or barley water. Do *not* give salt drinks. They are inefficient for making the patient vomit, and they can themselves be poisonous.

Keep the patient lying in the Recovery Position (see page 188).

Throughout you must keep a close watch. The conscious patient may become unconscious; the breathing patient may collapse and stop breathing; the suicide may intend to try again. It is more important to get the patient rapidly to hospital than to make him vomit. Try to induce vomiting only if the following conditions are all fulfilled:

(a) The attempt in no way delays the ambulance.

(b) The patient is conscious and cooperative.

(c) The poison is not a corrosive (e.g. bleach, strong acid or alkali) and not a petroleum product. They would cause more harm if vomited.

After the soothing drinks have been given, rub the back of his throat with your fingers or with the blunt end of a spoon handle round which you hold folds of a handkerchief. Send the vomit (or a sample) to the hospital.

Poisoning by gases and fumes

Immediately get the victim out of the contaminated area. It may be dangerous for you to venture into it unless you have a respirator and, in the hands of other helpers, a lifeline.

SHOCK

See page 176.

SNAKE BITES

The only biting snake in the UK is the adder and fortunately his bite, though painful and causing distress, is only very rarely fatal.

Victims do not know this and need reassurance.

The adder is *about* 75 cm long and must not be confused with the harmless grass snake (120 cm) or the smooth snake (60 cm) which have smaller heads and a more 'streamlined' look.

General colour is grey, yellow, brown or reddish

Get the victim at rest, lying down. Wash the wound, or wipe it clean, and put on a clean dry dressing. Now treat this part more or less as if it were fractured; immobilizing it reduces the spread of the poison. Get the victim to hospital as soon as possible. Because the pain may be intense it would be right to give aspirin or paracetamol.

You do *not* suck or cut the wound; you do *not* put chemicals in the afflicted area; you do *not* apply a tourniquet.

The back has a wide zig-zag marking

Adder

The head is broad, heavy, spadelike, widening from the neck

The sides bear heavy black spots

SPRAINS

A sprain is the wrenching of ligaments at a joint. If there has been a blow it might be accompanied by a fracture and should be treated accordingly.

If you see it within half an hour of the incident apply cold compresses for half an hour (cloths thickly folded, soaked in cold water then wrung out to be just moist). This helps reduce the swelling.

Then support the joint by thick padding of cotton wool interleaved in firm turns of bandage. Avoid tightness which could compress nerves and blood vessels which often lie close under the skin near joints.

STINGS

See Insect Bites (page 186).

STRAINS

These are wrenched muscle fibres, and generally occur after a heavy effort and usually not in the region of a joint. But treat them as Sprains.

STROKE

A stroke results from sudden damage to a blood vessel in the brain. The consequences therefore vary according to which part is affected, and can show as numbness or weakness of a hand, paralysis of one side of the body or difficulty of speech. Some are progressive, beginning with quite slight symptoms before serious ones develop. If you suspect a stroke get the victim to bed or at least lying down, with clothes loosened, and call a doctor. It is wise to have him in the Recovery Position (see page 188) lest he become unconscious.

TOOTHACHE

Aspirin or paracetamol and an early dental appointment are the main actions. But oil of cloves applied to the tooth (not on the gum and not repeatedly) can be temporarily helpful while waiting for treatment.

TOOTH SOCKET BLEEDING

The socket may bleed heavily some hours after a dental extraction. Do not plug the socket itself but let the patient bite hard on a thick gauze pad (or handkerchief) placed over the area. He should maintain this pressure for at least 15 minutes. It will be easier for him if he sits, with his elbow on a table and a hand cupped under the chin to give counter-pressure.

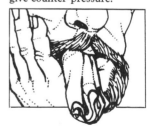

UNCONSCIOUSNESS

In first aid the cause of the person's unconsciousness is less important than the fact that he may choke and die if left on his back with his head bent forward. Blood, saliva or vomit could then flow back into the air tube. Also the tongue, floppy in the patient's unconscious state, can fall back and block the throat.

In all cases:

1 Check whether the victim has stopped breathing and needs artificial respiration (see page 177).

2 If he is breathing but with obvious difficulty in getting air in and out, quickly sweep his mouth with your finger to get out any obstruction, including dentures, then gently and smoothly bend his head well back and keep it thus; this will move the tongue clear of the throat. (Do not twist the head at the neck; see the note on fractured spine on page 185.)

3 Once you are satisfied about the breathing make sure there is no point of severe bleeding to be controlled. Also quickly cover any wounds.

4 Now you have to turn him into the Recovery Position,

Recovery position
Head bent back and face tilted down

Hand near face, bent at right angle at elbow

Upper leg bent at right angle at hip and knee

Lower arm and leg stretched out

but first do your best to check any likelihood of a fracture. This should be protected against movement as you turn him.

5 The Recovery Position safeguards the patient. It makes him lie firmly on his side, ensuring a clear airway and helping any fluid which comes into his mouth to flow out. Before you turn him over empty the pockets of anything which would be uncomfortable to lie on. As you turn him over, cup one hand over his head to protect it from the possibility of a hard blow on the ground.

6 Cover the patient loosely with a blanket or coat. Please realize that the apparently unconscious person sometimes can hear and register what is said around him. Guard your speech.

Never try to give anything by mouth to an unconscious patient. He cannot swallow and you would risk choking him.

The Recovery Position is not only for the completely unconscious. It is suitable for those who feel weak and faint, and essential for those who might suddenly lose consciousness.

WOUNDS

Severe bleeding must be controlled immediately (see page 178). Mild bleeding is likely to stop when the wound is dressed.

Before beginning put a temporary clean cover over the wound, wash your hands and collect your equipment. Wash with soap and water the area *round* the wound (not the wound itself) using a succession of moist swabs or clean cloth. Each stroke moves from the wound edge, away from it. Put on a clean dressing (e.g. gauze or see page 182). This must be big enough to extend well beyond the wound. A thick pad is then bandaged over it. Do not use antiseptics if a doctor or nurse is to give further attention. Otherwise you may use commercial preparations, provided you make sure you have the correct strength for open wounds and have read the manufacturer's instructions.

Object embedded in the wound

Do not try to pull it out. After the dressing has been lightly put over the wound, and the object, build up a protecting 'frame' of padding around the object's position, high enough to keep off the pressure of the ordinary pad and bandage which now follow.

Tetanus (lockjaw)

This infection is always a risk, in wounds, especially those contaminated with soil (the penetrating rose thorn, the road accident, the potato scraping knife, the animal bite). Consult your doctor for advice about protection. Refer also to Abdominal Wounds (page 177); Chest Injuries (page 180), and Eye Injuries (page 183).

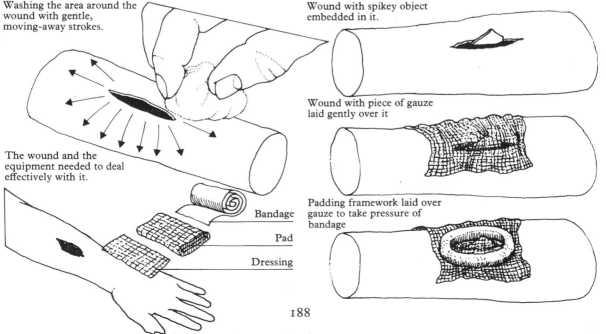

Washing the area around the wound with gentle, moving-away strokes.

The wound and the equipment needed to deal effectively with it.

Bandage

Pad

Dressing

Wound with spikey object embedded in it.

Wound with piece of gauze laid gently over it

Padding framework laid over gauze to take pressure of bandage

FIRST AID KIT

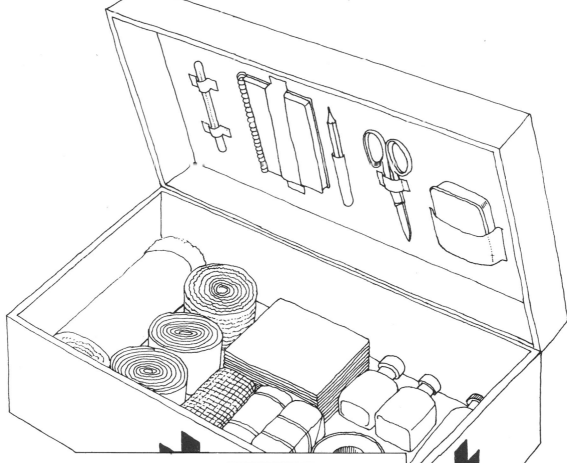

If you have a car, keep two kits. One stays permanently at home, the other stays in the car. First aid material should be housed in firm plastic or metal boxes with well-fitting lids. You can use the inside of the lid of the car box as a tray to hold objects cleanly when you are working on the road. Clearly label your boxes; do this on several sides of the car kit so that it can be easily spotted in any position, e.g. in the back of the car or the boot. At home keep the kit in an immediately accessible, dry place, out of the reach of children (therefore not in the bathroom). If you have a Home Medicine Cupboard (see page 173), the Home Kit can be kept in it. Do not retain any part of used dressings but replace them as soon as possible with new ones in intact wrappings.

First Aid Kits		Home	Car
Paper tissues		small pack	small pack
White gauze	1 metre pack	1	2
Cotton wool	15 g pack	1	2
Plain bandages	5 cm wide	2	2
	7½ cm wide	1	2
Crêpe bandages	7½ cm wide	1	2
PFA dressings	10 × 10 cm	2	3
(see page 182)	10 × 20 cm	1	2
Prepared sterile dressings	medium	1	1
	large	1	2
Adhesive dressing strip	5 cm wide	1	–
	7½ cm wide	–	1
Adhesive strapping	2½ cm wide	1	1
Safety pins		4	8
Scissors		small pair	large pair
Clinical thermometer		1	–
Soluble aspirin or paracetamol tablets		small pack or bottle	–
Oil of cloves		very small bottle	–
Pencil or pen		–	1
Notebook		–	1

In addition the car should carry:
Red warning triangle, Fire extinguisher, Large standing torch

PART 5
SURVIVAL
EMERGENCIES THAT CAN THREATEN LIFE, IN THE HOME AND IN THE WILD

You fall into a predicament that you must escape from by your own efforts, or die if you do not. That is the dramatic but not unrealistic scenario we mainly explore in this concluding chapter. We also look at some fairly common crises, occurring in and out of the home, which involve others, possibly your children or other members of your family, possibly strangers. Your house catches fire and people in it are trapped, or you come across someone in deep water who cannot swim. In such instances you are cast in the role of rescuer, and may have to place your own life at risk.

If you are a weekend or holiday adventurer, say a mountaineer or hang-glider, and take pleasure from overcoming natural hazards, then this chapter will not be satisfactory to you since it does not try to encompass the techniques required to pursue a dangerous hobby in reasonable safety. Your chosen pastime probably has a national association and its own specialized literature, and you should consult them for detailed advice.

Here we are concerned with the everyday killers—water, fire, exposure, attacks by animals, and hazards in the home. One common instruction applies to them all. Be decisive. If you see, or think you see, an emergency developing, don't wait for it to become a real emergency. Act promptly to curtail the danger. If the emergency has already arisen, don't hesitate. Decide quickly what to do. Then do it.

Should that sound so obvious as to be hardly worth saying, remember that it takes only seconds for someone to drown, or be overcome by smoke. In an emergency, there is *never* any time to spare.

CHILDREN IN THE HOME

This section looks at ways to prevent emergencies. It covers the precautions that parents would be wise to take to protect growing children in the home.

Children under 14 do not have the same kinds of accidents in the home as adults. A Government survey in 1974 showed that while many more adults were admitted to hospital for fractures (46.6 per cent) than from any other cause, with poisoning second (20.7 per cent), children as a whole—aged 0–14—were more susceptible to poisoning. This, by medicinal and non-medicinal agents, was the most frequent cause (31.1 per cent), followed by head and brain injuries (26.7 per cent), burns (13 per cent) and fractures (12.8 per cent).

Most parents with a child of pre-school age—and especially first-time parents—are inclined to be over-anxious about their child's health and safety. In periods of stress, perhaps after the child has fallen, cried a lot and suffered visible injuries such as cuts and bruises, the parents may complain of the difficulty of 'just keeping him/her alive'. Their anxiety, and tendency to be over-cautious, is borne out by the investigations of the Government-sponsored Home Accident Surveillance System. These show that, with infants aged 0–9 months, it is common for parents to take their child to hospital after an accident in the home—falls, at 60 per cent, being the most common category—and for the child then to be diagnosed as having 'No injury'. The tendency to over-caution is not unreasonable. Falls, producing bumps on the head, *can* be more damaging to very young children.

At that very young age, injuries to the head occur much more often than any other kind of injury. Burns and scalds are the next most common category, with hot water and hot drinks the most likely agents, followed by burns from hot objects or fires which the baby encounters as it begins to crawl about the home. So take special care:

1 When you, the baby and a hot drink are close together. Be wary of carrying a baby and a hot drink at the same time. Try to keep the baby out of range of hot drinks or other liquids which it can upset with a sudden movement.

2 Keep all fires guarded.

The next age group—nine months to four years—is the most accident-prone of all. Increased mobility leads to more cuts and bruises, burns and scalds, and to a far higher incidence of poisonings. Lessons for this group are:

3 Keep all poisons locked up or, at least, out of reach. That means the bleach, paintbrush cleaner, etc., often found under the sink (put them somewhere else!) as well as the weedkiller in the shed, the lavatory cleaner, and the pills and bottles in the medicine cupboard. Not all containers of, say, cleaning fluid or polish warn the user that they are dangerous. If in doubt, keep them out of sight. And keep your drinks cupboard locked.

4 Watch out for hot saucepans and kettles that can be tugged off a stove, or teapots, cups and mugs that can be knocked over.

5 Make sure that toys, tricycles and bicycles are safe.

After the age of five, accidents decline in number and more closely resemble the adult pattern. More accidents take place in the garden or outside play area, and more involve tools and pieces of adult equipment such as nails, screws, tacks, kitchen knives, cans and can-openers. Make sure that your child understands how to use equipment safely before setting him/her loose with it. Use your common sense and expect your child to do the same. As a refresher, have another look at the hazards diagram on page 131 in the chapter on Ageing.

The most dangerous years

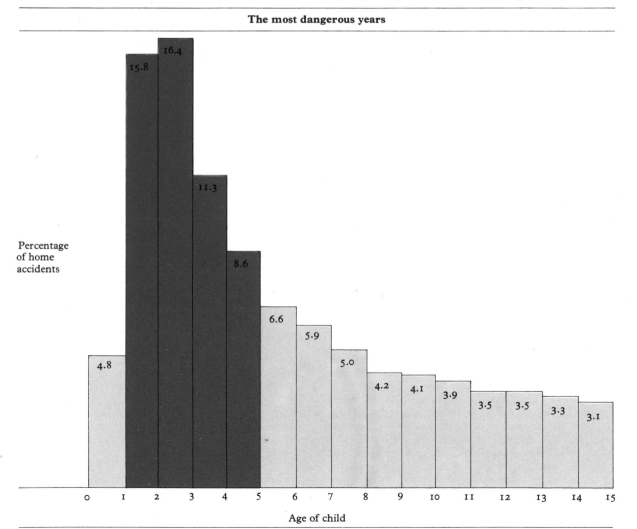

Percentage of home accidents

Age of child

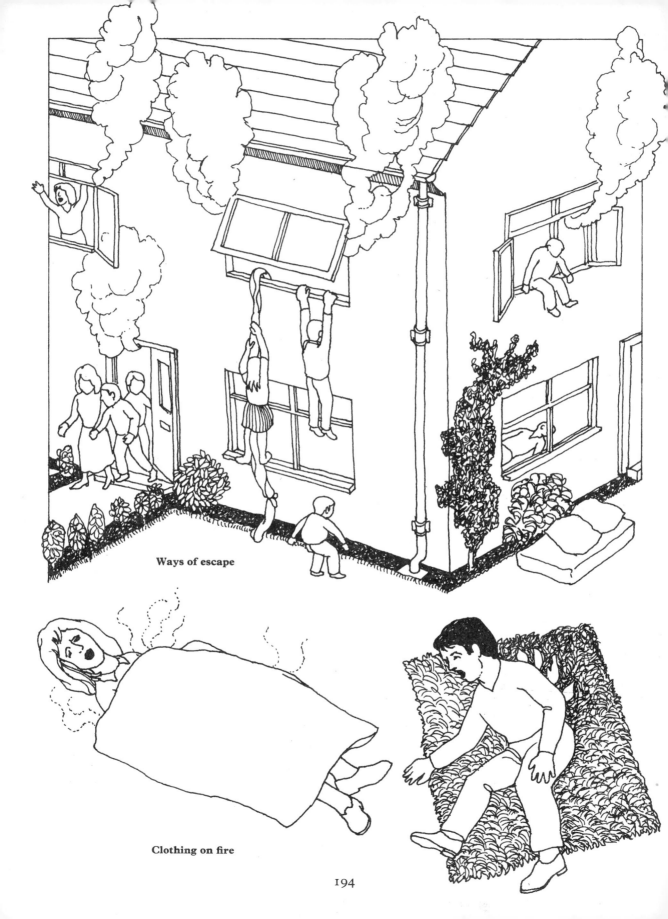

Ways of escape

Clothing on fire

HOUSE ON FIRE

Extensive research into the causes and behaviour of fires in the home has made it possible to formulate a fairly precise drill. Parents and other householders would be well advised to *learn* this drill so that they can put it into operation at a moment's notice. Your first task is to make sure that everyone in your house –including lodgers and other families–knows what to do should a fire break out. To establish what to do, read this section and adapt its general instructions to the lay-out of your home. Draw up a simple plan, and discuss it with everyone concerned.

FIRE! When a fire starts, get everyone down to the ground floor and help them to leave the building. Do not allow people to start gathering possessions together. Get them out of the building.

Call the fire brigade immediately (999 and ask for Fire), or ask a neighbour to do so. Don't assume that someone else will make this essential call.

Now, and not before, is the time to assess the size and spread of the fire. Try and limit it by closing all doors and windows, even in rooms away from the fire.

TRAPPED BY FIRE If the fire has cut you off from the usual exit, go back to a suitable room and shut the door and any other openings such as hatches, fanlights, etc. Fill up any cracks with bedding, cushions, etc., so that the room is reasonably sealed. Go to the window and try to attract attention.

Despite your efforts, the room may fill with smoke. Seek air by leaning out of the window, or, if smoke and flames from below prevent this, get down close to the floor. Here the air should be clearer. See if you can now hold out in the room until the fire brigade arrives.

You may have to make your escape before the fire brigade can get to you. If you are upstairs, say in a bedroom, make a rope by rolling sheets or other materials and knotting them together at the ends. Tie one end to a bed or heavy piece of furniture and climb down hand over hand to safety.

The rope solution may be impossible, and your next resort is to jump. Try to soften your landing by throwing down cushions or bedding. Climb out of the window feet first, and lower yourself to the full extent of your arms before dropping the rest of the way.

From heights above the first floor, dropping is dangerous and should only be done if no other solution offers itself. Try to land with knees bent, then break the impact by rolling forwards or sideways.

CLOTHING ON FIRE If you see someone whose clothes are on fire, make him lie on the floor with the flames uppermost and smother him in blankets, rugs or a thick coat. If it happens to you, and no one is there to help, put out the flames by rolling vigorously on the floor –preferably one covered with rugs or a carpet.

ATTACKS BY ENRAGED ANIMALS

Your tactics for escaping from a sudden attack by an animal will depend on two factors: the nature of the escape route, and the presence or otherwise of cover.

Clearly, your best move is to put some form of barrier between yourself and the animal as quickly as possible: a door, or a farm or garden gate may be sufficient to prevent or deter the animal from further pursuit. If you can get through or over one of those before the animal, say a bull, catches you, then instant flight is recommended. The chief drawback to running away is that your eyes are turned away from your pursuer. So, every few seconds, look back and check its position. If it is catching you up too fast, you must change your plans before it *does* catch you.

If clear-cut escape is out of the question, you must rapidly exploit any cover that may be available. Even if you can't climb that nearby tree, you may at least be able to run round it in an effort to slow the animal and perhaps halt it. Once it has been brought to a stop, there is every chance, provided you also remain quite still, that the animal will grow bored and in time walk away.

The same principle applies to close-quarter attacks, say by an enraged dog. Even though it may have attacked and bitten you, even drawn blood, you should remain still and silent. Do not take your eyes off the animal. Your steady gaze is your best line of defence. It may take time, and you must be patient, but with luck you will notice the dog showing signs of boredom. It lowers its gaze, or its eyes may flick towards other objects. It may even walk away–though if it is protecting a house or piece of land this is unlikely. Now is the time to consider a careful withdrawal.

Without taking you eyes off the animal, move slowly back to a safe position. If there is no obvious point of safety, e.g. on the other side of a door or fence, move away from the territory that the animal seems to be protecting. Once at a reasonable distance–say not less than 30 paces–you may be able to turn and walk away at a normal pace. But, until you are fairly sure of yourself, all your movements should be slow and cautious.

EXPOSURE

Anyone, not just the seasoned hiker, can be at risk to exposure. It only takes a sudden change in the weather, or the less likely but not impossible misfortune of a plane crash, to produce circumstances that can lead to exposure and so demand that you must act if you are to stay alive.

Properly, exposure is an injury which no lone survivor can treat. Your skin goes pale and cold, you feel tired and without energy, your mind wanders, your limbs do not work adequately, your hands and feet may swell. If you are on your own, the best you can do is try to ensure that you don't fall victim to exposure.

SURVIVAL RESOURCES It is a first principle that you must maximize all available resources. If you have survived a plane crash, or are stranded in your car by, say, a heavy snowdrift, make every effort to gather about you all possible aids. Most aircraft, and passenger planes in particular, should have good supplies of food and water, blankets and first-aid equipment. Your luggage, and that of other passengers, may well produce many useful items. If you are in a car, don't forget the contents of the boot, or delay collecting them

until you are walled in. A commercial traveller in ladies' underwear saved himself during a Northern blizzard recently by raiding his samples case and pulling on layers of tights, which gave him much valuable overnight insulation.

CLOTHING The three main agents of exposure are cold, wet (from rain, snow, fog, even your own sweat) and wind. Together they can chill the blood and drain away body warmth. Your extremities are most at risk—the head, hands and feet. Conserve body heat by getting the most from your clothes, as follows:

1 Fasten your clothing at the neck, wrists and ankles. Wrap trouser bottoms in socks to seal in warmth. Use spare socks as gloves.

2 Warmth is trapped by insulating layers of still air between your clothes. Add an extra layer with plastic sheeting or newspaper.

3 Keep your body and clothes as dry as possible. Wriggle your toes and move your feet at the ankles at regular intervals to keep the circulation going.

4 Let sweat escape. If you start building an emergency bivouac, you may sweat. Do not let this sweat soak into your clothes and rob you of body warmth. Keep a flow of air running in at the neck. If you are sweating a lot, keep your shirt untucked to admit more air.

Ways to conserve body heat

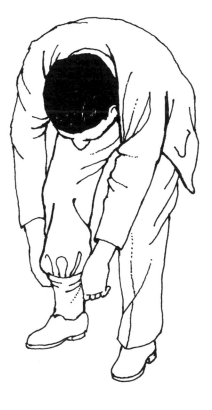

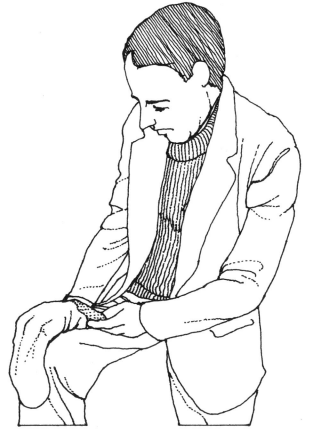

SURVIVAL KIT

If you hike or travel a lot in a climate which has hostile periods, it is well worthwhile carrying with you or keeping in the car a pocket survival kit. It won't keep you alive by itself, but it will save you a great deal of time and energy on your road to survival. The container can be small, something like a tobacco tin being especially useful since it can double as a container for heating food and fluids, and as a signalling device. Keep it waterproof when not in use by wrapping it in a sealed plastic bag.

Contents:

1 Matches and striker. To save space, wrap 20 matches in a small plastic bag. Remove the striker from a matchbox and wrap it separately in plastic. Fasten the two packages together with a strip of sticking plaster.

2 Candle. Mainly to act as a fire-lighter.

3 Whistle. For signalling to rescuers.

4 Compass. A simple magnetic compass, though made less accurate by the tin container, will nonetheless give a useful idea of direction.

5 Penknife or razor blade. If the former, make sure it's good and sharp; if the latter, wrap well when not in use.

6 String. Roll up 2–3 metres.

Supplement with shoelaces as necessary.

7 Sheet of notepaper. For lighting fires or leaving messages.

8 Pencil. Cut to fit tin.

9 Aspirin or paracetamol tablets. 4–6 in tinfoil to help overcome pain and keep the survivor active.

10 Basic First Aid materials. Adhesive dressing $7\frac{1}{2}$ cm wide. Plain bandage, $7\frac{1}{2}$ cm wide. Gauze pad. Safety pins. Seal the tin in a plastic bag.

SHELTER AND WARMTH

We will assume that your first efforts to get away or be rescued have come to nothing. It will soon be dark. Your next moves must be to seek shelter, keep yourself warm, and wait. The natural shelter is the simplest type, since it comes ready-made or nearly so and you can quickly adapt it to suit your needs. Try to find a large fallen log. Exploit any hollows in the ground under the log, or concentrate on the protected area on the lee side. Collect firewood and light a fire on the place where you propose to spend the night. While the ground is drying out, collect more firewood for the night's supply, stones for your permanent fire, and plant material and leafy branches to make a mattress. If you need protection from rain, collect poles and more leafy branches to make a roof. After your first fire has been burning for about 30 minutes, dismantle it carefully and use the embers to build your second fire about 1.5 metres from the log. Make sure that no burning embers remain on your bed-site, then lay down the plant mattress close to the log; the thicker you can make it, the further you will be from the cold ground. Cover yourself with more plant material if you wish; the extra layer of trapped air will help to maintain body warmth.

Types of fire

1 Star fire
This is a good fire if fuel is scarce. Start with small sticks then introduce four logs as shown. Push them into the centre as they burn.

2 Camper's fire
The all-purpose fire to cook on and sleep beside. Keep stones open on the side facing your bivouac. Close up when cooking.

3 Altar fire
Build up a dry base when the ground is wet, muddy or covered in snow.

To keep off rain, build a roof as shown with poles and leafy branches, placing the latter butt-ends upwards. Use vines, creeper or fibrous roots as binding material. Wedge the poles against stones on the windward side. This kind of shelter allows you to enjoy the benefits of the fire during the night.

The other main type of natural shelter is the cave. Mountain caves are the least complicated since all you have to do is find a dry place near the entrance and build your fire and mattress as for the log bivouac, above. If the cave has a wide, draughty entrance, you can partly block it with poles and leafy branches or with a heap of stones.

Caves on the sea coast are to be treated with suspicion. Only if you are sure the sea will not come into it should you use a cave situated at or near shore level. Signs of a dry, usable cave are a dry, sandy floor inside the cave, vegetation growing outside, and a line of seaweed and driftwood *lower down* the shore which indicates the high-water mark. Signs of a wet, dangerous cave are the presence of seaweed and other washed-up objects inside it, and the absence of a high-water mark outside.

Log bivouac
Poles and cross-poles covered with leafy branches

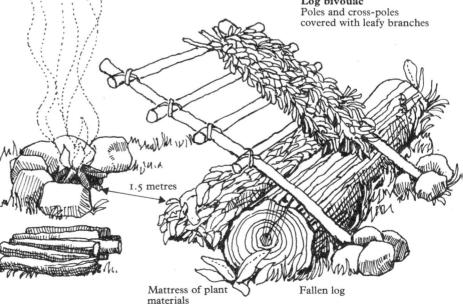

1.5 metres

Mattress of plant materials

Fallen log

Snow burrow

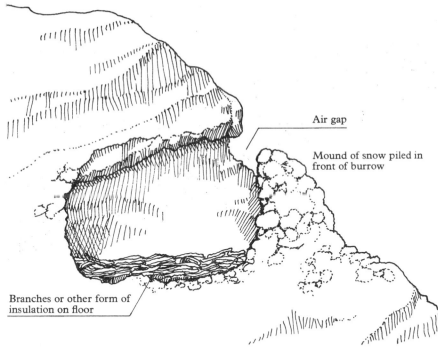

Air gap

Mound of snow piled in front of burrow

Branches or other form of insulation on floor

SNOW SHELTERS

Snow is a good insulator, and the primitive snow burrow can be an efficient form of shelter. Dig into a drift and create a cave which you wall up on the outside, leaving a gap for air to get in. This is important because the air inside your burrow will quickly turn stale if you seal it off. If fresh snow falls, clear it away from your air gap. The same principle applies if you are cut off in your car in a snowdrift. Use a stick or umbrella to keep open an air-tunnel.

In the snow burrow, be sure to line the floor with some insulating material such as a sheet of plastic, leafy branches, a rucksack or even a sheet of newspaper. Your body warmth will tend eventually to melt the walls and floor of the burrow, so all the insulation you can provide will be helpful to you. If your exertions in building the burrow cause you to sweat, take care to regulate for loss of body warmth, as described earlier.

WATER AND FOOD

Although you can live for several days without food and suffer no great discomfort, you must have water to replace the considerable amounts lost each day from your body by natural processes. In mild climates about 2.5 litres are lost each day, and in hot climates the figures can be 5 + litres.

You can go without water for the first 24 hours, after which you must try to replenish. In hot climates try to stay cool by staying in the shade and moving as little as possible. The cooler periods occur before sunrise, in the late afternoon and at night. Keep clothes *on* to reduce the amount of moisture lost through sweat. Rain is a good source of water. Collect it by making a hole in the ground and lining this with waterproof material such as a plastic sheet. Or capture it in a piece of clothing and wring this out into a container. A piece of clothing, e.g. a cotton shirt, can be used to collect early-morning dew by dragging it through grass and wringing it out as above.

Snow and ice are less good because in very cold conditions you can waste a lot of time and precious fuel melting them. Ice is more useful than snow, but if you suck lumps of it you will lose valuable body warmth for only a small return in water.

Look for ground water near the base of cliffs, inside caves (be wary of going far into them if you have no light), and dig for water in dry river beds. Another possible source of water is the fluid in plants, in particular in the vines, roots and branches of trees. Cut lengths, hold vertically and squeeze. Do not drink the fluid if it is milky. It must be clear unless you are certain it is safe, as is the milk from coconuts.

Sometimes, when their will to resist is weakening, people are tempted to drink fluids that in normal circumstances they would not dream of taking. Do *not* drink any of the following liquids:

Sea water
Urine
Petrol, fuel oil, anti-freeze
Plant or other liquids with a salty or soapy taste.

If you have a plentiful supply of water, drink more than you may think you need. Even if it is very cold and you do not feel thirsty, you should still drink plenty of water. If you do not have more than 1 litre of water per day, try not to eat food. When your hunger forces you to start looking for food, there are some ground rules you should remember:

1 Plant foods are quite adequate for survival, and you need not spend long unnecessary hours trying to catch fish, birds or other forms of mobile food.

2 The edible parts of plants can include the leaves, shoots, pith, bark, roots, tubers, bulbs, flowers, nectar, pollen, fruits, berries, nuts, seeds, gums and resins.

3 Treat all unfamiliar plant foods with suspicion. Test for edibility by tasting briefly on the tongue, or biting off a portion and spitting it out. If the taste is bitter, acid or like almonds, reject the food. Test further by boiling in water for 15 minutes and tasting again (soak in running water for 1 hour if you have no means of lighting a fire and boiling water). Hold a small amount in your mouth for 5 minutes, and then swallow if no burning sensation is felt. Take a small portion, then wait for at least 8 hours. Provided you have had no ill effects by then, you can assume that the food is edible.

RESCUE

The great question that soon plagues the lost or stranded is: Should I stay put, and wait to be rescued, or should I leave my shelter/camp/car/ crashed aircraft and try to get through to some form of human habitation?

Each case must be judged on its merits, but on the whole it is better to stay where you are. The main reason is that it is more than likely that people will be out searching for you. A crashed plane or a car is easier to spot from the air than a lone human being, and probably offers better camping resources than you would find in the wild. If the weather is bad enough to make travelling dangerous, that is another reason for staying put.

It can nevertheless be safer to move on. If no searchers have been in the area for 7 days, or if your camp is dangerously or obscurely situated – at very high altitude, for example, or in a dense forest – then you might do better to leave.

If you leave, write a note giving your name and the date, and briefly explaining what has happened to you, the compass course you propose to take, and what supplies you have with you.

SIGNALS

Once you have weathered your first night, you should prepare signals that can be understood by searchers approaching you either on the ground or in the air. The chief types are:
1 Sound signs.
2 Visual signs.
In a forest, or in fog on a mountainside, your problem may be to attract the attention of rescuers you have heard but who haven't heard you. If you have a whistle (there should be one in your Survival Kit), then the International Mountain Rescue Code procedure is as follows:
Blow once every 10 seconds for 6 blasts. Wait for 1 minute and repeat. Wait for an answer.
The answer should come in the form of 3 blasts, 1 being delivered every 20 seconds, followed by 1 minute's silence, followed by a further set of 3 blasts.
If you have to shout a sound signal, get the best out of your voice by learning the Far-Call. This is delivered in two breaths. First take a deep breath and shout 'Fah-ah-ah-ah-ah-ah' as you exhale. Follow with a second deep breath and the sound 'Caw-aw-aw-aw-awl'. Cup your hands round your mouth to channel the sound more efficiently. Repeat at 1-minute intervals for up to 5 minutes. If there is no response, give your voice a rest and repeat later.
If you have a torch, a simple visual signal is to flash the International Mountain Rescue Code, described above. You can also flash signals using a reflecting surface to bounce sunlight in a given direction. Use a can lid or the lid of your Survival Kit to do this. Follow the method described in the diagram below.

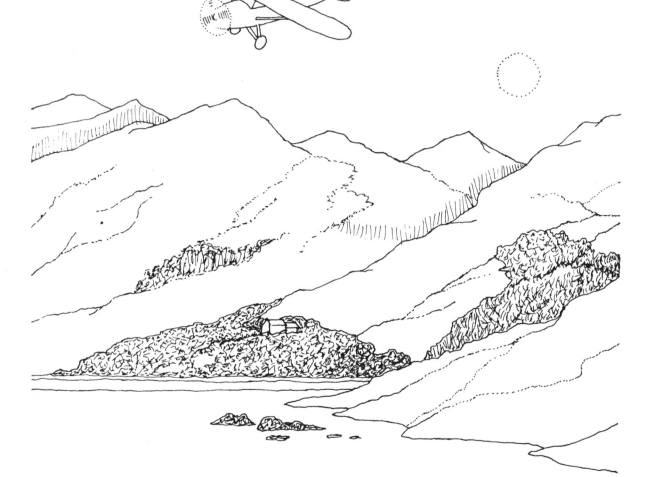

Flashing signals by heliograph
Take a can or the lid of your Survival Kit and bore a hole in the centre. Using the tip of your pencil as a fore-sight, collect the sunlight and reflect it on to your forward hand. As you look through the hole in the reflector you should see a dark spot on your hand. Now swivel this dark spot upwards until it shines on the tip of your pencil-sight. Aim at your rescue target.

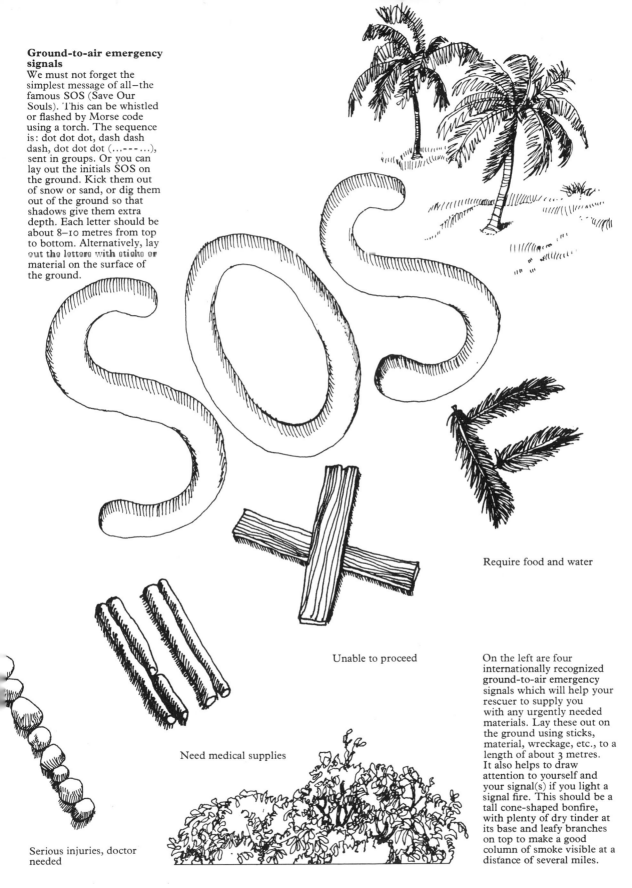

Ground-to-air emergency signals

We must not forget the simplest message of all—the famous SOS (Save Our Souls). This can be whistled or flashed by Morse code using a torch. The sequence is: dot dot dot, dash dash dash, dot dot dot (...---...), sent in groups. Or you can lay out the initials SOS on the ground. Kick them out of snow or sand, or dig them out of the ground so that shadows give them extra depth. Each letter should be about 8–10 metres from top to bottom. Alternatively, lay out the letters with sticks or material on the surface of the ground.

Require food and water

Unable to proceed

Need medical supplies

Serious injuries, doctor needed

On the left are four internationally recognized ground-to-air emergency signals which will help your rescuer to supply you with any urgently needed materials. Lay these out on the ground using sticks, material, wreckage, etc., to a length of about 3 metres. It also helps to draw attention to yourself and your signal(s) if you light a signal fire. This should be a tall cone-shaped bonfire, with plenty of dry tinder at its base and leafy branches on top to make a good column of smoke visible at a distance of several miles.

SURVIVAL IN WATER

This section offers outline advice on what to do if you yourself are stranded in deep water, and how you can help others in this predicament.

PERSONAL SURVIVAL

The need for personal survival may arise if you are swept out to sea by the tide, or downstream by a dangerous current, if you develop a bad attack of cramp, or if you fall overboard from a ship or have the misfortune to be involved in a sailing accident.

In the first instance, once you have established that the tide is running faster than you can swim, you must try and attract attention as rapidly as possible. But make sure you get the attention you want. If you just wave an arm, it is horribly likely that people on the beach will simply wave back, thinking that you seek only acknowledgment. No, you must send out the equivalent of a distress signal so that bystanders can see that you *are* in distress. Do this by beating stiff-armed on the water and kicking up an irregular pattern of splashes. And by shouting for help as best you can. Try always to direct your actions at a particular person or group on the beach or bank.

In the meantime try to stay calm. Beating about on the water is tiring, so conserve your energy if there is no immediate response. If no one seems to be about, wait until someone appears. Few British beaches or river banks remain unpopulated for long. If no one comes after a minute or two, have another go at splashing and shouting. There may be someone about, in a house, for example, who will see or hear you even if you can't see them.

Don't give up. Provided you have the ability to swim or float, you may be able to ride out the tide or escape from the fast current when it flows close to a bank. In the sea, rest by floating on your back like a starfish with arms and legs spread wide. Keep yourself facing the beach, and adjust your position by sculling with your arms. Be patient. Believe that you will be alright.

If, following some kind of accident, you find yourself in deep water with floating driftwood, grab the largest piece and use it as a float. Other aids to floating can be made from clothing. Remove shoes and heavy outer garments and discard them, but keep wellington boots or, failing these, trousers.

To convert your wellingtons into floats, take them off and empty them of water. They will then fill with air. Seal the tops by folding over once, and use them as floats held out on either side. With trousers, the procedure is to take them off and knot each leg at the foot. Then, holding them behind your head by the waistband, fling them forward over your head to fill them with air. Wrap them up at the waist and hold the two-legged 'bag' behind your head to act as a floating pillow.

Cramp is a painful condition, but you can usually treat it by alternately rubbing the afflicted area—usually in the calf or thigh—and floating on your back to rest the leg. It is also not difficult to swim to safety using a one-legged version of the side-stroke, with the cramped leg trailing beneath while you flex and kick with the other. Again, rest from time to time and massage the cramped leg until the pain passes.

Aids to floating

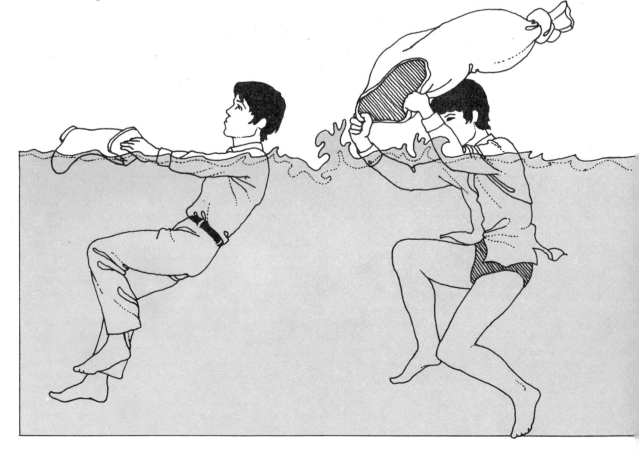

HELPING OTHERS IN DISTRESS

If you are on dry land when you see someone in distress in the water, look first for a life-belt and throw it out to the person, aiming for a point beside him that he can reach. In this way you reduce the chances of stunning him with a direct hit (life-belts of the type found on beaches and beside rivers are surprisingly heavy). Tell the subject to get inside the belt while you look for a suitable length of rope. Coil this neatly over one hand, hold one end firmly and throw the rest out to the subject, telling him to grab the rope and hold on to it with both hands while you haul him in to safety.

If no such aids are available, or the subject is unconscious, and you decide to enter the water, be careful how you do so. Reeds, jagged objects and glutinous mud can wreck the best of rescue intentions. When you reach your subject, do not let him grab wildly at you. From a stand-off position 2 metres away, reassure him, tell him to be quite still and you will take him in tow. Swim behind him and take up one of the towing positions illustrated below. Proceed as in the diagrams. Whichever method you use, always keep the subject's head well back and chin up. If the subject continues to struggle, warn him that you will leave him there if he does not calm down. If that has no effect, try to bring him to his senses with a sharp blow.

If you come into land at a raised bank, tell your subject to remain still and swivel him round until he is facing the bank. Quickly place your arms through his, as shown, and 'jump' him upwards on to the bank, pushing until his centre of gravity is on land. Lever his legs on to the bank to complete the rescue. Apply artificial respiration if necessary (see page 177 for details).

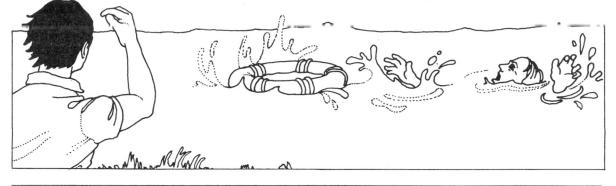

Chin tow
Best for unconscious subjects. Hold him under the chin with head well back, keeping the nose and mouth out of the water. Towing arm should be *straight*. Swim using a one-armed side-stroke.

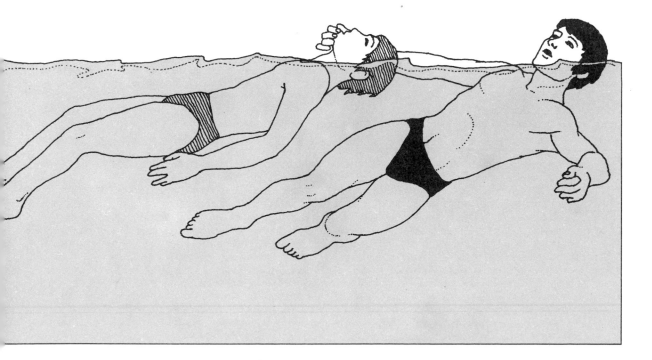

Orthodox tow
Hold the subject firmly under the chin as shown, his head pulled well into your shoulder, chin up and nose and mouth out of the water. Swim on your back using a breast-stroke kick. Scull with your free arm if you can. The subject, though conscious, should not attempt to propel himself.

Side tow
Hold the subject across his chest with one arm and support his body on your hip. Swim with an adapted side-stroke.

Landing
Swivel the subject to face the bank, place your arms through his and 'jump' him over the side. Quickly push his legs up to complete the landing.

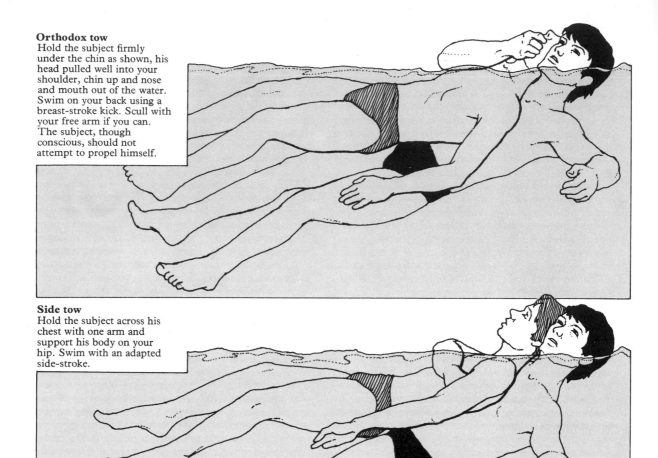

SUBMERGED CAR

If you are in a car that topples into water and is submerged, there is a special drill to follow. It requires you to wait while the water pressures inside and outside the car become more or less equal. The first rule, therefore, is:

Don't panic.

It is *normal* to wait while the car fills up with water. This is your best means of escape, and you must allow time for the right circumstances to build up. Cars do not always sink immediately in deep water. If yours floats for a short while, then try to get out as fast as possible. Once the car is submerged, the outside water pressure will prevent you from opening the door until later.

Water will enter the car through many apertures as it sinks, usually with the heavier engine-end leading. Try to control the rate of entry by winding up all windows. (If you have electric windows these should continue to function.) Release your seat-belts, check that your chosen escape door is unlocked, and lift the head of children or injured people above the water level Switch on all lights to help rescuers to find you. Reassure everyone and tell them what you are going to do next.

When the water reaches chin-level, the water pressures will have begun to even out and you may be able to open the door. If not, keep trying by pushing at regular intervals. Keep calm. When the door does open, hold it open, and get the others to form a human chain. Tell everyone to take a deep breath and swim out. The purpose of the chain is to ensure that no one is left behind and trapped when the door closes again. It is generally simpler if the person holding the door leaves last.

First steps

In a submerged car, these are the first actions to take as the passenger compartment fills with water:
1 Wind up windows.
2 Release seat belts.
3 Keep all heads above water.
4 Choose unlocked escape door.
5 Switch on lights.

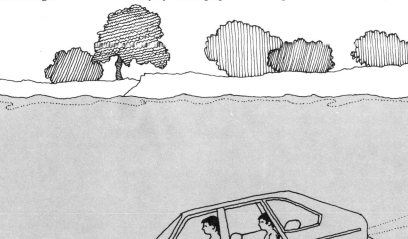

Escape

As soon as you can force open the door, form a human chain and swim out. Last to leave should be the person responsible for keeping the door open.

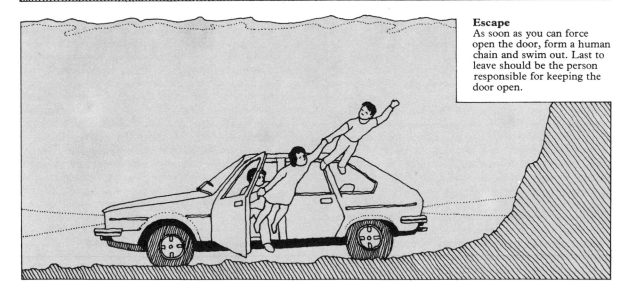

INDEX

Page numbers in bold type refer to principal entries,
those in italics to illustrations

A

Abdomen 26, 153
  pain in 153, 159
Abdominal wounds 177,
  177, 179, 179
Accidents
  home 130, *130*, 192–193,
  193
  prevention of *131*,
  192–193
  see also First aid
Acidity, of stomach 151
Acne 104, *104*
Acrobat 66
Acute retention, of urine
  169
Adder 187, *187*
Adhesive dressing strip
  182, *182*
Adrenal gland 37, *37*, 88
Adrenaline 37
Adult Evening Centres
  124
'Afterbirth', see Placenta
Ageing **122-137**
Aid, First 173, **174-189**
Aids for the handicapped
  132–135, *132, 133, 134,*
  135
Ailments, common
  138-173
Alcohol 49, 53, 88, 110,
  114-117, 119, 147, 152,
  159, 163, 176, 186
Alcoholics Anonymous
  117
Alcoholism 116–117
  National Council on 117
Alimentary canal 150
Allergic rhinitis (hay
  fever) 161
Allergy 144, 160–161
  food 161
Alpha rhythms 91, *91*
Amino acids 46, 48, 49
Amphetamines 119
Anaemia 60, 147, 161
  iron deficiency 60
Analgesics 170
Angina pectoris 58, 149
Angio-neurotic oedema
  150
Animals, attacks by 195
Ankle 157
  sprained 157
Antibiotics 118, 142, 164,
  .166
Anti-depressants 114
Anti-histamine cream 165
Antiperistalsis 25
Anus *24*, *105*, 154
Anxiety neurosis 159
Aorta 18, 147
Aphthous ulcers 150
Appendicitis 59, 153
Appendix *24*

Aqueous humour *33*
Arm 155
  fractures 184, *184*
  movement of 17, *17*
Arteriosclerosis 148
Artery 20, *21*
Arthritis 156
  rheumatoid 156
Artificial respiration 149,
  176, **177**, *177*
Asthma 161, 178
Athlete's foot 104, *104*,
  145, 156
Atlas vertebra 14, *14*
Atrium 20, *21*
Auditory nerve *34*
Autonomic nervous
  system 30, 33
Axis vertebra 14, *14*

B

Babies, and diet 60
Back, the 157, 158
  common ailments
  157–159
  fractures 185, *185*
Backbone 14, *14*, 15
Bacteria 18, 26, 98, 104,
  142, 163, 169
Badminton 83, 84, *84*
Balancing ability 68, *68*
Baldness 100
Bandages, emergency
  178, *178*, 180, 181, 189,
  189
  see also Dressings
Bannister, Roger 86
Barbiturates 90, 119, 162,
  163
Barium meal X-ray 151,
  153
Basic Home Exercise
  Programme 70–73
Basketball 83, 84–85
Bath, aids for
  handicapped users *133*
Bed
  bug 104
  correct design of 127
Bedsore 127
Bed-wetting 168
Benzodiazepine drugs
  118, 163
Bereavement, problems
  of 137
Biceps *17*
Bile 26, 39, 152
Biopsy 151, 172
Bivouac, emergency 196,
  198, *198*
Blackheads 104
Bladder 17, 26, *26*, 27, 35,
  105, 128, 152, 153, 168,
  169
  stone 128
Bleeding 161, 176, **178**,

178, 187, 188
  ear 186
  nose 186, 187
  tooth socket 187, *187*
Blisters 145, 179, *179*
Blood **18-19**, 155
  cells 12, 18, *18*
  circulation 18, *19*, 28
  platelets 18, *18*
  plasma 26
  stream 12, 162
  test 18
  see also Bleeding
Blood cholesterol 57
Blood pressure 20, 58
  diastolic 20, 147
  high 147, 149
  systolic 20, 147
Body
  heat 100, 196
  temperature 98
  weight, and fitness 66
  workings of **10-39**
Boil 145
Bone
  composition 12, *12*
  fractures 156, 184, *184*,
  192, 193
  marrow *12*, 18, 27
Bowel 26, 128, 153
  impacted 128
Bowls 83
Boxing 66, 86
Brain **28-31**, 124
  fore- 29, *29*
  hind- 28, *28*, 30
  injury 186, 192, 193
  mid- 28, *28*
  stem 15
  tumour 141
Breast, female 109, 171
Breastbone *13*
Breast-feeding 60
Breath, holding 68
Breathing 28, 180
  see also Artificial
  respiration
Breathlessness 146–147
British Red Cross
  Society 132, 176, 177
Bronchiole 142
Bronchiolitis 142
Bronchitis 112, 142, 144
Broncho-pneumonia 148
Bronchus (pl. bronchi)
  23, *23*, 142, 145
Bruise 145, 186
Bug, bed 104
Bunions 126
Burns **179**, *179*, 192, 193
  chemical 180
Burrow, snow 199, *199*

C

Caecum *24*
Calcium 12, 39, 46, 51,

53, 60, 124, 165
Calories 46, 53, 54, 60,
  61, 66, 67, 80
Cannabis 119
Cancer
  of colon 59
  of lung 112, 113
Capillary system 18, *19*
Car accidents 180
  submerged 205, *205*
Carbohydrates 45, 48–49,
  55, 61, 161
Carbon chain 48, 49
Carbon dioxide 18, *19*,
  24, 92
Carbuncle 145
Cartilage 12
Cataract 126
Catheter 128
Caves, as shelter 198
Cellulose 52
Cereals, energy values of
  62
Cerebellum 28, *29*, 30
Cerebrospinal fluid 31
Cerebrum 29
Cervix 36, *36*, *105*, 106
Check-up, medical 68
Cheiropompholyx 145,
  156
Chemical burns 180
Chest
  common ailments
  146–149
  injuries 180, *180*
  pains 144, 146
Chickenpox 163, 165
Childbirth, helping at 180
Children
  and accidents 192–193,
  193
  and sex 109
  growth rates of 166, *167*
  illnesses of 163–168
Chloral 163
Chlorphenazone 163
Choking 144, 176, **181**,
  181
Cholecystitis 152
Cholelithiasis 152
Cholesterol 26
Cigarettes
  consumption of 110–112
  effects of 112
Cirrhosis 114, 117
Citizen's Advice Bureau
  136
Climbing, for exercise 78
Clothes 98, *99*, 100
Cocaine 119
Coccyx *13*, 14, 158
Cochlea *34*
Cold, see Hypothermia
Cold, common 141, 142,
  144, 163, 164
Colitis 153
Collagen 124
Collar bone 15, 156, 184,
  184

SUMMARY OF ADDRESSES

Alcoholics Anonymous,
11 Redcliffe Gardens,
London, SW10 9BG
(or see local telephone directory)

National Council on Alcoholism,
45 Great Peter Street,
London, SW1P 3LT

Disabled Living Foundation,
346 Kensington High Street,
London W14 8NS

U and I Club,
9e Compton Road,
Islington,
London, N1
(for sufferers of cystitis and other
urinary and vaginal disorders)

British Red Cross Society,
9 Grosvenor Crescent,
London, SW1
(or see local telephone directory)

St John's Ambulance Association,
1 Grosvenor Crescent,
London, SW1
(or see local telephone directory)

St Andrew's Ambulance Association,
Milton Street,
Glasgow, C4
(or see local telephone directory,
Scotland only)

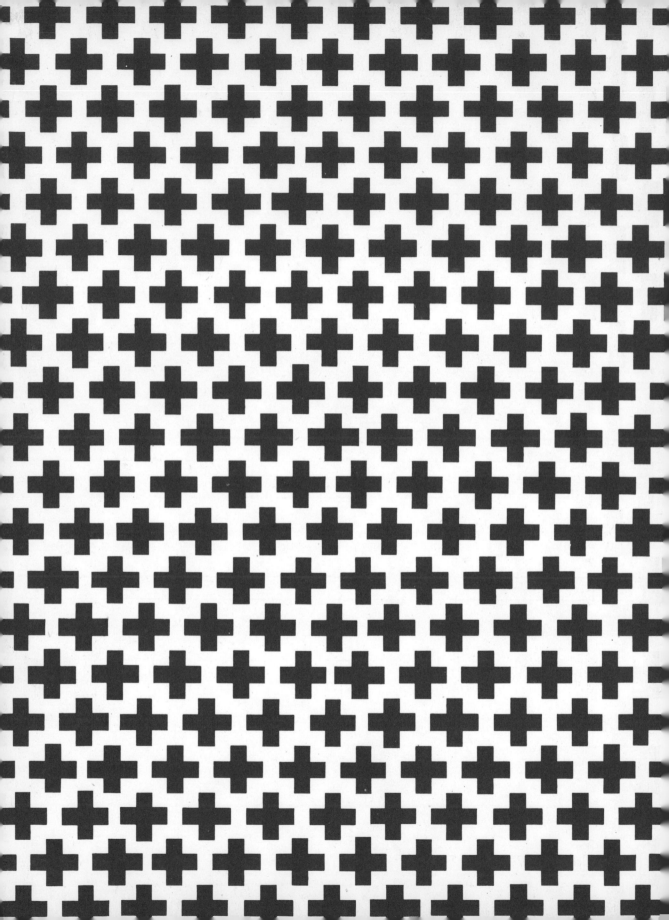